THE COMPLETE BOOK OF

Cancer
Prevention

FOODS, LIFESTYLES & MEDICAL CARE TO KEEP YOU HEALTHY

BY THE EDITORS OF
Prevention® Magazine Health Books

Rodale Press, Emmaus, Pennsylvania

Printed in the United States of America

Book design by Acey Lee
Cover design by Acey Lee

If you have any questions or comments concerning this book, please write:

Rodale Press
Book Reader Service
33 East Minor Street
Emmaus, PA 18098

Library of Congress Cataloging-in-Publication Data

The Complete book of cancer prevention.

Includes index.
1. Cancer—Prevention. 1. Prevention (Emmaus, Pa.)
[DNLM: 1. Diet—popular works. 2. Life Style—popular works. 3. Neoplasms—prevention & control—popular works. QA 201 C737]
RC268.C64   1988

616.99′4052   87–26594

ISBN 0–87857–740–8   hardcover
ISBN 0–87857–874–9   paperback

Distributed in the book trade by St. Martin's Press

2 4 6 8 10 9 7 5 3   hardcover
2 4 6 8 10 9 7 5 3 1   paperback

Contributors to *The Complete Book of Cancer Prevention:*

Editor:	**Carol Keough**
Part One	Ellen Michaud
	Stephen Williams
	with Jane Sherman
Part Two	Sharon Faelten
	Diane Fields
	Marcia Holman
	Ellen Michaud
	Sally Novack
	Cathy Perlmutter
	Carole Piszczek
	Jennifer Whitlock
Part Three	JoAnn Brader
	Nancy Zelko
	The Rodale Food Center
Part Four	Martha Capwell
	Marcia Holman
	Gale Malesky
	Thomas Shealey
Glossary	Jane Sherman
Copy Editor:	Lisa Baker Andruscavage
Research Staff	**Susan Nastasee**
	Holly Clemson
	Martha Capwell
	Jan Eickmeier
	Ann Gossy
	Alice Harris
	Jill Jurgensen
	Cemela Dee London
	Paris Mihely
	Sally Novack
Office Staff	**Roberta Mulliner**
	Kelly Trumbauer
	Kim Mohr

Executive Editor, Prevention® Magazine Health Books: William Gottlieb
Group Vice President, Health: Mark Bricklin

Contents

PART THREE

PART FOUR

How to Use This Book to Prevent Cancer

Welcome to *The Complete Book of Cancer Prevention*. It's complete because it thoroughly details the risk factors for 19 different lifestyle cancers, provides quizzes that enable you to evaluate your risk of getting the disease, and recommends specific cancer prevention plans that can maximize your health and minimize your risks. Nothing is left out. We've even included more than 50 recipes packed with the nutrients known to put your body in cancer-fighting trim.

Say you're concerned about lung cancer. Flip through the alphabetically ordered chapters in part 1 until you come to Lung Cancer. Then sit down and read. What causes lung cancer? Who usually gets it? Who doesn't? Take the quiz Are You at Risk for Lung Cancer? and find out whether or not you are. Do you smoke? Do you work with asbestos or radioactive materials? Do you usually leave green, yellow or orange fruits and vegetables to hamsters?

If you answered yes to any of those questions, you may be at increased risk for lung cancer. So we'll suggest you flip to these entries in part 2 of the book: Early Detection, Fruit, Heredity, Indoor Pollution, Marijuana, Outdoor Pollution, Prescription Drugs, Tobacco, Vegetables, Vitamin A, Vitamin C and Vitamin E. Each one will tell you how to make changes in your life that will minimize your risk of cancer.

Vitamin A, for example, is a substance that one researcher describes as a kind of cellular "shock absorber" in the way it protects your body. Does it actually prevent lung cancer? How? Should you get it from supplements? From diet? How much is enough? How much is too much?

The Complete Book of Cancer Prevention will tell you. And it won't leave you wondering how to work prevention into your life. Since a key finding by the cancer researchers consulted for this book is that 30 percent of all cancer deaths can be prevented by diet—and many of the researchers and cancer specialists we interviewed have changed their diet to reflect this—we've included recipes loaded with nutrients like vitamin A in part 3, Cancer-Fighting Recipes. Use them as a part of your overall cancer prevention plan.

Nor have we forgotten those of you who have already had one bout with cancer. Congratulations on your win. Part 4, Preventing a Recurrence, is for you. You'll get the latest information on chemotherapy, hormone therapy, immunotherapy, mind/body healing, radiation therapy and surgical treatment. What are they? What do they do? What will you feel? How can you maximize treatment effects and minimize side effects?

Use the information to understand your doctor's advice and put your options into perspective. Then fight. And, remember, we're fighting, too.

Preventable
Cancers

Planning Your Anticancer Program

You can prevent cancer. You can get up tomorrow morning, put on your slippers, pull on your bathrobe and decide not to get it. Sounds almost too simple, doesn't it? Too undramatic? According to cancer specialists across the country, it's not. It's not because, along with your robe and your slippers, you can also put on a new attitude toward your health, your body and your life. And that new attitude—a determination to produce an internal and external environment conducive to good health—can alter the course of your life. Literally.

You can make a real and significant improvement in your odds against cancer because between 80 and 90 percent of all cancers are the result of things we do to ourselves. We eat too much fat. We drink too much alcohol. We douse the world with bug spray. We smoke. We lie in the sun till we blister.

Why do such activities cause cancer? The answer to that question is the focus of millions of dollars of research at cancer centers around the country. But it starts, scientists believe, somewhere in our genes. Each and every cell contains the genetic codes that determine so much of what the cell does.

We have thousands of genes, doctors tell us, but at least 20 of them can be altered by a shaft of radiation, a blast of smoke or a viral attack that resets the intricate "grow/don't grow" codes of a cell. And once those codes are reset, a single cell can grow uncontrollably. Like an alien inhabitant, it can grow and multiply and travel until it colonizes your entire body. It can jam your body's highways, eat its food and shut off its air. It can—and does—kill.

There's not much we can do about our genes. Not today. But we can, scientists tell us, control many of the triggers that start them down the road to our destruction. Tobacco smoke, for example. Ever wonder why U.S. Surgeon General C. Everett Koop, M.D., gets so mad about it? If you think his warnings printed on cigarette packs are scary, you should see him in action at a press conference. His beard bristles. His eyes narrow. His hands grip the sheet of paper in front of him.

Why? Why does the nation's chief health officer look so deeply angered whenever tobacco smoke is mentioned? Maybe it's because he knows that every puff we take is putting us at risk for a painful, lingering disease. And death. Maybe because he knows that we can prevent it. By not smoking. By avoiding smoke-filled rooms. By demanding that our legislators ban tobacco in the same way they banned asbestos. (Asbestos is responsible for 2 percent of all cancer deaths. Tobacco is responsible for 35 percent.)

But why is it so important to *prevent* cancer? Doesn't science have a fusillade of magic bullets with which to treat it? Magic guns to zap it? What about all the headlines heralding new discoveries?

If you talked to the generals in the "War on Cancer"—the massive, government-backed effort to blitz the disease—they might say yes. They might tell you the War on Cancer is almost over. You might even believe them. Just look at the weapons in their arsenal, they'd say. There's immunotherapy, the use of chemicals that push your body's own molecular defenses into anticancer overdrive. There's chemotherapy, the use of super-strong drugs that squelch cancer. There's precision surgery, where the disease is cut out of the body. There's radiation therapy, where powerful rays zap renegade cells. Cancer is retreating, they'd tell you; health will soon hoist the flag of victory.

That's the news from the battlefield. But behind the lines—where scientists analyze statistics and so-called breakthroughs are tested in the laboratory of time—there's not so much enthusiasm for cancer treatment. In fact, there's doubt. With a capital "D" that could also stand for defeat.

Publicly, government officials report that advances in the detection and treatment of cancer from 1950 to 1982 have been "limited." Privately they're more pessimistic, even angry. Reports of increasingly successful cancer treatments have been, except in a very few instances, a "cruel fraud," says one former high-ranking official at the National Cancer Institute. And much of the scientific community seems to agree.

"We are losing the war against cancer," write two researchers in the *New England Journal of Medicine*, one of the nation's most respected magazines for doctors. That doesn't mean we can't win, they say, but the tools of victory aren't new, space-age treatments. Or perfect understanding of cancer-cell mechanics. Or anything that happens in a hospital. No, the best way to beat the disease, say these scientists, is "a shift in research emphasis, from research on treatment to research on prevention."

Clearly, beating cancer is in *your* hands. And, indeed, you can do it. Read on to find out how.

Bladder Cancer

You hardly ever hear a peep from your pancreas or an ouch from your adrenals. But when the bladder is bothered, you know it—that urgent ache is a clear signal this organ is being overtaxed. About 40,000 people every year receive another, more urgent message from their bladder—they find out it's been inhabited by a malignant tumor.

Most of the people are white men over 65, and it's likely they're suffering from either papillary or transitional-cell carcinoma, the two kinds of tumors that have accounted for 88 percent of all bladder cancer.

Papillary bladder cancer is the most common type of all. Fortunately, it's also the type that is most easily cured. When this condition develops, abnormal cells grow out from the bladder wall, reaching into the bladder cavity. This kind of growth makes this cancer fairly easy to see and easier to remove.

Transitional-cell carcinoma, on the other hand, penetrates the bladder wall and is more likely to become ulcerated and infected. Most deaths from this type of cancer are due to infection rather than directly from the cancer itself.

DETECT IT EARLY

While some cancers are known for spreading quickly throughout the body, bladder cancer tends to spread slowly. When symptoms do appear, they can be dramatic. The most common should be enough to make people rush to their doctors immediately: blood in the urine. This symptom will usually strike suddenly and painlessly.

Even though bloody urine is most often caused by some other condition—infection, benign tumor or bladder stones—no one should discount the possibility of cancer when they suffer this symptom. Even if the bleeding stops for a few days, or weeks, cancer might be spreading in the bladder, so don't think that a sudden disappearance of the symptom means there is no problem. See a doctor right away if you have blood in your urine.

Fortunately, bladder cancer is often cured if it is detected at an early stage. Chemotherapy, radiation therapy and surgery are the common forms of treatment. Among men who have localized tumors at the time of treatment, 70 percent are alive and healthy after five years. For women, this figure is 76 percent. And when the cancer is so advanced at the time of treatment that long-term survival isn't likely, the symptoms and pain of bladder cancer can often be relieved.

So the best bet is to prevent the cancer or catch it very early. There are several risk factors for bladder cancer that people have a lot of control over. One of the most controllable is smoking, which many scientists and doctors say is linked directly to bladder cancer. According to the American Cancer Society, smokers are twice as likely as non-smokers to get bladder cancer.

Another group of people at risk are those who suffer chronic bladder infections. Anyone in this group should be sure to ask their doctor to do a thorough examination to find and treat the cause. Otherwise, changes in the bladder from chronic infections might raise the risk of cancer.

The artificial sweetener saccharin does not appear to be a dietary link to bladder cancer. Products that contain saccharin are sold with the warning that the artificial sweetener has been shown to cause cancer in laboratory rats. But even though saccharin is considered to be a low-level carcinogen, recent studies show there is no increased risk of bladder cancer for people who consume artificial sweeteners.

Employment in a place where specific chemicals are used in rubber, leather and dye manufacturing is also a risk factor. Benzidine and

2-naphthylamine are now known to be carcinogens. Other workers who are suspected of having slightly increased risks of developing bladder cancer due to their jobs are housepainters, hairdressers, truck drivers, textile workers, chemical workers, metalworkers, machinists and printers. However, the cause isn't necessarily the same in each profession.

ARE YOU AT RISK FOR BLADDER CANCER?

White men over age 65 and people with a history of chronic bladder infections are at greater than average risk for bladder cancer. However, there are other risk factors that are controllable. Answer these questions to see if you are doing all you can to prevent bladder cancer, or at least ensure early detection.

- Do you abstain from smoking?
- If you have chronic bladder infections, do you seek treatment promptly each time one occurs?

If you answered no to either of these questions, you may be at increased risk for bladder cancer. For more information that may help you prevent it, please read these chapters in part 2 of this book:

- Chapter 42, Indoor Pollution
- Chapter 59, Sugar and Artificial Sweeteners
- Chapter 63, Tobacco

CHAPTER 3

Breast Cancer

Scars, disfigurement, amputation, sex appeal, suckling, fondling, beauty. Breast cancer is a disease that brings out a range of fully charged, contrasting emotions—much like the words above. But breast cancer is that kind of disease, a harrowing compound of fear and loss and pain that strikes 115,000 new victims and kills 38,000 every year.

The statistics, too, are dramatic—but perhaps unnecessarily so, because breast cancer is one of the most controllable cancers there is. According to the American Cancer Society, the five-year survival rate could be increased if breast cancer were detected early and received prompt treatment. In addition to early detection, there's a lot you can do to avoid breast cancer altogether.

The female breast is mainly made up of supportive connective tissue and fat, laced throughout with a network of glands that work together to produce milk after a child is born. A group of ducts connects the glands to the nipple. Changes in the breast, such as the development of a hard lump, are the most common signs of breast cancer (although lumpy breasts are often caused by problems other than breast cancer). Swelling, puckering, dimpling, redness, skin irritation that persists, pain or tenderness are other signs to be on the lookout for. Also a nipple discharge or a nipple that inverts or takes a strange shape may be signs of breast cancer. Any woman with these symptoms should see a doctor.

You should know the uncontrollable risk factors for breast cancer, because if you have any of them, prevention and early detection become that much more important.

Family history. Women whose mother or sister have had breast cancer run a much greater risk than other women of getting the disease.

Cancer history. Women who have had previous breast cancer have a four to five times greater risk of developing a second cancer.

Menstrual history. Women who began to menstruate early (before age 12) or whose menopause began later than average (after age 55) are at an increased risk for breast cancer.

Pregnancy. Women who've never had a baby or didn't have one until they were over 30 years old are at greater risk.

Age. Two-thirds of all breast cancer develops in women who are older than 50.

DETECTING CANCER EARLY IS VITAL

Ignorance is probably responsible for more deaths due to established breast cancer than any other controllable risk factor. While examination of the breast itself won't stop cancer from forming, it is definitely the most important thing you can do to reduce the danger of death from breast cancer.

Self-examinations are the first step. These simple home examinations should be done by every woman once a month. If there are any changes in how the breast feels from month to month, you should see a doctor. There's really no excuse for not examining your breasts regularly. If you find that you are too squeamish to do the monthly exam, find a doctor or nurse to do it for you.

Also, the American Cancer Society recommends that women aged 20 to 40 have their doctor do a thorough breast exam every three years. In addition, women between the ages of 35 and 40 should have a baseline mammogram (a breast x-ray to which future mammograms will be compared). Women over age 40 should have a breast exam by their doctor every year and a mammogram every one or two years until they are 50 years old, when they should start having a mammogram every year.

Most women and doctors can first feel a lump only after it has grown to more than ½ inch in diameter. By this time, cancer cells have been present for many months or even years. There is a real risk that these dangerous cells have spread beyond the breast to the lymph nodes under the arm and possibly to other parts of the body. Mammography, on the other hand, can find lumps that are just half this size, or even smaller. The chance that breast cancer has spread is significantly reduced if it's caught at this early stage.

PREVENTING BREAST CANCER

There are several factors in the way you live that you can alter to help prevent breast cancer. People concerned about breast cancer might want to evaluate their diets first. Some experts believe that consuming too much fat may increase your risk of cancer. One reason for this risk may be that excessive fat may lead to being overweight. And body fat could be a vital link in the development of breast cancer and other reproductive cancers, according to Rose E. Frisch, Ph.D., a Harvard School of Public Health professor in Boston.

"We've known from other research for some time that fatter women make more estrogen and more potent forms of estrogen that have been related to increased cancers of the reproductive system. It's possible that the leaner women make less estrogen and less potent estrogen, and we hope to do research that clarifies this." (Hormones, like estrogen, were also for some time considered to be the link between breast cancer and women who took high-dose birth control pills. However, most of the pills now dispensed have very low doses of hormones, and the cancer risk is minimal.)

Another possible dietary factor influencing breast cancer is the consumption of the trace mineral selenium, found in soil and certain foods, according to Oliver Alabaster, M.D., author of *The Power of Prevention* (Fireside) and associate professor of medicine and director of cancer research at George Washington University in Washington, D.C. Dr. Alabaster says the exact *way* that selenium protects against breast cancer isn't known, but its protective factors are definitely known. For example, in New Zealand, where the soil is low in selenium, people have one of the highest breast cancer rates in the world. Dr. Alabaster cites this fact to support the connection between the mineral and breast cancer. Because selenium can be toxic if taken in too large amounts, it would be wise to speak with your doctor before taking any supplements. Selenium is found naturally in good quantities in seafood, liver and kidney. It's also found in other meats and whole grains.

A third possible factor is how much alcohol a woman drinks. In a study done at the Harvard Medical School, Boston, researchers discovered a correlation between drinking and the incidence of breast cancer. The study was based on a survey of 89,000 women's eating and drinking habits. Researchers concluded that women appear to place themselves at increased risk of developing this form of cancer by consuming as few as three alcoholic drinks a week. And those women who take a drink or more a day may have a 50 percent chance (or higher) of developing breast cancer than women who never drink.

ARE YOU AT RISK FOR BREAST CANCER?

Women who have a family or personal history of breast cancer, those who began menstruating before age 12 or began menopause after age 55, those who have never had a child or had a first full-term pregnancy after age 30, and women over age 50 are at greater than average risk for breast cancer. However, there are other risk factors that are controllable. Answer the following questions to see if you are doing all you can to prevent breast cancer, or at least ensure early detection.

- Do you keep your weight down?
- Do you follow a low-fat diet?
- Do you limit your consumption of alcohol?
- Do you exercise regularly?
- Do you perform a breast self-exam every month?
- Do you follow the American Cancer Society guidelines for breast examinations (ages 20 to 40—breast exam by a doctor every three years; ages 35 to 40—breast exam by a doctor every three years and a baseline mammogram; ages 40 to 50—breast exam by a doctor every year and mammogram every one or two years; over 50—breast exam by a doctor and mammogram every year)?
- If you think you are in a high-risk group, does your doctor take that into account during checkups?

If you answered no to any of these questions, you could be at increased risk for breast cancer. For more information that may help you prevent it, please read these chapters in part 2 of this book:

- Chapter 21, Alcohol
- Chapter 24, Breast Self-Exam
- Chapter 25, Breastfeeding
- Chapter 30, Early Detection
- Chapter 31, Estrogen Replacement Therapy
- Chapter 32, Exercise
- Chapter 33, Fat
- Chapter 40, Heredity
- Chapter 49, Obesity
- Chapter 54, Prescription Drugs
- Chapter 55, Protein
- Chapter 64, Vegetables
- Chapter 69, Vitamin E
- Chapter 71, X-Rays

A second study, this one by the National Cancer Institute, also concluded that women who consumed moderate amounts of alcohol ran a 50 to 100 percent higher risk of developing breast cancer.

In addition to diet, exercise may also prove to be an unexpected ally in the fight against breast cancer, according to Dr. Frisch and other researchers at Harvard University, Cambridge, Massachusetts. They compared a group of former college athletes with a group who were nonathletes in their college years to examine the relationship between breast cancer and exercise. "We found that the nonathletic women had almost twice the risk of breast cancer than did the former athletes," says Dr. Frisch. "Exercise started early in life seems to have a long-range protective effect, as this finding illustrates.

"I think that in the long run, what may really make a difference is body composition—the amount of fat versus the amount of muscle you see on these women," Dr. Frisch says. "We think it's very likely that the former college athletes had been lean for a long time, although that was something we could not measure."

Women who begin exercising at a later age may still reap some protective benefits, Dr. Frisch believes. "We know cancer usually takes a long time to develop and that the highest risk is in the menopausal years. Women who begin exercising in their twenties or thirties have 25 years to get in good shape and stay that way."

Protective effects don't come easy. What's required is two to three hours a week of intensive activity.

Cervical Cancer

Even though cervical cancer is becoming less common, there are still about 61,000 new cases a year. Fortunately, cervical cancer is almost completely curable if it's caught early. And there are many things a woman can do to prevent this cancer.

The cervix is the neck of the uterus, which protrudes into the vagina. It serves as a canal between the two.

The treatment for cervical cancer depends on how advanced the cancer is. If it is caught early, minimal surgery can often cure it, leaving the woman able to have children. Extensive cancer usually requires removal of the uterus and cervix—a total hysterectomy—which makes it impossible to have children. Radiation therapy may also be used in some cases.

Clearly, it's best to avoid getting this cancer in the first place, or at least to try and catch it early, when treatment is relatively simple and effective.

SELF-CARE IS THE KEY

But catching it early requires some vigilance, and it appears that many women aren't aware of that fact: only half who get cervical cancer are cured. The low rate is due mainly to the fact that many women put off visiting their doctor for too long.

Most cell changes in the cervix follow a long, slow course. Cervical cancers usually take many years to develop. Women who end up with invasive cancer usually either have not been getting a yearly cancer screening (Pap smear) or are among the unlucky few who develop a rapidly growing cancer.

When a doctor does a Pap smear (named after George Papanicolaou, the Greek-American who invented it), he takes a scraping of cells from the cervix. The Pap smear can usually detect inflammation or disordered growth of the cells of the cervix—possibly precancerous changes—before any signs are visible to a doctor's eye. These changes are known as cervical dysplasia (the abnormal development of cells).

The results of Pap smears are categorized and classified according to the severity of the tissue change. Or the cellular changes are simply described in detail. Changes of the cells that are detected by the Pap test can indicate that the cervix is reacting to various vaginal problems. It may reveal, for example, that the cervix has been exposed to one of the viruses (herpes or papilloma) that have been associated with cancer. However, not all cervical dysplasia will become malignant if left untreated.

STARTLING NEW FINDINGS

The whole school of thought concerning cervical dysplasia, which can lead to cancer, has been turned upside down recently as the result of findings that many of these tissue changes are caused by a group of sexually transmitted viruses known as human papilloma virus (HPV) or, commonly, as the condyloma virus. If they are allowed to flourish, all these viruses will cause abnormal tissue growth or breakdown. Some will form tiny flat warts that can grow undetected on the cervix or in the vagina (or on the penis, in men). Others form large, cauliflower-shaped warts.

There are about 40 of these viruses, and 3 of them are often associated with cancer. The main sign of exposure to these viruses is the development of flat genital warts, which often go undetected until they're discovered during a gynecological examination in women or a penile exam in men.

The most important risk factor for these viruses is a history of many different sexual partners. Each time a person has sexual intercourse with a new partner, the odds of being infected with a virus increase. Intercourse is by far the most prevalent way the viruses are spread.

This risk is illustrated by the fact that nuns rarely ever get cervical cancer, but prostitutes consider it almost an occupational hazard. And if a woman is monogamous but her partner strays to visit prostitutes, the woman is at greater risk for cervical cancer. The frequency with which a woman has sex with just one partner isn't a risk factor.

There's another disturbing risk factor for some women. The wife of a man whose previous wife died of cervical cancer is three times more likely than normal to develop cervical cancer.

Having intercourse at a young age is also a risk factor, because the cervical tissue may be more sensitive during puberty and thus may be more vulnerable.

Obviously, if a woman is diagnosed as having cervical dysplasia, she should have her husband get a checkup, too, and treatment, if necessary. Checking the spouse is especially important if a woman finds herself having repeated bouts with the virus.

While researchers believe the papilloma virus initiates most symptoms of cervical dysplasia—indeed, some doctors believe it's the cause of most cervical cancers—they also think other risk factors may make some people more vulnerable to the virus, or that there are forms of dysplasia which are not virus-related.

In some women, the lesions just disappear of their own accord, but in others they develop into cancers. No one knows exactly why some of the lesions turn into cancer.

There are some other known risk factors for the cancer. Smoking is one. In one study women who reported ever smoking cigarettes regularly had a 50 percent elevated risk of invasive cervical cancer compared to nonsmokers.

It's true that there have been two British studies linking the use of birth control pills with cervical dysplasia, but many top researchers contest these findings. Other birth control methods may offer some protection. Women who use a diaphragm or whose partners use a condom have lower than usual cervical cancer rates, possibly because the devices protect the cervix from infection.

Researchers are also finding that nutritional status apparently plays a role in the development of cervical cancer. Poor nutrition may make cervical cells less able to withstand the mutagenic effects of some viruses or the carcinogens found in the cervical mucus of women who smoke. It can also weaken the body's immune system, making it less able to fight infection.

Some women with newly diagnosed cervical cancer have been found to have lower than normal intake of vitamins C and A and the B vitamin folate. This last vitamin seems to play a role in dysplasia, especially in women who use birth control pills, according to researchers at the University of Alabama at Birmingham.

All of this indicates that women should make sure that they are getting plenty of fresh fruits and vegetables that are rich in vitamins C and A, and folate-rich dark leafy greens.

But perhaps the most important preventive measure is to get a regular Pap smear. The American Cancer Society recommends that most women have a Pap smear only once every three years, after they've gone two years in a row with normal results. The American College of Obstetricians and Gynecologists recommends one Pap smear a year. Women should have these tests even if they've had a hysterectomy.

There are two good reasons for an annual Pap smear. One is the remote possibility that you may develop a fast-growing cancer. The other is that the Pap smear isn't always accurate—occasionally it suggests that the cervix is normal when it isn't, and vice-versa. More frequent tests minimize the chances of walking around with undetected dysplasia or cancer.

ARE YOU AT RISK FOR CERVICAL CANCER?

Women who became sexually active during puberty, those who have had multiple sex partners and those who are married to a man whose first wife died of cervical cancer are at greater than average risk of cervical cancer. However, there are other risk factors that are controllable. Answer the following questions to see if you are doing all you can to prevent cervical cancer, or at least ensure early detection.

- Do you have regular Pap tests?
- Do you avoid being sexually promiscuous?
- Do you abstain from smoking?
- Do you eat a balanced diet that includes vitamin A, vitamin C and the B vitamin folate?
- If you think you are in a high-risk group, does your doctor take that into account during checkups?

If you answered no to any of these questions, you may be at increased risk for cervical cancer. For more information that may help you prevent it, please read these chapters in part 2 of this book:

- Chapter 22, Allergies
- Chapter 30, Early Detection
- Chapter 49, Obesity
- Chapter 50, Oral Contraceptives
- Chapter 52, Pap Tests
- Chapter 54, Prescription Drugs
- Chapter 57, Selenium
- Chapter 58, Sex
- Chapter 63, Tobacco
- Chapter 64, Vegetables
- Chapter 65, Vitamin A
- Chapter 66, Vitamin B
- Chapter 67, Vitamin C

C H A P T E R 5

Colorectal Cancer

If your Toyota were a person, it might get cancer. That's because when Japanese people export themselves from their country to America, they (or their descendants) have a higher risk of cancer of the colon and rectum. But it's not part of a revenge plot by Detroit executives. Most likely, it's diet. The Japanese typically switch from a low-fat diet to the high-fat, low-fiber Western diet. And that's a little like committing hari-kari with a knife and fork. But these new citizens aren't the only victims of dietary mayhem.

Colorectal (large bowel) cancer has been linked to the high-fat, high-protein and low-fiber diets characteristic of industrialized, urban countries the world over, including western Europe, Australia, New Zealand and the United States. It is less common in Africa and most third world countries, where a diet that's high in fiber and low in fat is the norm.

It seems, at least in relation to diet and cancer of the colon, that progress hasn't necessarily been for the better. In the United States, perhaps the most developed country on earth and the one richest in processed food, about 138,000 people get cancer of the large bowel each year.

It makes sense that diet would play a major role in the health of the large bowel—after all, the organ's only real function is to process the food we eat and hold waste products. The colon is the last five or six feet of the intestine. The rectum, which is located at the end of the colon, is five or six inches long and leads to the outside of the body where waste is expelled. The main purpose of these two sections of the bowel—together called the large bowel or large intestine—is to absorb water and minerals from what's left of food that's been digested and to hold on to the waste until the body gets rid of it.

FIGHT FAT IN YOUR DIET

While no one knows exactly which carcinogens in the diet cause most colorectal cancer, evidence suggests that it somehow involves dietary fat. Many experts now believe that fats we eat interact with bacteria that live in the large bowel, leading to either bacterial formation of carcinogens or a failure of the body's ability to break down carcinogens. This process takes a long time—you don't just get cancer one day after eating something fatty—so it's generally believed that reducing the overall fat in the diet will reduce a person's chances of getting colorectal cancer.

Fiber is thought to be another significant factor in colorectal cancer. But it's not a cause, it's a preventive factor. Again, the relationship isn't clear, but research suggests that fiber might actually absorb the carcinogens that are formed when fats meet bacteria in the bowel, then carry them more rapidly out of the body with other waste products. The benefits of a high-fiber diet are supported by the fact that vegetarians and Seventh-Day Adventists in the United States who eat high-fiber, low-fat diets have lower rates of bowel cancer than people who eat the typical American diet.

Calcium is another substance that people should be sure they are getting enough of if they want to reduce their risk of colorectal cancer. Get at least your Recommended Dietary Allowance (RDA) of calcium (800 milligrams), and consider asking your doctor if you should take more than that.

REGULAR EXAMS ARE ESSENTIAL (AND NOTHING TO FEAR)

Regular medical exams won't prevent the colorectal cancer from forming. But they can prevent it from *spreading* by detecting it early—

ARE YOU AT RISK FOR COLORECTAL CANCER?

People over age 40, those who have a history of ulcerative colitis and those who have a family history of polyps in the bowel are at greater than average risk for colorectal cancer. However, there are other risk factors that are controllable. Answer the following questions to see if you are doing all you can to prevent colorectal cancer, or at least ensure early detection.

- Do you follow a low-fat diet?
- Do you eat plenty of whole grains, vegetables, bran and other sources of fiber?
- Do you consume at least the RDA of calcium?
- If you are over 40 or if you think you are in a high-risk group, do you have routine digital rectal examinations?

If you answered no to any of these questions, you could be at increased risk for colorectal cancer. For more information that may help you prevent it, please read these chapters in part 2 of this book:

- Chapter 26, Calcium
- Chapter 28, Colorectal Examination
- Chapter 30, Early Detection
- Chapter 32, Exercise
- Chapter 33, Fat
- Chapter 34, Fiber
- Chapter 38, Fruit
- Chapter 40, Heredity
- Chapter 42, Indoor Pollution
- Chapter 49, Obesity
- Chapter 51, Outdoor Pollution
- Chapter 64, Vegetables
- Chapter 67, Vitamin C
- Chapter 68, Vitamin D
- Chapter 72, Yogurt

before it has a chance to take over. An American Cancer Society study concluded that everyone over 40 years old should have a digital rectal examination every year. The recommendation applies to both men and women, because the cancer strikes with no sex preference. During a digital rectal examination the doctor inserts a rubber-gloved finger into the rectum to feel for any changes that might indicate cancer, and takes a stool sample to test for hidden blood. People with ulcerative colitis, polyps or a family history of colon cancer should have even more thorough and more frequent exams. These usually involve a proctosigmoidoscopy, whereby your doctor can examine the rectum and lower colon, or a fiberoptic colonoscopy, which allows an examination of the entire colon.

TWO BIG RISK FACTORS

Aside from lifestyle factors, there are two main health problems that can make a person more susceptible to colorectal cancer. One is a history of ulcerative colitis. The other is a family history of polyps in the large bowel (sometimes called Gardner's syndrome). People with either of these problems should be sure that their doctor regularly examines them carefully.

The symptoms of colorectal cancer can be as dramatic as blood in the stools or as seemingly innocuous as constipation or a change in bowel habits that persists for more than a couple of weeks. Diarrhea, abdominal pain, pain in the lower back and bladder symptoms can be other signs. While these are frequently also symptoms of more minor problems, such as hemorrhoids, anyone who notices a persistent change in bowel habits should see their doctor.

Treatment most often includes surgery to remove the affected part of the colon, depending on the type and severity of the disease. Sometimes the colon will continue to work much as it always did. If cancer is in the rectum, a surgical procedure called a colostomy is performed to make an opening (stoma) in the abdominal wall, through which body wastes are removed. Fortunately, this type of surgery is the exception, not the rule. With good screening for early colorectal cancer and good care, many more than the present 50 percent of all colorectal cancer sufferers could be cured.

Esophageal Cancer

Cancer of the esophagus is a relatively rare cancer in this country, but it's also one of the deadliest. There are about 9,400 new cases each year and about 8,000 deaths. To put it bluntly, the prognosis for cancer of the esophagus is almost always bad, no matter how sophisticated the medical treatment is.

But this cancer doesn't just take its toll indiscriminately. While good nutrition plays a role in preventing this cancer, there are two key steps you can take to greatly reduce your risk for cancer of the esophagus: Drink only moderately, if at all, and don't smoke. It's that simple.

DON'T DOUBLE YOUR PLEASURE

Studies in the United States, Denmark and France have found that smoking a lot and drinking a lot are the most important risk factors. A major study of black men in Washington, D.C., (which has the highest rate of esophageal cancer of all cities in the United States, at 28.6 per 100,000 black men) implicated overindulgence in alcohol as the main risk factor responsible for 80 percent of esophageal cancers. And doubling the "pleasure" won't double the fun: People who both drink and smoke are 30 times as likely to get esophageal cancer as people who do neither.

A healthy diet has been linked to a healthy esophagus. Some studies point to deficiencies in vitamins C and A, riboflavin and zinc as risk factors for esophageal cancer. Eating pickled foods may also increase your risk. So make sure your diet is healthy, in addition to not smoking and drinking only moderately.

THE WARNING SIGNS

It makes sense that things you swallow and smoke have an effect on your esophagus. It's the tube that connects your mouth to your stomach. It also makes sense that the main sign of cancer of the esophagus is trouble swallowing. Other signs include choking on food that you'd expect to swallow easily, pain and spasms following meals and recurring indigestion.

Unfortunately, by the time these symptoms appear, esophageal cancer has usually spread beyond control. The cancer can spread directly to surrounding parts of the body or to other areas via the lymph system and blood. Surgery and radiation are the usual treatments for cancer of the esophagus.

ARE YOU AT RISK FOR ESOPHAGEAL CANCER?

Answer the following questions to see if you are doing all you can to prevent esophageal cancer.

- Do you abstain from smoking?
- Do you drink alcohol only moderately, if at all?
- Do you eat a balanced diet that includes adequate vitamins and minerals?

If you answered no to any of these questions, you may be at increased risk for esophageal cancer. For more information that may help you prevent it, please read these chapters in part 2 of this book:

- Chapter 21, Alcohol
- Chapter 42, Indoor Pollution
- Chapter 48, Nitrites and Nitrates
- Chapter 63, Tobacco
- Chapter 66, Vitamin B
- Chapter 67, Vitamin C

C H A P T E R 7
Eye Cancer

Eye cancer is a rare disease compared to a lot of other cancers, striking about 2,500 people and causing about 400 deaths each year. Even though it's rare, it's still worthwhile to know what you can do to help lower the odds of getting eye cancer.

When doctors speak of eye cancer, they're referring to one of three main types that are found in various parts of the eye—the eyeball itself, the eye socket and the eyelids, along with a membrane called the conjunctiva that covers the eyeball and lines the inside of the eyelids.

At least three kinds of cancer can occur in the eyeball. One cancer of the eyeball tends to develop in the iris—the colored part of the eye. Another takes place in the whitish tissue on the outside of the eye, and about 60 percent of people with this eyeball cancer are still alive five years after diagnosis. One other cancer of the eyeball is retinoblastoma, which is inherited in 40 percent of the cases and usually strikes infants and young children. Treatments for this cancer are becoming more successful.

There are several types of cancers of the eye socket, and the treatment depends on the type. The same is true of cancer of the eyelid and conjunctiva.

The symptoms that should send you to a doctor to check on cancer of the eye include double vision or a decline in vision, swelling, pain, squinting or changes in the eyelid. If you have these symptoms, see an ophthalmologist, because early detection is the one of the best ways to prevent death from eye cancer.

EYE COLOR INFLUENCES CANCER RISK

Researchers have recently uncovered some information that may help you avoid eye cancer in the first place. Apparently, the color of your eyes is an uncontrollable risk factor for developing eye cancer. People with blue eyes are more susceptible to this disease, which really is a melanoma that develops on the retina. But a *very* controllable factor is how much time you spend in the sun, according to research done for the National Cancer Institute.

Probably for that very reason, people born in the South are three times more likely to get the disease than other people. Those who get intermittent, intense exposure to ultraviolet (UV) light while sunbath-

---

ARE YOU AT RISK FOR EYE CANCER?

People who live in sunny areas, those who have blue eyes and those with a family history of eye cancer are at greater than average risk for eye cancer. However, there are other risk factors that are controllable. Answer the following questions to see if you are doing all you can to prevent eye cancer, or at least ensure early detection.

- Do you protect your eyes from ultraviolet rays?
- Do you know the warning signs that should send you to an ophthalmologist?
- If you have a family history of eye cancer, do you have regular medical and/or ophthalmological checkups?

If you answered no to any of these questions, you could be at increased risk for eye cancer. For more information that may help you prevent it, please read these chapters in part 2 of this book:

- Chapter 40, Heredity
- Chapter 60, Sunglasses

ing, gardening and vacationing in sunny climes are also at a greater risk for this cancer.

A National Cancer Institute study of more than 400 patients was the first to link exposure to the ultraviolet radiation in sunlight to a risk of eye cancer. (It's already been tied to skin cancer.) And according to one theory, the reason for having greater risk if your eyes are blue is that the protective pigment of the eyes is distributed unevenly.

But all people should practice prevention to keep UV radiation out of their eyes. While everyday sunglasses offer some protection, the best sunglasses filter out all but 5 percent of UV radiation—a label on the glasses should tell you how well they filter. If you're still in doubt, ask your optician for help. In addition to sunglasses, hats can help, too. And if you're doing something like gardening, wear sunglasses to guard against a strong reflection from the soil.

Kidney Cancer

The kidneys are extremely hardworking organs, and without them our blood would very quickly begin to resemble the water supply of a city where all the municipal water treatment employees are on vacation—awfully dirty. That's because the kidneys process all the blood in the body every three or four minutes, filtering out toxins and other things the body has no use for.

Considering that it takes most people a couple of minutes just to brush their teeth and wash their face, that's a remarkably short time to clean up the entire body's blood supply. But the kidneys do it 24 hours a day, seven days a week. The waste they filter goes to the bladder where it is stored until let out of the body in the urine.

Because they filter the blood, the kidneys are exposed to many by-products of the body's metabolism. Despite this exposure, cancer of the kidneys isn't very common. However, unless it is caught early, the survival rate for kidney cancer can be quite low. It accounts for about 8,900 deaths in the United States every year and afflicts three times as many men as women.

TWO TYPES OF KIDNEY CANCER

There are two main types of kidney cancer. The most common is renal-cell cancer, and it usually affects men 40 to 75 years old. The usual warning sign for this cancer is bloody urine, but a dull backache, a feeling of fullness or a lump in the upper abdomen are also symptoms. Some people also have high blood pressure, fever, loss of appetite (with or without nausea and vomiting), constipation, weakness and fatigue.

Treatment is usually surgical removal of the affected kidney. If the cancer is caught early, the five-year survival rate can be as high as 78 percent.

The other main type of kidney cancer is the renal-pelvic tumor, which accounts for about 1,500 cases a year and affects mostly people who are 60 to 80 years old. Blood in the urine is the principal symptom, and backache may also be present. Again, surgery is the preferred treatment. Survival rates depend on when the cancer is caught. A person's chances are greatly improved if the cancer is detected early, so it's important to get regular checkups and heed the warning signs.

ARE YOU AT RISK FOR KIDNEY CANCER?

Men between the ages of 40 and 75 are at greater than average risk for renal-cell cancer, and people between the ages of 60 and 80 are at greater than average risk for renal-pelvic tumors. However, there are other risk factors that are controllable. Answer the following questions to see if you are doing all you can to prevent kidney cancer, or at least ensure early detection.

- Do you abstain from smoking?
- Do you limit your exposure to cadmium on the job (if applicable)?
- Do you avoid using saccharin regularly?
- Do you avoid eating a high-protein diet?

If you answered no to any of these questions, you could be at increased risk for kidney cancer. For more information that may help you prevent it, please read these chapters in part 2 of this book:

- Chapter 59, Sugar and Artificial Sweeteners
- Chapter 63, Tobacco

Certain steps also help to prevent kidney cancer, even though its direct causes are not known. Studies implicate tobacco in its development, so don't smoke. A high-protein diet also has been linked—although not conclusively—to kidney cancer. Saccharin too, has been associated with kidney cancer in animals. And, if you are a rubber worker, an alkaline-battery maker or an electroplater, try to avoid exposure to cadmium while on the job.

Laryngeal Cancer 9

The larynx is located just above the trachea, or windpipe. It's the Adam's apple, the organ that allows a person to talk. Cancer here can have devastating effects on a person's health and ability to communicate.

Cancer of the larynx is more common among men than women, and among blacks than whites. There are about 11,500 new cases a year. It is a very rare cancer among nonsmokers.

Cancer of the larynx exists in two main types. One, cancer of the glottis, is slow-growing and takes a long time to spread to the lymph system and other parts of the body. The main symptom of this type of cancer is hoarseness—not surprising since the cancer is in the vocal cords. Although hoarseness usually means something other than cancer, like infection, allergy or some sort of injury, any hoarseness that lasts more than a few weeks should be checked by a doctor.

The other type of cancer of the larynx occurs in the supraglottic region, which is above the vocal cords. It doesn't cause many early symptoms, other than possibly an unclear, uncomfortable feeling deep in the throat.

Supraglottic cancers can be treated with radiation alone if they are caught early. Otherwise they also require surgery.

When caught early, more than 85 percent of cancers of the larynx can be managed with radiation therapy only. Laser surgery is sometimes used for selected early tumors. And sometimes major surgery is required to remove the whole larynx, but only in very advanced cases. This kind of surgery usually cures the disease, but also takes away a person's voice. Fortunately, many people who retain a part of their larynx after surgery can learn to speak again with therapy.

Some minor risk factors for cancer of the larynx are exposure to asbestos and nickel. By far, however, the main factors are cigarette smoking and alcohol. People who smoke run about ten times the risk of getting cancer of the larynx than people who don't smoke. Heavy drinking also increases the risk, especially if the heavy drinker also smokes.

There are no uncontrollable risk factors for cancer of the larynx.

ARE YOU AT RISK FOR LARYNGEAL CANCER?

Answer the following questions to see if you are doing all you can to prevent laryngeal cancer, or at least ensure early detection.

- Do you avoid exposure to asbestos and nickel?
- Do you abstain from smoking?
- Do you drink alcohol only moderately, if at all?
- Do you avoid using alcohol and tobacco together?

If you answered no to any of these questions, you may be at increased risk for laryngeal cancer. For more information that may help you prevent it, please read these chapters in part 2 of this book:

- Chapter 21, Alcohol
- Chapter 30, Early Detection
- Chapter 63, Tobacco
- Chapter 67, Vitamin C

Liver Cancer

The liver is a remarkably adaptable and tough organ that does a lot of work and at times takes a lot of abuse. Its duties include boosting energy by storing glycogen for blood sugar, storing vitamins A and D and making bile, cholesterol, digestive enzymes and complex proteins. As if that weren't enough, the liver also detoxifies alcohol and other chemicals that can harm the body.

Given the liver's important functions, humans are lucky that the liver's regenerative powers are strong enough to almost strain belief. In some cases 80 percent of the liver can be surgically removed and, if the liver is given enough medical assistance to keep going, it will start to rebuild within days and will totally regenerate itself in two to four months. But such a near-miracle is possible only when the liver is healthy. By the time a liver becomes cancerous, unfortunately, it's often too damaged to allow for successful surgical removal of the affected part, not to mention regeneration.

Liver cancer is diagnosed as one of two main types—primary, which starts in the liver itself, and secondary, which spreads from a cancerous organ such as the breast, lung or colon. Liver cancer frequently doesn't cause any noticeable symptoms during the early stages. But as liver cancer develops it can result in loss of appetite, weight loss, malaise, abdominal swelling, pain, fever and jaundice. The cancer occurs most often in the elderly and is more common in men and blacks. The good news is that primary liver cancer is becoming less common.

Unfortunately, secondary liver cancer *is* common because, according to some estimates, 50 to 60 percent of all cancers may spread to the liver eventually. The treatment is usually surgery or chemotherapy. The survival rate depends on the type of original cancer and the extent to which it has spread.

Primary liver cancer is relatively rare in the United States, accounting for 1 or 2 percent of all cancers (it's still very common in some developing countries), but it is also very often fatal. And there are several lifestyle factors that greatly contribute to a person's chances of getting primary liver cancer.

The greatest influence on the development of liver cancer in the world is hepatitis B virus, but this isn't a great problem in the United States due to effective screening of blood products for the virus. However, hepatitis B remains a serious problem for hemophiliacs and intravenous drug abusers.

DON'T PICKLE YOUR LIVER

Cirrhosis of the liver is linked closely to liver cancer. Cirrhosis commonly results from alcohol abuse, but also can come from viral and parasitic infections, hepatitis, nutritional deficiencies and other illnesses. In this country someone with cirrhosis is 40 times as likely to get liver cancer as someone who has never had cirrhosis. If you get viral hepatitis, there's not much you can do to turn back the clock, but remember that most people who get the illness do not develop liver cancer. If you drink alcohol in excess, you're increasing your chances of cirrhosis and liver cancer—and there's only one thing you can do to reduce your risk: moderate your drinking.

Other risk factors include exposure on the job to vinyl chloride, which is used to make plastics. This risk is rare.

Thorotrast, a chemical used in x-ray exams between 1930 and 1955, is another cause of an increased risk of liver cancer, though it's no longer used.

Aflatoxins, which develop from a fungus that grows on peanuts and other foods that aren't stored properly, can lead to liver cancer, at least in animals. But the Food and Drug Administration (FDA) controls the amount of these aflatoxins that can be present in food products such as peanut butter.

For women who have a history of liver disease, oral contraceptives are a possible risk factor.

ARE YOU AT RISK FOR LIVER CANCER?

Black men, elderly men and hemophiliacs are at greater than average risk for liver cancer. However, there are other risk factors that are controllable. Answer the following questions to see if you are doing all you can to prevent liver cancer, or at least ensure early detection.

- Do you drink alcohol only moderately?
- If you are exposed to vinyl chloride on the job, do you have regular medical checkups?
- If you are a woman with a history of liver disease, do you avoid the use of oral contraceptives?
- Do you abstain from abusing intravenous drugs?
- If you have hemophilia, do you have regular medical checkups to discover possible exposure to hepatitis B virus?

If you answered no to any of these questions, you could be at increased risk for liver cancer. For more information that may help you prevent it, please read these chapters in part 2 of this book:

- Chapter 21, Alcohol
- Chapter 42, Indoor Pollution
- Chapter 43, Iron
- Chapter 50, Oral Contraceptives
- Chapter 51, Outdoor Pollution
- Chapter 58, Sex

Lung Cancer

11

Each year, about 140,000 people get lung cancer, and about 125,000 people die from it. The vast majority of these deaths could be considered just a slow form of suicide. That's right, suicide, because more than 90 percent of deaths due to lung cancer could be prevented if people would take just one simple step: Give up cigarettes.

This is the key to preventing lung cancer. People who smoke may find it hard to own up to the fact that cigarettes are greatly increasing their risk of lung cancer. A common thought is, "It'll never happen to me." But a smoker has no reason to feel so confident. The risk of death from lung cancer is 15 to 25 times greater for a person who has smoked two or more packs a day than it is for someone who hasn't smoked. The risk rises with the number of years of smoking.

WOMEN ARE CATCHING UP

Lung cancer isn't just a macho disease anymore. Statistics show that as cigarette consumption rises in a group, so does the lung cancer rate.

ARE YOU AT RISK FOR LUNG CANCER?

People who live in polluted cities or work with asbestos are at a greater risk for lung cancer, especially if they smoke. Answer the following questions to see if you are doing all you can to prevent lung cancer, or at least ensure early detection.

- Do you abstain from smoking?
- Does your diet contain daily servings of green, yellow or orange fruits and vegetables for beta-carotene?
- If you are exposed to asbestos or radiation on the job, do you have regular medical checkups?

If you answered no to any of these questions, you may be at increased risk for lung cancer. For more information that may help you prevent it, please read these chapters in part 2 of this book:

- Chapter 30, Early Detection
- Chapter 38, Fruit
- Chapter 40, Heredity
- Chapter 42, Indoor Pollution
- Chapter 46, Marijuana
- Chapter 51, Outdoor Pollution
- Chapter 54, Prescription Drugs
- Chapter 63, Tobacco
- Chapter 64, Vegetables
- Chapter 65, Vitamin A
- Chapter 67, Vitamin C
- Chapter 69, Vitamin E

Women as a group began smoking in the 1940s, and now lung cancer has surpassed breast cancer as the leading cause of cancer deaths.

How do cigarettes ruin the lungs? Certain cells in the bronchi (air passages to the lungs) produce mucus to wash out foreign matter and keep the lungs clean. Other cells are equipped with cilia—little hairs that sweep the mucus toward the throat. Cigarette smoke causes the cilia to disappear. When that happens, mucus collects in the bronchi. A "smoker's cough" is really an attempt to force out the mucus and clear the lungs, but it doesn't clear them well enough. Continued smoking causes the cells to grow abnormally and eventually turn into cancer cells. So don't smoke.

Smoking isn't the only thing that's murder on your lungs. A small percentage of lung cancers are probably related to occupational hazards such as asbestos (among smokers especially), radiation and various chemicals. And while some research shows that people who live in polluted cities may get more lung cancer than people who don't, the increased risk is found only among smokers.

The early symptoms of lung cancer include coughing, loss of appetite and weight loss. Some symptoms are hard to recognize in a smoker because they aren't much different from the symptoms many long-term smokers have anyway: chronic coughing and wheezing. Others are harder to ignore—blood in the sputum, bout after bout of pneumonia, fever, weight loss and weakness.

There are three basic treatments for lung cancer: surgery, chemotherapy and radiation therapy. But in general these treatments are ineffective. The prognosis for lung cancer is dismal. Only 5 to 10 percent of lung cancer patients are alive and well five years after treatment.

So clearly, the best way to avoid lung cancer is to not smoke. After you stop, your risk of lung cancer is halved during your first 5 nonsmoking years, and it approaches that of someone who has never smoked after 15 years. If you don't smoke but do work in a hazardous occupation, you should let your doctor know, so that he can check your sputum and give you regular chest x-rays that can detect lung cancer early.

And anyone concerned about cancer, whether they smoke or not, should try to eat more dark green, deep yellow and orange fruits and vegetables. There is evidence that the beta-carotene in them can help reduce the risk of lung cancer.

Oral Cancer

12

Cancer of the tongue, pharynx, tonsils and oral cavity or mouth can be especially frightening because the mouth is so visible and so useful. And everyone is usually aware of what goes on in their mouth. Fortunately, however, some oral cancers respond well to treatment.

There are several important lifestyle factors, including smoking, drinking alcohol and not getting enough vitamin A and the B-complex vitamins, that can influence your risk of oral cancer, so there's a lot you can do to prevent it.

When people speak of oral cancer, they mean a cancer that can strike the lips, the insides of the cheeks, the gums, the soft palate, the tonsils, the floor of the mouth and the tongue. These cancers affect about 20,100 people a year, and 70 percent of them occur in men over age 45.

There are two important medical conditions that can sometimes lead to oral cancer. One, called leukoplakia, can appear anywhere in the mouth as a white, cracked plaque; the other, called erythroplakia, shows up in the mouth as a velvety, reddened area.

Oral cancer first appears as small, painless ulcers that cause the surrounding tissue to swell. As the sore grows, it often becomes infected and painful. It will continue to spread unless treated.

The mouth is subject to various types of ulcers, from cold sores to canker sores, and just because there's an ulcer in the mouth doesn't mean there is cancer. But any ulcer that doesn't heal in about two weeks should be checked by a doctor.

Because cancer can often be successfully treated if it is caught early, it's a good idea for everyone to be aware of ulcers or lumps that might indicate cancer.

SIMPLE SELF-EXAMINATION

Here's a list of symptoms that may indicate the presence of oral cancer:

- White, smooth or scaly spots on the lips or in the mouth.
- Swelling or lumps in the mouth or on the neck, lips or tongue.
- Numbness, burning, dryness or pain for no known reason.
- A sore or red spot that doesn't heal in two or three weeks.
- Repeated bleeding in the mouth with no known cause.
- Trouble speaking or swallowing.

Here is an exam that you can do by yourself with a mirror. The self-test is adapted from one developed by the American Dental Association.

1. Tilt your head back and look at the jaw and neck for any unusual bumps or masses.
2. Drop your head back to its normal position and feel the right side of your neck and under your jaw. Do this for the left side to see if both sides feel the same.
3. Look at the outside of your lips and feel them with your fingers. Pull your lower lip down and feel the inside and outside of it. Do the same on the upper lip. Look for color changes or lumps.
4. Pull your lips out, look at your gums and touch them with your forefinger to see if anything has changed since your last inspection.
5. Pinch your cheek lightly and pull it away from your teeth. Keep your mouth a little closed and look at the cheek and feel it with your fingers. Do the same on the other cheek, looking for differences or changes.

6. Stick out your tongue and grasp the end with a piece of gauze. Look at and touch the top surface of the tongue. Then pull the tongue to the right and left and examine each side for lumps or growths.

7. Put the tip of your tongue to the back of the roof of your mouth and examine the bottom of the mouth and tongue, touching it with your forefinger.

8. Open your mouth and say "Ahhhh." Tilt your head back and look at the roof of your mouth and the tonsil area and feel it. Note any white patches or lumps. (You'll need good room light or a flashlight.)

INCREASE YOUR CHANCES OF BEATING THE PROBLEM

There are several preventive steps that you can take to help ensure that your self-test will come up negative and to reduce your risk of mouth cancer. Your lifestyle plays a key role in oral cancer.

The primary lifestyle factor influencing cancer of the mouth is tobacco in all its forms—from inexpensive snuff or chewing tobacco to the most expensive Havana cigar. In terms of oral cancer, tobacco is always spelled P-O-I-S-O-N. It puts you at 4 to 15 times greater risk of getting cancer of the mouth, depending on the type and amount of tobacco used.

Heavy smokers who polish off more than one pack a day are 1.5 times more likely than light smokers and 6 times more likely than nonsmokers to get mouth cancer.

Where the cancer develops depends primarily on the site of maximum exposure to tobacco. People who stick snuff in their cheek get cancer of the cheek or gums. Pipe smokers are more likely to get lip cancer.

Alcohol is also a problem when it comes to oral cancer, but because most heavy drinkers also smoke, the exact action of the alcohol is not clear. Some experts estimate that people who drink more than seven drinks a week double their risk of mouth cancer. And when cigarettes and liquor are combined, the risk increases substantially. Drinking 1½ ounces of liquor and smoking two packs of cigarettes a day puts a person at 15 times the normal risk for oral cancer.

As for diet, a deficiency in vitamin A and the B-complex vitamins has been associated with oral cancer (these deficiencies are more common in heavy drinkers than in nondrinkers).

Finally, irritation and infection of the mouth from dental problems or broken teeth can cause an increased risk of cancer, especially if a person smokes and drinks.

ARE YOU AT RISK FOR ORAL CANCER?

Men over age 45 are at greater than average risk for oral cancer. However, there are other risk factors that are controllable. Answer the following questions to see if you are doing all you can to prevent oral cancer, or at least ensure early detection.

- Do you abstain from using tobacco in any form?
- Do you drink alcohol only moderately, if at all?
- Do you avoid using tobacco and alcohol together?
- Do you consume at least the RDA for vitamin A and the B vitamins?
- If you have dental problems that may cause irritation and/ or infection, do you seek treatment promptly?

If you answered no to any of these questions, you may be at increased risk for oral cancer. For more information that may help you prevent it, please read these chapters in part 2 of this book:

- Chapter 21, Alcohol
- Chapter 30, Early Detection
- Chapter 63, Tobacco
- Chapter 65, Vitamin A
- Chapter 66, Vitamin B
- Chapter 67, Vitamin C

CHAPTER 13

Ovarian Cancer

Ovarian cancer is the most serious gynecological cancer a woman can have, and the fact that it sometimes remains hidden so long before detection can make it frightening. This problem of early detection is serious. The survival rate is only about 40 percent, largely because it is rarely caught soon enough for effective treatment. About 1 in 100 women will develop ovarian cancer, but there are ways to lower the risk, including changes in diet.

The symptoms of ovarian cancer, if they appear at all, can be easily mistaken for symptoms of less serious illnesses. But constipation, flatulence, water retention, a frequent need to urinate, pain, swelling, nausea and abdominal discomfort are symptoms that shouldn't be taken lightly, especially if there seems to be no clear reason why they are occurring.

These symptoms are especially important when they occur in a woman who is over 40 years old (though most ovarian cancers hit women between age 55 and 59) or who has a long history of ovarian dysfunction. Some experts say that all women between the ages of 40 and 60 should have routine pelvic exams, even though these tests sometimes miss cancers. In the near future, however, a blood test may be approved as a screening test for ovarian cancer.

Ovarian cancer is rare in women under age 35, and is more easily cured when it affects a woman before she experiences menopause. It more often affects women who have few or no children, who have a history of menstrual difficulties or who have had previous breast, intestinal or rectal cancer. Just because a woman fits one of these categories doesn't mean that she will get ovarian cancer, but it might be an added reason to be aware of the warning signs that sometimes come with ovarian cancer. Treatment involves surgery, chemotherapy and hormonal therapy.

ARE YOU AT RISK FOR OVARIAN CANCER?

Women who are 55 to 59, those who have a history of menstrual problems, those who have never had a child and those who have had previous breast, intestinal or rectal cancer may be at greater than average risk for ovarian cancer. However, there are other risk factors that are controllable. Answer the following questions to see if you are doing all you can to prevent ovarian cancer, or at least ensure early detection.

- Do you follow a low-fat diet?
- Do you have regular pelvic exams, especially if you are over 40?
- If you think you are in a high-risk group, does your doctor take that into account during checkups?

If you answered no to any of these questions, you may be at increased risk for ovarian cancer. For more information that may help you prevent it, please read these chapters in part 2 of this book:

- Chapter 33, Fat
- Chapter 49, Obesity
- Chapter 63, Tobacco

Pancreatic Cancer

Though the pancreas is one of the body's most indispensable organs, chances are most people couldn't locate it on a body map any more easily than they could pin a tail on a donkey while blindfolded. It doesn't beat like the heart, inflate like the lungs or gurgle like the stomach to let you know where it is.

For the record, the pancreas resides to the rear of the stomach, just in front of the kidneys. And the things it accomplishes from its anonymous position are very important—namely, the manufacture of insulin and digestive juices. Without your pancreas, you would need injections of insulin to control blood sugar levels, and you would have to eat digestive enzymes to process food.

Pancreatic cancer usually hits people between 50 and 70 years old, and it hits black people and men more frequently. The rate of this cancer has been increasing over the last 30 years, and it is now the fifth most common cause of cancer deaths in the United States, killing about 23,000 people a year.

THE "CURE" ISN'T A CURE-ALL

Pancreatic cancer is often inoperable by the time it's diagnosed. And, unfortunately, the vast majority of pancreatic cancer patients die—current treatments can cure only 1 or 2 percent.

A person's chances are improved if the cancer is caught early, especially if the tumors are still small. So it's important to know the warning signs of pancreatic cancer: jaundice (yellow eyes and skin from bilirubin that's building up in the body), abdominal pain, loss of weight and loss of appetite. But these symptoms may not be present (they don't always indicate cancer, either). In any case, it's always a good idea to try to prevent cancer with the right lifestyle.

One important risk factor for pancreatic cancer is cigarette smoking. Moderate or heavy smokers have two to four times the risk of pancreatic cancers as nonsmokers. And the only way to reduce the risk is to quit smoking. Don't wait until tomorrow; quit today.

ARE YOU AT RISK FOR PANCREATIC CANCER?

Black men between the ages of 50 and 70 are at greater than average risk for pancreatic cancer. However, there are other risk factors that are controllable. Answer the following questions to see if you are doing all you can to prevent pancreatic cancer, or at least ensure early detection.

- Do you abstain from cigarette smoking?
- Do you follow a low-fat diet?
- Do you eat plenty of fruits and vegetables?
- Do you eat fried or grilled foods in moderation?
- Do you watch for the warning signs?
- Do you drink alcohol only moderately, if at all?

If you answered no to any of these questions, you could be at increased risk for pancreatic cancer. For more information that may help you prevent it, please read these chapters in part 2 of this book:

- Chapter 21, Alcohol
- Chapter 33, Fat
- Chapter 37, Food Preparation and Cooking
- Chapter 38, Fruit
- Chapter 49, Obesity
- Chapter 55, Protein
- Chapter 63, Tobacco
- Chapter 64, Vegetables
- Chapter 66, Vitamin B

A high-fat diet also has been associated with pancreatic cancer. One study showed that the rate of this particular cancer rose in Japan when fat in the diet was increased. And in Sweden, a two-year study done by the National Institute of Environmental Medicine revealed that certain kinds of fats and certain cooking techniques also appear to increase the risk of developing cancer of the pancreas. The risk appeared higher for people who frequently ate fried or grilled meat, but did not appear to increase if the meat was prepared in another way. Risk also increased with the consumption of margarine, but not with the consumption of butter. Low risk was associated with eating lots of fruits and vegetables, especially carrots and citrus fruits.

Other factors that may come into play in the development of pancreatic cancer include chronic alcoholism, pancreatitis, diabetes, working in the dry-cleaning business and having a job for ten years or more at a place where you are closely exposed to gasoline. While no single risk factor can be held directly responsible for pancreatic cancer, all of these may play a role.

C H A P T E R 15
Prostate Cancer

The prostate is a chestnut-size gland that hardly serves any purpose other than to contribute most of the fluid that combines with a man's sperm to make semen. A simple chore, right? Yes, but somehow this molehill of an organ manages to make a mountain out of itself.

One in ten men eventually seeks surgical relief from prostate problems ranging from difficulty in urinating, because the gland has enlarged, to cancer. And cancer of the prostate is a real problem, second in incidence only to lung cancer among American men, and is responsible for 18 percent of all male cancer. Each year there are about 86,000 new cases and 25,500 deaths. Only 2 percent of all cases occur in men under age 50. Black men have a much higher rate of prostate cancer, possibly due to high-fat diets as well as other lifestyle factors.

Symptoms of prostate cancer, when they occur, can include difficulty in urinating (because the prostate enlarges and cuts off the urethra), the need to urinate frequently, blood in the urine or a change in the flow of urine. Back pain, or a feeling of back bone pain, is also a common symptom. (But these symptoms are quite common, and they don't necessarily indicate cancer.)

The majority of prostate cancers are "silent," meaning they go unnoticed. In fact, autopsies of the prostates of men who died of various other causes showed that slow-growing, "silent" cancer was present in the majority of men over age 80. And the percentages increase with age.

SOME CANCERS ARE NO PROBLEM

These slow-growing cancers aren't much to worry about. When doctors find them in elderly men they just leave them alone, because the surgical treatments can be more risky than the disease.

Scientists are now working on better ways to diagnose the cancer early so it won't get out of hand. The simplest method is still the tried-and-true rectal exam done in the urologist's office. During this exam the doctor inserts a gloved finger into the rectum and actually feels the prostate for enlargement or growth that may be cancerous. That's why one of the most important things a man can do to prevent problems with prostate cancer is to have a digital rectal exam (which is not as uncomfortable as it may sound) once a year after the age of 40. There is also a new blood test for prostate cancer, called "prostate specific antigen," that you might want to ask your doctor about.

Whatever the test, if the doctor suspects cancer, he'll then have to do a biopsy to find out what kind of cancer it is. Treatment is usually radiation, hormones, or surgery. New methods have reduced the risk of impotency, which used to be a primary concern of men facing hormonal or surgical treatment for prostate problems.

The survival rate for this cancer is 78 percent for men with early stage cancer. But advanced cancers are harder to cure. Fortunately the survival rate has increased greatly since 1950, and will probably continue to get better.

STOP CHEWING THE FAT

There's considerable evidence that diet plays a role in prostate cancer. A low-fat diet might be a good preventive measure against prostate cancer (and it will help prevent other cancers, too). Studies in Asia and South Africa show that where people eat a very low-fat diet, men are at lower risk for developing enlarged prostates and prostate cancer. And scientists at Loma Linda University in California found that Seventh-Day Adventist men who ate a lot of fatty foods like meat, cheese and eggs were 3.6 times more likely to have fatal prostate cancer than Adventist men who didn't make these foods a major part of their diet (most Adventists are vegetarians). In fact, this same study also showed that obese men were 2.5 times more likely to have fatal prostate cancer than men who were closer to their desirable weight.

That fat may be associated with increased prostate cancer mortality is supported by a 35-year study of Japanese men, who (like many Japanese these days) adopted a diet higher in fat than they had previously followed. The study showed that the mortality rate for prostate cancer rose along with the fat intake.

Another substance that may cause prostate cancer is cadmium, which rubber workers, welders, electroplaters and alkaline-battery makers can be exposed to.

ARE YOU AT RISK FOR PROSTATE CANCER?

Black men and men over age 50 are at greater than average risk for prostate cancer. However, there are other risk factors that are controllable. Answer the following questions to see if you are doing all you can to prevent prostate cancer, or at least ensure early detection.

- Do you follow a low-fat diet?
- Do you limit your exposure to cadmium on the job (if applicable)?
- If you are over 40, do you have your doctor perform regular prostate examinations?

If you answered no to any of these questions, you may be at increased risk for prostate cancer. For more information that may help you prevent it, please read these chapters in part 2 of this book:

- Chapter 30, Early Detection
- Chapter 33, Fat
- Chapter 49, Obesity
- Chapter 54, Prescription Drugs
- Chapter 64, Vegetables

C H A P T E R 16
Skin Cancer

In 365 sunrises, 422,000 new cases of skin cancer.

They're getting cancer on the beach. At the pool. On the slopes. In the garden. Wherever they're burning or tanning, people are increasing their risk of getting skin cancer, making it more common than all other cancers combined. Fortunately, it's also readily cured, except for the rarest form of the disease, called melanoma, which is more serious but is still highly curable if detected and removed early. But why depend on treatment when skin cancer is so easy to prevent—first by knowing your skin type, second by protecting your skin from sun damage?

WHAT'S YOUR SKIN TYPE?

Your risk of skin cancer is determined to a great degree by your type of skin. After 30 minutes in the noonday summer sun, Type One skin always burns and never tans; Type Two always burns or tans less than average; Type Three gets a mild burn and tans; and Type Four skin never burns and tans more than average. People with Types One and Two are at greater risk from the sun than those with Types Three and Four and should take extra care to protect themselves from the sun's rays. People with Types Three and Four are much safer. For obvious reasons, fair-skinned white people have the most risk from the sun, and black people have the least risk. Light-colored eyes and hair can always indicate that a person is at risk. One survey found that skin cancer develops in 3.4 people per 100,000 blacks but in 232.6 people per 100,000 whites. Skin cancers usually strike older white people who have worked outdoors most of their lives—like farmers and construction workers. Melanoma more often hits younger people with indoor jobs who get large amounts of sun once in a while—like those who vacation at the beach.

THE CANCER BELT

The sun's importance is highlighted by the fact that the southern and southwestern areas of the United States have more than twice as many skin cancer cases as the northern states have. Tucson, Arizona, has experienced a great jump in the number of skin cancer cases recently because it's a very sunny place that's had a big influx of fair-skinned people. Most skin cancers hit the body in the same places the sun does—the face, the backs of the hands, the tops of the ears and even (as if they didn't already get enough abuse) the scalps of bald men.

But the sun isn't the only risk factor for skin cancer. A group of chemicals called polycyclic aromatic hydrocarbons has been linked to cancer in animals. Exposure to these hydrocarbons may pose a risk for people who work with coal tars, pitch, asphalt, soot, creosote, and lubricating and cutting oils.

Two treatments for psoriasis, crude tar ointments and chemicals called psoralens, which make skin more sensitive to light, also predispose people to skin cancer.

In blacks, burn scars and chronic infections can make skin more susceptible to cancer.

OUTWITTING THE SUN

Some risk factors for skin cancer are hard to reduce. Burned, you can't get rid of the scar. Employed as a highway worker, you can't avoid the asphalt. But too much sun is the major risk factor. And for most of us—even for those whose fair skin would make Snow White jealous—

ARE YOU AT RISK FOR SKIN CANCER?

People who have light skin that is more likely to burn than tan, fair hair and light-colored eyes and those who live in the Sun Belt are at greater than average risk for skin cancer. However, there are other risk factors that are controllable. Answer the following questions to see if you are doing all you can to prevent skin cancer, or at least ensure early detection.

- If you have an outdoor job, do you protect your skin from overexposure to the sun?
- Do you avoid intermittent, heavy exposure to the sun, such as weekends at the beach?
- Do you avoid contact with coal tars, pitch, asphalt, soot, creosotes and lubricating and cutting oils on the job (if applicable)?
- If you are being treated for psoriasis, have you talked with your doctor about the risk that may be posed by any drugs he has prescribed?
- If your skin is black and you have burn scars or a history of chronic skin infections, do you have regular medical checkups?
- Do you avoid even brief but concentrated exposures that result in sunburn?
- Do you avoid the use of tanning salons and home sun-lamps?
- Do you avoid frequent x-rays?

If you answered no to any of these questions, you may be at increased risk for skin cancer. For more information that may help you prevent it, please read these chapters in part 2 of this book:

- Chapter 30, Early Detection
- Chapter 40, Heredity
- Chapter 44, Jewelry
- Chapter 51, Outdoor Pollution
- Chapter 57, Selenium
- Chapter 61, Sunscreens
- Chapter 68, Vitamin D
- Chapter 71, X-Rays

sun damage can be avoided. Here are some guidelines from the Skin Cancer Foundation in New York City to help you reduce the damage:

- Avoid exposing yourself to the sun between 10:00 A.M. and 2:00 P.M., when it's the strongest (11:00 A.M. to 3:00 P.M. during daylight saving time).

- Choose tightly woven clothing and wear a hat, long-sleeved shirts and long pants for greater protection.
- Use a sunscreen with a protection factor of 15 or more before you go out in the sun and every two hours thereafter. Keep in mind that the sun is stronger nearer the equator and at high altitudes. A sunscreen is just as important on an overcast day as on sunny days.
- Check with your doctor to see if any medicine you are taking makes you more sensitive to light, and follow his recommendations on what to do about spending time in the sun.
- Remember that reflective surfaces like snow, water, cement and sand can reflect burning sun rays onto your skin, even if you are sitting in the shade.
- Stay away from tanning parlors. The ultraviolet light they use will increase your risk of skin cancer.
- Be careful about exposing your children to too much sun.

FIVE WARNING SIGNS OF SKIN CANCER

If all these precautions don't work, the next best step is catching the cancer early. And that's not hard to do either. Just give your skin an occasional once-over, looking for these warning signs: a sore that doesn't heal in six weeks; lumps or growths that keep bleeding or enlarge (especially if they are firm to the touch); any mole that looks splotchy, brown or black, or has an uneven border (like a maple leaf); a mole or other growth that changes size or shape; and a mole that itches or feels sensitive.

C H A P T E R 17
Stomach Cancer

There's good news about stomach cancer: The number of people in the United States developing this disease has dropped to about one-fourth of what it was 50 years ago. No one knows exactly why the rate has declined, but it's a welcome development. In America in the 1930s, stomach cancer was the main cause of cancer death in men and the third leading cause in women. Despite the good news in 1985, about 24,700 Americans got stomach cancer, and 14,300 people died from it. And it's still a scourge in other countries, including the United Kingdom, China, Chile, Iceland and especially Japan (which has a much higher rate than the United States, probably due to diet.)

No one knows for sure what the causes of stomach cancer are. But cigarette smoking is thought to be a risk factor. And diet seems to be implicated, too.

It seems likely that a diet that's high in fruits and vegetables may protect against stomach cancer. Studies have shown that people who eat more raw vegetables, such as cabbage, lettuce, celery and green and yellow vegetables, or a diet that's rich in both fruits and vegetables have lower rates of stomach cancer. The decrease in the rate of stomach cancer in the United States over the years might be the result of a rise in the consumption of citrus fruits and lettuce, as well as better food storage methods.

VITAMIN C PROTECTS AGAINST STOMACH CANCER

This decline in stomach cancer might be due to the vitamin C contained in fruits and vegetables, because this nutrient can counteract the formation of carcinogens called nitrosamines in the stomach. These

---

ARE YOU AT RISK FOR STOMACH CANCER?

People who have type A blood and those who have had pernicious anemia are at greater than average risk for stomach cancer. However, there are other risk factors that are controllable. Answer the following questions to see if you are doing all you can to prevent stomach cancer, or at least ensure early detection.

- Do you eat smoked, salted, pickled and high-nitrite foods only rarely, if ever?
- Do you eat daily servings of fruits and vegetables that are rich in vitamin C?
- Do you frequently eat foods that are rich in vitamin A?
- Do you abstain from smoking?
- If you think you are in a high-risk group, does your doctor take that into account during checkups?

If you answered no to any of these questions, you could be at increased risk for stomach cancer. For more information that may help you prevent it, please read these chapters in part 2 of this book:

- Chapter 30, Early Detection
- Chapter 37, Food Preparation and Cooking
- Chapter 38, Fruit
- Chapter 42, Indoor Pollution
- Chapter 48, Nitrites and Nitrates
- Chapter 51, Outdoor Pollution
- Chapter 56, Salt
- Chapter 57, Selenium
- Chapter 64, Vegetables
- Chapter 67, Vitamin C

nitrosamines are generated when other chemicals, called nitrites and nitrates, are present in the stomach. The theory suggesting a link between these two agents and cancer has not been fully established. If it is true, the problem may be very serious because these chemicals are in everything from bacon to well water, and it would be hard to avoid ingesting some at least once in a while.

Eating foods rich in vitamin A, like liver, sweet potatoes, carrots and spinach, also might reduce your risk.

The ways people preserve food have also been indicated as possible causes of stomach cancer. Salt-preserved, smoked and pickled foods have all been associated with stomach cancer, and this may explain why the rate of this disease is so high in Japan, where these methods of curing food are popular.

There are also some uncontrollable factors that make a person more likely to get stomach cancer. Pernicious anemia, a rather uncommon disease of the red blood cells that is associated with low stomach acidity, is a risk factor for stomach cancer. Having type A blood is another risk factor.

Most people with stomach cancer experience very few symptoms. The most common are weight loss and loss of appetite.

Surgery is usually the most successful treatment. For those few patients whose cancer hasn't spread to other parts of the body, there's about a 75 percent chance of a cure. But most cases are so advanced by the time they are diagnosed that the overall five-year cure rate for stomach cancer is about 10 percent. With this dismal cure rate, it's clearly best to try to prevent stomach cancer in the first place. Fortunately, there are positive steps a person can take to reduce the risk of stomach cancer.

C H A P T E R 18
Testicular Cancer

One cancer that is exclusively a male problem is testicular cancer. Testicular cancer accounts for only 1 percent of all cancer in men and only 3 percent of cancers of the male urogenital organs. But among men aged 18 to 32 years old, a group that's not normally plagued by cancer, testicular cancer is one of the most common malignancies. Men over age 60 also have a greater than normal chance of getting the cancer, as do those whose testicles didn't descend properly into the scrotal sac shortly after birth. (Because the condition can be easily corrected in male infants, the American Cancer Society recommends that parents have male babies checked for this problem.)

Some men might be comforted by the fact that few men get the disease, but it should be taken very seriously. If untreated, it can spread quickly to other parts of the body. And testicular cancer can be fatal.

Fortunately, the savage effects of testicular cancer can largely be prevented if the problem is caught early. Even men who aren't in the high-risk age groups should do a monthly self-exam.

The first sign of testicular cancer is usually a slight enlargement of one testicle, along with a possible change in its consistency. Pain may be absent, but often there is a dull ache in the lower abdomen or groin, together with a sensation of dragging and heaviness. Symptoms such as these indicate that a visit to your physician is in order.

SELF-CARE SAVES LIVES

But even if you have no pain or sluggishness, it is a good idea to perform a monthly three-minute exam to check for lumps on the testicles. These lumps can be an early sign of cancer.

When a lump is found, the affected testicle must be surgically biopsied—that's the only way to check if the lump is malignant. If the biopsy is positive, as with any cancer, your doctor will advise a series of investigations to determine whether the disease has spread before deciding on a treatment. Malignancies are almost always confined to one testicle. If that testicle must be removed, the remaining testicle will be perfectly capable of maintaining sexual potency and fertility. And in the very rare cases where both testicles have to be removed, any potency problems can be corrected with testosterone injections.

Though the risk of testicular cancer is low, the self-exam is simple, and if it detects the cancer early, the effort will have been well worth your time. If you find a cancer early enough, the chance of a cure is very high.

ARE YOU AT RISK FOR TESTICULAR CANCER?

Men between the ages of 18 and 32, those over age 60 and those who have an undescended testicle are at greater than average risk for testicular cancer. Whether or not you fall into any of these categories, you should perform a testicular self-exam every month to ensure early detection.

If you are at risk for testicular cancer, please read the following chapter in part 2 of this book.

- Chapter 62, Testicular
  Self-Exam

Thyroid Cancer

The thyroid gland is a tiny organ with a big job: It controls growth and body metabolism. Without a thyroid, our bodies would gradually slow down so much that they'd come to a stop—a dead stop.

The thyroid is located in the neck, just below the Adam's apple. But it was not always located there. Before birth, the thyroid actually migrated from another part of the neck as the embryo developed in the womb. But sometimes the thyroid gland—or part of it—doesn't complete the migration. This failure to develop properly accounts for those rare cases of thyroid tumors that develop in places where the thyroid isn't supposed to be, such as in the upper part of the chest.

Benign thyroid tumors don't cause any great problems except in rare cases where they get so big that they make it difficult for a person to swallow or breathe. But sometimes thyroid tumors are cancerous, and these must be treated.

Whichever type, they are usually discovered when a person looks in the mirror while shaving or applying makeup and spots a bulge in the neck, below or next to the Adam's apple. Sometimes they're noticed by family or friends. Usually the tumors don't cause any other obvious symptoms. The tumors strike women five times more frequently than men and are especially common in women of childbearing age. People who are diagnosed as having localized thyroid cancer (one out of two people will discover the cancer at this "localized" stage) have an excellent prognosis after treatment, which usually consists of surgery, radiation or hormonal therapy.

The primary risk factor for the development of a malignant thyroid tumor is radiation exposure. The most common source of overexposure is from outdated medical practices, like treating infant and adolescent illnesses such as mastoiditis, tonsillitis and breathing difficulties with x-rays. Others, such as the inhabitants of the Marshall Islands who were exposed to fallout when an atomic bomb was detonated on the Bikini atoll in 1954, and the Japanese at Hiroshima and Nagasaki, have also been exposed to radiation and, as a result, are at an increased risk for thyroid cancer. Because doctors quit using x-rays for everyday medical treatment in the 1950s (and hopefully no one will be exposed to accidental radiation or bombs in the future), cancer from these types of radiation exposure will no doubt decline steadily from now on.

Iodine works as a preventive factor against thyroid cancer, and is distributed in emergency situations—such as the Chernobyl meltdown. On a day-to-day basis, however, too much iodine can be dangerous. In fact, it is yet another risk factor for a certain type of thyroid cancer.

ARE YOU AT RISK FOR THYROID CANCER?

People who have been overexposed to radiation as a result of medical treatment with x-rays, probably during childhood, or through proximity to a nuclear accident or nuclear testing are at increased risk for thyroid cancer.

If you think you are in a high-risk group, please read the following chapter in part 2 of this book.

- Chapter 71, X-Rays

Uterine Cancer

When doctors speak of uterine cancer, they're usually referring to cancer of the endometrium—the lining of the uterus, which plays such a key role in reproduction. During the time of the menstrual cycle when there is no blood flow, the endometrium grows and thickens in anticipation of a fertilized egg. If no egg ever shows up, the thickened endometrium is shed during menstruation. This happens over and over, each month from menarche until menopause. If an egg is fertilized, it makes its home in the endometrium, where it develops into a fetus. Later, the endometrium helps make the placenta, which nourishes the fetus until it is born.

Unfortunately, cancer of this life-giving organ is becoming more and more common. There are about 39,000 new cases each year and about 6,000 deaths, a great increase since the 1940s. This cancer accounts for 9 percent of all cancers. The rise in the number of cases might be due to the fact that women live longer now than they used to, the increased use of hormone therapy to treat menopause, high-fat diets, obesity and cigarettes.

THE PROGNOSIS IS GOOD

Whatever the reason, there is cause for optimism: If a woman exercises good self-care and the cancer is caught early during a checkup, the odds are overwhelming that the woman will survive.

Uterine cancer usually strikes women who are older than 50 and younger than 65. Women who have a history of infertility are more likely to be victims of this cancer. It most frequently strikes women who are well-off financially (probably because of high-calorie, high-fat diets). Overweight women seem to be at more risk, as are women who began menstruating at an early age. Diabetes and high blood pressure are more common among women with this cancer. Smoking is also a risk factor. Women who get the cancer after menopause tend to have continued menstruating after age 50 or had excessive bleeding during menopause. Among women who get uterine cancer before they experience menopause, many have had problems with frequent periods, excessive menstrual flow at the onset of puberty or times when they didn't menstruate at all.

The hormone estrogen is thought by many to be a serious factor in cancer of the endometrium. This might be responsible for the increased risk overweight women face. While all women produce estrogen in their ovaries until menopause, overweight women have excess estrogen. And while no one knows the direct relationship between estrogen and cancer of the endometrium, women who have had estrogen therapy have been shown to be at greater risk for the cancer. The risk rises with the dosage and the length of treatment. Finally, estrogen causes cancer in laboratory animals.

Because of this risk, the experts recommend that women take estrogen, which they can get only with a doctor's prescription, in low doses when necessary for the symptoms of menopause. And even these low doses should be stopped and reevaluated after six months, and not continued for more than a year.

Estrogen is not all bad. In fact, the benefits can outweigh the risks if the hormone is administered carefully. But women who are undergoing estrogen therapy should be extra careful to do two important things to reduce the risk of uterine cancer: Have regular gynecological examinations and ask the doctor about combining estrogen with progestin. If you experience any of the symptoms of cancer of the endometrium, which in the early stages are bleeding between menstrual periods, excessive bleeding during periods and bleeding after menopause, see your doctor immediately.

If your doctor suspects cancer, you'll have to undergo some tests. The Pap test is only 60 percent accurate for this type of cancer, and the doctor might have to take a tissue sample directly from the endometrium to confirm the diagnosis.

The treatments for cancer of the endometrium are the hormone progesterone, radiation and surgery. Fortunately, if endometrial cancer is caught early, the five-year survival rate is over 90 percent.

ARE YOU AT RISK FOR UTERINE CANCER?

Women who are between the ages of 50 and 65, those who began menstruating at an early age or began menopause after age 50, those who have a history of infertility or a history of menstrual problems and those who are on a high socioeconomic level are at greater than average risk for uterine cancer. However, there are other risk factors that are controllable. Answer the following questions to see if you are doing all you can to prevent uterine cancer, or at least ensure early detection.

- Do you keep your weight down?
- Do you follow a low-fat diet?
- Do you abstain from smoking?
- If you think you are in a high-risk group, does your doctor take that into account during checkups?
- If you are undergoing estrogen replacement therapy, do you have frequent checkups, and have you and your doctor explored other methods of treatment?
- Do you know the warning signs that should send you to a doctor immediately?

If you answered no to any of these questions, you may be at increased risk for uterine cancer. For more information that may help you prevent it, please read these chapters in part 2 of this book:

- Chapter 30, Early Detection
- Chapter 31, Estrogen Replacement Therapy
- Chapter 32, Exercise
- Chapter 33, Fat
- Chapter 49, Obesity
- Chapter 63, Tobacco

An Encyclopedia
of Preventives
and Risks

C H A P T E R 21
Alcohol

Most people are familiar with the short-term effects of drinking too much. Speech becomes slurred, walking turns into staggering, vision doubles, and, on that infamous "morning after," the head pounds. The effects of alcohol—a combination of carbon, hydrogen and oxygen—are dramatic. Should you imbibe one too many all too often, drinking can lead to liver, heart and brain disease.

But does alcohol alone cause cancer? Science has not given us an absolute yes or no answer. Ethanol (pure grain alcohol) has not been shown to cause cancer in laboratory animals—and the rat test is one of the hallmarks of a carcinogen. But studies of people's drinking habits do link alcoholic beverage consumption with an increased risk of cancer. For example, researchers at the Harvard Medical School in Boston linked alcohol consumption to an increased risk of breast cancer. They based their conclusion on a survey of 89,000 women's eating and drinking habits. They found that women who drank one drink or more a day increased their risk by 50 percent compared to nondrinkers. In another study done by the National Cancer Institute, moderate drinking was associated with an increased risk of up to 100 percent. However, the danger isn't limited to daily or heavy drinking. Taking as few as three drinks a week appears to increase the risk for breast cancer. Heavy drinkers are also known to develop certain additional kinds of cancer—notably of the mouth and throat. If alcohol doesn't cause cancer in the lab, why should it seem to cause the disease elsewhere? One reason may be that most people don't drink *pure* ethanol. They drink alcoholic beverages containing other, nonalcoholic components that may be responsible for the added risk. Or alcohol may act as a cocarcinogen, that is, it may allow other harmful substances an opportunity to do their dirty work.

THE BUTT OF THE ISSUE

For example, a series of studies linked alcohol with cancer of the mouth and throat. But these studies also revealed that many of the people with cancer drank *and* smoked. And close analysis of statistics shows that alcohol and tobacco work together, like partners in crime. Together, they make each other more carcinogenic than either would be alone.

One study, for instance, found that heavy drinkers were 2 to 6 times more likely than nondrinkers to get mouth and throat cancer. Heavy smokers experienced a twofold to threefold increase in risk. But people who drank and smoked heavily had a risk more than 15 times that of abstainers. In another study, women who smoked one pack of cigarettes a day, in addition to consuming at least one drink daily, were 18 times more likely to have cancer of the tongue and mouth than women who did neither.

The fact that a definite connection between heavy use of alcohol and tobacco has been made with the development of head and neck cancers implies that these kinds of cancers may be the most preventable, according to scientists from Case Western Reserve University School of Medicine, Cleveland, Ohio.

Many scientists have found a similar link between alcohol and smoking and cancer of the mouth, throat and esophagus, the tube leading from your throat to your stomach. One study of moderate smokers estimated that those who are also heavy drinkers are 25 times more likely to get esophageal cancer.

Alcohol has also been suspected as a risk factor in cancers of several other sites, including the stomach, rectum, prostate and pancreas. However, evidence for these associations is sparse and conflicting.

HOW ALCOHOL ALLEGEDLY DOES ITS DIRTY WORK

Scientists are increasingly convinced that alcohol, especially when consorting with tobacco, might cause cancer. But ask them *how* these substances create such havoc, and the best they can do is guess. Here are the most intriguing theories.

The solvent theory. The person inhales cigarette smoke. Each puff draws in chemicals that are known or suspected carcinogens. These substances stick to the mouth, nose and throat in a coating of burnt resins called tar. Then, when the smoker takes a drink of alcohol, it dissolves the tar and passes the chemicals into his body's cells.

The busy liver theory. If a person downed ten martinis in one night, his liver would have to work overtime to detoxify all that alcohol. Some scientists suggest that this hypothetical person's liver would be so busy, it wouldn't have enough enzymes left to detoxify other dangerous substances—such as those resulting from smoking.

The activated carcinogen theory. Another theory is that liver enzymes are stimulated under the influence of alcohol. These enzymes are the ones that convert procarcinogens (like those found in tobacco smoke) into dangerous carcinogens. This action supposedly makes the chemicals even more likely to alter cell activity and cause cancer.

The irritated tissue theory. Anybody who has ever slugged a shot of straight whiskey should have no trouble believing that it can irritate your body's tissues. It is so strong a drink that you can *definitely* feel it going down. Some scientists suggest that alcohol can irritate the cells and change them in such a way that carcinogens can have a greater impact. To make matters worse, alcohol reportedly decreases saliva production, thus prolonging the exposure of a carcinogen, such as tobacco tar, to the tissues in the mouth area.

The weakened immune system theory. According to one cancer theory, we are constantly being bombarded by thousands, maybe millions, of possible carcinogens. We constantly stave them off, thanks to our elaborate immune system. However, alcohol may weaken these defenses, leaving us more vulnerable to the noxious agents.

The malnutrition theory. Chronic alcoholics often consume one-third to one-half of their daily calories in alcohol. And while alcohol has the *calories* of food, it does not have the nutrition. As a result, even a heavy person may be malnourished. Malnutrition alone has been associated with esophageal cancer, regardless of a person's smoking or drinking habits. Some doctors have put these bits of information together and suggested that alcohol may cause cancer indirectly, by encouraging malnutrition.

The secret ingredient theory. Pure alcohol might not be related to cancer. Rather, the culprit could be a contaminant found in alcoholic beverages that causes the problem. For example, ingredients in African maize beer and Puerto Rican "moonshine" rum have been associated with high rates of esophageal cancer.

Whether or not American alcohol has dangerous levels of contaminants is debatable. Several by-products of fermentation and distillation of alcoholic beverages have been shown to act as cancer-causers. These substances are more prevalent in spirits such as bourbon and Scotch than in vodka.

If this theory holds water, then vodka, which is essentially diluted pure alcohol, may be the least risky drink.

HOW TO CUT YOUR RISKS

No matter whether you drink imported French champagne or Kentucky "moonshine", no matter if contaminants are swirling around the ice cubes in your glass, the key to cancer prevention may be *quantity*.

A little alcohol goes a long way. Some doctors feel that a small amount of alcohol might even be good for you. One to three drinks a day may protect against heart disease. Anything more than that, and you might be headed for trouble. One study showed that people who regularly drank three to five drinks a day were likely to die earlier than those who drank less. The risk rose sharply for those who had six or more drinks a day.

"You shouldn't smoke at all. But if you are a smoker, the more you smoke, the less you should drink," says Oliver Alabaster, M.D., director of cancer research at the George Washington University Medical Center, Washington, D.C., author of *What You Can Do to Prevent Cancer* (Simon & Schuster). "The data isn't precise enough to show an exact cut-off point, but I'd say if you smoke more than ten cigarettes a day, you should have no more than one drink a day, and you should stay away from strong spirits."

All things considered, alcohol plays a minor role in America's cancer scene. According to Dr. Alabaster, an excessive indulgence in alcohol, especially when combined with smoking, is thought to cause about 3 percent of all cancer in the United States.

That statistic isn't meant to imply that alcohol is safe. Heavy drinkers, especially those who smoke, do have a greatly increased risk of getting cancer of the mouth and throat. Some 76 percent of oral cancer in men could have been eliminated if they had used neither alcohol nor tobacco, estimates Kenneth J. Rothman, Dr.P.H., a professor of family and community medicine at the University of Massachusetts Medical School.

CANCER PREVENTION PLAN: ALCOHOL

- Limit drinking to one to three drinks a day.
- If you smoke more than ten cigarettes a day, you should have no more than one drink a day, and you should stay away from strong spirits.

C H A P T E R 22
Allergies

The runny nose, the itchy eyes, the persistent sneeze—it's enough to wear out any allergy sufferer. But take heart, something *good* may be going on inside your body. It seems that allergies give your immune system a rousing workout, possibly making it a strong defender against cancer.

As odd as it may seem, studies are now showing that allergies could be your ally against this dreaded disease. In one Montreal study, allergist Roman Rozencwaig, M.D., looked at 100 families and found a much lower rate of cancer in those with allergies than in those without allergies.

In yet another study closer to home, researchers at the State University of New York in Buffalo interviewed more than 17,000 patients, including those with and without cancer. What they discovered was that among those patients who reported suffering with allergy-related diseases, such as hives, hay fever and asthma, there was a low risk of various forms of cancer.

What was their strong weapon? Researcher John E. Vena, Ph.D., believes it may be a well-developed immune system. "A person with allergies has an immune system that has gotten good at recognizing foreign things in the body and getting rid of them," says Dr. Vena, assistant professor of social and preventive medicine at State University of New York. "Such 'foreign things' could include the first cancer cells that develop."

Perhaps even more revealing about the study is that it showed that allergies appeared much more protective against certain types of cancer, particularly the virus-related cancers of the reproductive system. "Most notable in our study was the decreased risk for cancer of the cervix, associated with a history of asthma, hives and other allergies," reports Dr. Vena. Since cervical cancer is thought to be caused by the herpes virus and human papilloma virus, it may be that a well-developed immune system is capable of successfully attacking these viruses.

Another interesting finding is that certain types of allergies seem to be more protective than others. "We found that a history of hives was more strongly related to a reduced risk of cancer than was asthma." Why the difference? No one knows at this point, admits Dr. Vena. "It could be that the study relied on self-reporting and, very simply, hives are more easily identified and defined than asthma, an allergy disorder that can mean different things to different people."

If you are itching to find out just which allergies may protect against which types of cancer—stay tuned. Dr. Vena's follow-up studies plan to zero in on these questions and will use more sophisticated means of defining allergies, such as skin tests.

Barbecued Foods

It's a summertime scene that's as typically American as a Norman Rockwell painting: kids splashing in the plastic pool, grownups chatting on lounge chairs, the host sending up mouthwatering smoke signals from the grill.

There's just one problem with this scene. Those smoke signals may spell cancer. True, the risk of cancer from grilling is *very* slight, even somewhat theoretical. But it's a risk you should know about, because it's easily reduced or eliminated—with a cup of soy protein, for instance, or a sheet of aluminum foil. To that end, here's a guide to cooking out without scorching your health. But before we get to those tips, let's take a close look at these carcinogens—the substances that accent the "ill" in grill.

PAH, HUMBUG

Scientists discovered the possible connection between cooking and cancer almost 25 years ago when they found cancer chemicals—

polycyclic aromatic hydrocarbons (PAH)—in beef grilled over a charcoal fire. But research since then shows that the PAH scare was mostly humbug. "The risk from PAH is so low that it can't be measured," says Michael Pariza, Ph.D., director of the Food Research Institute at the University of Wisconsin, Madison.

But the PAH-cancer connection led researchers to see if they could find other cancer chemicals in cooked food. And they did.

Dr. Pariza says that new studies raise concerns about what happens when high-fat, high-protein foods—the barbecue favorites like burgers, ribs and chicken—are grilled. According to some experts, the intense, close heat turns fat and protein into mutagens, chemicals that can damage the genetic material of cells and so cause cancer.

John H. Weisburger, M.D., Ph.D., vice president for research at the American Health Foundation in Valhalla, New York, also found that well-done foods—browned and charred—contained these mutagens, and that they caused cancer in rats. But this time it wasn't just meat that caused the trouble. Other foods also contained mutagens when they were browned. What this means, says Dr. Weisburger, is that "mutagenic activity occurs because of a browning reaction . . . in food and perhaps not just from the decomposition of fat [and] protein through high heat."

This doesn't mean you have to turn your hibachi into a planter. "Comparing hazards, I'd be more concerned about driving after having a couple of beers at a picnic than about having eaten barbecued burgers," comments Dr. Pariza.

EIGHT TIPS FOR HEALTHY GRILLING

Still, it can't hurt to be on the safe side. That means not charring so heavily and cutting back on the meat. Sound like a barbecue for wimps? Not so. With the tips that follow, you can have your grilled food and eat it, too.

Look for lean cuts. Use less fatty fare like chicken without the skin and lower-fat fish. Boil ribs for about 20 minutes to reduce fat. Mix hamburger with soybean protein, suggests Dr. Weisburger. Studies show that soy reduces the total amount of fat, making a burger less likely to produce mutagens—and making it more nutritious as well.

Prepare fewer protein foods. Try grilling vegetable and fruit kabobs, squash, even corn on the cob.

Slather on nonfat sauces. Instead of butter, margarine or oil, try marinades made from lemon juice, tomato sauce, vinegar or Worcestershire sauce.

Cover the grill. Use aluminum foil punctured with holes to allow fat to drip while protecting foods from flare-ups and smoke.

Don't char food. Avoid overbrowning by using a rotisserie for more even cooking. Set food higher off the grill and hold your hot dog further from the flame. If smoke becomes too heavy from burning fat, move the food to another section of the grill and reduce the heat. Remove any charring that does form on the food.

Precook indoors. It reduces cooking time and the amount of fat.

Be wise about woods. Researchers in the department of Food Science and Human Nutrition at Colorado State University in Fort Collins found that mesquite, the plant from the American Southwest that is fast becoming a fuel favorite, had a slightly higher formation of PAH due to its unique composition than did hickory wood. (And while PAH may not be much of a danger, there's no sense exposing yourself to any mutagen when you don't have to.) Also, recent studies indicate that PAH forms more readily when soft woods from conifers like pine or spruce trees are used as fuel.

Forgo the flames. Avoid grilling over a burning log fire. Instead, wait until embers form and there are no more flames.

CANCER PREVENTION PLAN: BARBECUED FOODS
- Limit consumption of barbecued foods.
- When you grill, avoid heavy charring and use lean meat.
- Barbecue fewer protein foods.
- Protect grilling foods from fat flare-ups and smoke.
- Precook foods to lessen grilling time.

24

Breast Self-Exam

Vicky, age 42, is a big believer in the value of breast self-exams (BSE for short). She's read the brochures and seen the technique demonstrated in educational films. She even knows someone who recently discovered a lump. So naturally, at her annual exam, when her doctor asks if she regularly examines her own breasts, Vicky nods her head yes.

"I lie," she confesses. "I know that BSE is something I should be doing for my own health, so I say I do it. The truth is, the whole thing scares me—so I end up avoiding it."

Unfortunately, Vicky is like most women. "Very few women examine themselves, and that includes women physicians," says Susan Love, M.D., director of the Breast Clinic at Beth Israel Hospital, Boston. In fact, although 96 percent of women have heard of BSE, only 29 percent perform this simple procedure—one that experts feel could prevent up to 20 percent of the deaths from breast cancer.

Why? Because they're afraid, like Vicky. Afraid of what they might find and afraid of what will happen once they find it. Yet that same fear—focused positively—could save lives.

Just ask Donna. A Philadelphia nurse in her late fifties, she, too, feared examining her breasts. Yet, unlike Vicky, Donna didn't let her fear keep her from performing the examination.

It was a good thing that Donna had the courage, for it was during a BSE that she noticed something different about her right breast. "I saw a dimpling and right away knew I should have it checked out," recalls Donna. Her doctor found a tumor under the dimpling, which was later determined to be cancerous.

Then she got the good news. Because the tumor was discovered at such an early stage, it was possible to remove just the lump, which spared Donna her breast—and her life. "If I hadn't noticed that tiny change and alerted my doctor, I might not be here today to tell my story," Donna says.

Studies bear out Donna's experience. Nearly 95 percent of all cancerous lumps are discovered by women themselves. In a National Cancer Institute-supported study of 246 newly diagnosed breast cancer patients, more than one-third of the patients who never practiced breast self-exam had advanced stages of cancer, compared to only 5 percent of those who had routinely done self-exams.

FIGHT FEARS WITH FACTS

To get more women to practice the self-exam, it's important first to change how the BSE is perceived. "Everyone thinks you're supposed to find some tiny grain of sand or a BB pellet, and this can make you crazy," says Dr. Love. The focus, instead, should be on *not* finding anything. "The idea is not to look for lumps but to familiarize yourself with your breasts in their normal state so you'll notice anything different," she says.

Gail Diem, Ed.D., a health promotions specialist formerly with the American Health Foundation, would agree that a better way to approach BSE is to believe the payoff is health, not cancer. "BSE is something positive we can do for ourselves, and it's a preventive measure we can control," she says.

The way you feel about doing a BSE can even affect how well you perform it, according to one study. Researchers found that women who admitted they were afraid of discovering breast lumps or who believed that lumps were best found by a doctor were much less successful in detecting lumps than women with the most confidence and positive attitudes.

If you are too scared of finding cancer to do a BSE, here are some facts that may help you to fight your fears.

FEAR #1: I may lose my breast.
FACT: Mastectomy (removal of the breast tissue) may not be the only

course of action against breast cancer. A study reported in the *New England Journal of Medicine* says that half of all women who discover lumps that are cancerous may now be candidates for lumpectomy, a relatively simple procedure that removes lumps by way of a small incision that leaves only a minor scar in most cases.

"The more vigilant a woman is, the better, because the smaller the lump found, the easier the operation and the greater the chances of success. In a few cases, a woman can be in and out of the hospital in a day with almost no disfigurement whatsoever," says C. Barber Mueller, M.D., of the McMaster University Medical Center in Hamilton, Ontario.

FEAR #2: I can't examine my breasts as well as a doctor can.
FACT: According to Roger S. Foster, Jr., M.D., director of the Vermont Regional Cancer Center, women who examine their own breasts find tumors at an earlier stage and are more likely to survive the disease. In his survey of 1,004 women with breast cancer, 90 percent who performed self-exams detected their own tumors, and doctors estimate that, on the average, their treatment was started a crucial six months sooner than that of women who did not examine their own breasts.

In another study, conducted at the University of North Carolina School of Medicine at Chapel Hill, 80 doctors—specializing in general medicine, family medicine, general surgery and obstetrics and gynecology—were tested on their skill at finding lumps using silicone breast models. The results? The doctors found an average of 8 lumps (out of a possible 18). What's even more revealing is that even the best lump finders, the general medicine specialists, found lumps only half the time.

The lesson here is that the doctor doesn't necessarily perform a better examination than you can—particularly if you have been trained and you perform the BSE often enough to know how your breasts usually feel.

FEAR #3: I'm afraid I won't do BSE right.
FACT: Studies have shown that women who are not good at examining themselves haven't been trained properly. But instruction and periodic reinforcement can boost confidence and help women stick to a BSE schedule.

"It's important to get hands-on instruction in BSE," says Maureen Looney, R.N., clinical nurse with the Breast Clinic at Beth Israel Hospital. "Brochures are not enough for all patients. You may need someone to show you what's normal tissue for you and what's not. You may need someone who will help distinguish the bumps from the lumps. This guidance is especially important if your breasts are naturally lumpy."

If your doctor or the nurse can't show you, check out your local hospital or community health center. Many now include BSE training (some even offer instruction on a walk-in basis) along with diagnostic services such as mammography. Some teach on lifelike breast models, while others literally take you by the hand and guide you in checking your own BSE technique.

LEARNING BSE TECHNIQUE

Most BSE instruction is based on the American Cancer Society recommendations, which instruct women to feel their breasts in a circular pattern and to observe changes in the mirror. Some doctors now feel that the standard BSE skips certain steps that could sharpen skills.

"We found that even when women are practicing BSE regularly, only one out of five of them is doing it correctly," reports Holly L. Howe, M.D., director of Cancer Surveillance, New York State Health Department. Women who were more successful at finding lumps in breast models, says Dr. Howe, were those who used the most sensitive part of their fingers (the finger pads between the joint and tip), who pressed very firmly, and who covered the entire area from the collarbone to the bra line and under the armpit. These points are not always emphasized during training.

Other experts claim that an up-and-down grid pattern improves surface coverage of the breast. Clinical trials are now in progress to determine the best method of teaching breast lump detection.

Until those results are in, don't abandon BSE. No matter what technique you use, practice makes for proficiency. "BSE should become a monthly habit, as automatic and routine as brushing your teeth," suggests Maureen Looney. Practice in your daily shower; soapy hands glide easily over your skin and can help you detect any small changes underneath the breast surface.

You can choose from a variety of BSE methods, but pick the one you feel most comfortable using. You may want to use the clock, or rotary, method described below, but if you prefer another method, by all means use it.

Perform the following steps at the same time each month (a week following your period or, if you are past menopause, the first of each month):

1. Observe breasts in the mirror for pulling in of an otherwise normal nipple, scaling or crusting of nipples, dimpling or any watery, yellow, pink or bloody discharge. (If any of these are present, see your doctor.)
2. Lean forward slightly to observe any changes in the breasts, like puckering of the skin.

3. Raise your arms slowly and evenly overhead and press your hands together in front of your forehead. Observe any changes.

4. Place your hands on your hips and tighten your chest and arm muscles by pressing firmly inward, again observing the breasts.

5. To palpate (feel) the breast, lie flat on your back with a folded towel or small pillow under your right shoulder. Raise your right arm overhead. Cup your left hand and use the finger pads, not the tips, to feel for any unusual lumps or changes in the texture of the skin of your right breast.

6. Either begin at the nipple, proceeding in a rotary direction around the nipple toward the outer regions of the breast, or examine one half of the breast at a time. Start with the inner half of the breast, examining the areas from the collarbone to the lower bra line and from the nipple to the breastbone (sternum) in the center of your chest. Use varying degrees of touch for each area you press.

7. Pay special attention to the outer area between the nipple and the armpit, as well as in the armpit and under the nipple itself. This is where the majority of breast cancers occur. Lower your right arm to your side, using your left hand to feel carefully for lumps. Be aware, however, that a ridge of firm tissue in the lower curve of each breast is normal.

8. Repeat steps 5–7, using your right hand to feel your left breast.

Chart any changes you find on a breast diagram that has been divided into four parts. Also include a description of how any changes feel. Compare these diagrams monthly.

In addition to performing a monthly BSE, be sure to get a regular breast checkup from your doctor (yearly, if you are over 40 or have a family history of breast cancer) as well as a baseline mammogram (which will be used to compare future mammograms) if you are between 35 and 40. If you are over 50, you should have annual mammography.

A LOOK AT LUMPS

A lump that occurs *on* the breast—that is, a bump that you can feel when running your fingers over the skin—is usually a sebaceous cyst or a boil. A sebaceous cyst is nothing more than a fluid-filled sac caused by a blockage in a sebaceous gland in the skin. This type of cyst is often found on the areola, the pigmented area around the nipple.

EDUCATING YOUR FINGERS

Although breast self-exam is one of the best weapons against breast cancer and literally at their fingertips, women who practice BSE may not be doing so successfully. One reason may be that they are working with a set of dumb digits—fingers that haven't been properly trained in the science of self-exam, fingers that can't really tell normal lumpy tissue from tumors.

That's where the MammaCare Method comes in. Developed by a group of researchers with a grant from the National Cancer Institute, MammaCare is a patented BSE method now being taught nationwide. The technique is based on the principles of braille, that is, training the fingers to read the breast. By using a horizontal and vertical pattern rather than circular motions, the technique is purported to improve finger sensitivity.

The founder of MammaCare is Henry Pennypacker, Ph.D., a professor at the University of Florida in Gainesville. He and his colleagues conducted a study that showed women trained in the MammaCare Method can detect breast lumps as small as ¼ to ½ inch in diameter (about the size of a pearl or pea). Those using the standard BSE can usually detect lumps that average ¾ of an inch (the size of a cherry). Women who have no BSE training of any type cannot usually find lumps until they have grown to 1½ inches, or the size of a golf ball. Of course, the smaller the lump, the better the chances of successfully treating breast cancer.

Should you want to learn the MammaCare technique, here's what to expect. At the MammaCare center at Mount Sinai Hospital in New York City, the instructor first explains that learning lump detection involves using a lifelike breast model. Covered by a thin silicone membrane, the model contains lumps of various sizes, both fixed and movable. It will be your job to find them.

You begin the actual learning by lying on an examining table and viewing a videotape overhead. As you watch, you practice the technique on the model as well as on your own breast. Step by step, the narrator demonstrates how to use the flat of the fingertips (the most sensitive part) to make three small circles, first using a light, then medium and then heavy touch in order to detect lumps at each tissue level, from the surface down to the rib cage. The same three circles are repeated about a finger-width apart, moving up and down the chest to cover every inch from collarbone to bra line and over to the armpit. As you find lumps on the model, you mark them with a sticker.

(continued)

EDUCATING YOUR FINGERS—*Continued*

At the end of the videotape, the instructor returns to see how well you learned the technique. In addition, she explains about diet and about lumpectomy, and finally provides a take-home kit complete with a training model and calendar.

The first lesson learned at MammaCare is that lump detection is no snap. Yet with immediate feedback from the instructor, you also learn that it's possible to find even the smallest lumps. At the end, you walk away feeling confident and a lot less scared about self-exams.

Still, MammaCare is not for everyone. Fees start at $85 for the two-hour session, and there are currently only two dozen centers nationwide. However, as more physicians become convinced of the merits of MammaCare's technique, a variation of that training could soon find its way into local doctors' offices. For more information, call 1-800-MAM-CARE, or write Mammatech Corporation, 930 N.W. 8th Avenue, Gainesville, FL 32601

If you find a lump, look at the other breast. Finding the same thing there means whatever you've found is probably normal for your breasts, since they are mirror images. Have your doctor check all unusual lumps as soon as possible.

And remember that 80 percent of all breast lumps found through self-examination do not turn out to be cancerous.

C	H	A	P	T	E	R	25

Breastfeeding

Breastfeeding not only gets baby off to a healthy start in life, it may have a health bonus for mom, too. It may protect women from developing breast cancer later in life, say researchers reporting on a cancer and steroid hormone study. Called CASH, it is a study of women, sponsored by the Centers for Disease Control (CDC) and the National Institute of Child Health and Human Development. In numerous centers across the United States, CASH researchers interviewed nearly 10,000 women aged 20 to 54 about their reproductive and breastfeeding histories, with the hope of uncovering the causes of female cancers.

One important clue to breast cancer may have emerged from investigators at the Fred Hutchinson Cancer Research Center, Seattle, Washington. When researchers compared histories of more than 300 women with breast cancer with those of women without breast cancer, one glaring difference became apparent. The women who had children and had breastfed for a long term reduced their risk of developing breast cancer compared with those women who had never breastfed. For the premenopausal women, the longer they had breastfed—either nursing one child at length or adding up the time spent nursing two or more children—the less risk of breast cancer they seemed to have.

What's even more intriguing about these results is that having breastfed seemed to help prevent breast cancer even for women with other commonly known risk factors, such as the age they started to menstruate, unusual adult weight or a family history of breast cancer.

PROTECTION LASTS FOR YEARS

The best news about this newfound bonus of breastfeeding is that it apparently keeps protecting you from breast cancer into the postmenopausal years. The most recent CASH studies, involving an impressively large number of women (about 9,000), have shown that protection extended past age 50, the normal age of menopause.

Not surprisingly, the women with the least risk of breast cancer were those who have had the most children and thus a longer breastfeeding experience. "We found that women who breastfed a total of two years or more had nearly a third less breast cancer than women who did not breastfeed," reports CASH researcher Peter Layde, M.D., coordinator of chronic disease activities with the CDC.

Still, even breastfeeding for a short time may be enough to reduce the risk of breast cancer later in life. Dr. Layde reports that among women who breastfed for a total of six months or less, there was 8 percent less breast cancer than among women who had not breastfed. Moreover, women who breastfed a total of about a year had 15 percent percent less chance of breast cancer, while women had nearly a fourth less risk if they breastfed up to a total of two years in their lifetime.

What this study suggests is that older women could consider their earlier breastfeeding experience a form of cancer insurance. "If, for example, you breastfed your two children for six months each, you would have given yourself some real protection against breast cancer," says Dr. Layde.

BREASTFEEDING GIVES YOU A BREAK

Just how does breastfeeding defend you from cancer? No one knows for sure. Probably the best explanation, says Dr. Layde, is that breastfeeding improves the hormonal "environment" of the breast; however, the details still need to be worked out. Lactation, for example, produces prolactin, a hormone that may help reduce the risk of breast cancer. Still others say that during breastfeeding the breast cells may change favorably or that nursing could mechanically serve to "flush out" carcinogens.

But no matter how the protective mechanism of breastfeeding works, it's a benefit that should not be overlooked, reminds Julie Stock, medical information liaison for La Leche League International. "For years, we've been telling women that breastfeeding has positive health benefits for them as well as their babies." Breastfeeding, she explains, contracts the uterus and helps a new mother get back into shape more quickly. And, by acting as a natural form of birth control, breastfeeding allows you more time to recover from pregnancy. The latest studies showing that breastfeeding protects against breast cancer only "add to the mounting evidence that doing what comes naturally has long-term benefits for the mother," says Stock.

CANCER PREVENTION PLAN: BREASTFEEDING

- Breastfeeding protects against breast cancer even to the postmenopausal years.
- Even short periods of breastfeeding provide some protection.

C H A P T E R 26
Calcium

Calcium. It's the glamour nu-
trient of the decade, a talked-about, sought-after, headlined star. National Dairy Board ads show sexy models swigging milk to get their
daily requirement of calcium. Antacid manufacturers push their products for their calcium content. A diet soft drink fortified with calcium is
being tested for its sales appeal.

People got hip to calcium because of hips—broken hips, to be
painfully exact. Scientists woke up to the fact (with a capital F) that a
lack of dietary calcium was behind the epidemic of osteoporosis, the
bone-robbing, bone-breaking disease that hit—and knocked down—
millions of American women. Calcium, said the experts, may be the
best way to prevent the disease. Millions of women who *didn't* want
osteoporosis listened—and the mineral was enshrined.

But calcium is a nutritional Ted Turner—it always wants to do
more. And like that brash businessman, it thinks big—in this case, The
Big C—Cancer. Calcium, scientists are now saying, may help prevent

colon cancer. And that's help wanted: Colon cancer is the second most common form of the disease, outranked in deadliness only by lung cancer.

CANCER WHERE THE SUN DON'T SHINE

The idea that calcium might help deter colon cancer got a boost when researchers noticed that the disease seemed to strike more frequently in latitudes far from the equator—places with less sunshine. The hypothesis was that since sunlight helps the body make vitamin D, and vitamin D enables the body to absorb calcium, it was this nutritional pair that reduced colon cancer.

On top of this, scientists reported that in Scandinavia colon cancer occurs least where consumption of milk is greatest. And that idea was milked for all it was worth when Cedric Garland, Dr.P.H., and his colleagues at the University of California, San Diego, School of Medicine in La Jolla, took a close look at the diets of more than 2,000 men from Chicago over a 19-year period. What Dr. Garland found was that men whose diets contained the least vitamin D and calcium had almost three times the risk of getting colon or rectal cancer. They suspect that calcium combines with harmful bile acids and fatty acids in the intestine and escorts them safely from the body.

Another study makes calcium's role in colon cancer even more convincing. Researchers from Memorial Sloan-Kettering Cancer Center and Cornell University Medical College in New York City gave 1,250 milligrams of calcium a day (more than the Recommended Dietary Allowance, or RDA) to people from families that had increased frequencies of colon cancer. In people predisposed to colon cancer, an early sign of the disease is increased cell "proliferation"—unusually rapid growth of the cells lining the inside of the colon. In this study, the researchers discovered that two to three months after starting supplementation, the cells reverted to a normal pattern that was nearly the same as in people at a low risk for colon cancer.

The researchers echo the conclusions drawn from Dr. Garland's study. "Calcium modifies the environment in the colon," says chief researcher Martin Lipkin, M.D. "We think that calcium binds bile and fatty acids, reducing their irritation to the colon lining and thus decreasing the proliferation of cells. The result is a lower risk of colon cancer."

This isn't to say that the calcium-cancer connection is chiseled in scientific stone, or that the first commandment of an anticancer diet is now "Thou Shalt Drink Milk." There's always a devil's advocate in science—another researcher conducted a study of 8,000 men that found *no* connection between the mineral and a reduced risk of colon cancer.

Still, there's enough evidence to allow some experts to suggest that calcium might be protective.

OVERCOMING THE CALCIUM SHORTAGE

But exactly how much calcium might you need to protect yourself from cancer? At this point, no one really knows. But we do know how much you need for other aspects of good health.

The government's National Institutes of Health (NIH), for example, say postmenopausal women should get 1,000 to 1,500 milligrams a day. The scientists who set the Recommended Dietary Allowances for nutrients plan to increase the current calcium RDA of 800 milligrams to somewhere between the current RDA and the newer NIH requirements. So it seems that 1,000 milligrams is about the appropriate number for bone health. Certainly, getting this amount each day couldn't hurt in your effort to thwart cancer.

That's what you're getting every day—if you're a Siamese twin. Most Americans get about 500 milligrams a day. That means you probably have to *double* your intake.

So, it sounds like Americans have one more big problem to worry about—The Calcium Crisis. But this is a problem with a simple solution—in fact, a *lot* of solutions. There are super-easy ways to get more of this mineral. Let's look at absorption first. And let's do that by answering some questions.

Do I lead a shady life? If you don't get enough sunlight (the main source of vitamin D), calcium may not be absorbed. But it doesn't take two weeks on the beach to get your D. "Just 15 minutes a day, with sunlight on your hands and face, should be enough in most cases," advises Dr. Garland.

Other ways to get enough vitamin D include drinking milk (low-fat, please) or taking a supplement (200 International Units is the RDA for adults).

Am I a coffee or cola lover? Caffeine disrupts the kidneys' ability to reabsorb calcium. Researchers at Washington State University, Pullman, reported that people who drank caffeinated coffee lost twice as much calcium as those who drank decaf. Not only that, the coffee drinkers tended to drink fewer calcium-rich dairy products.

It's possible to counteract your calcium losses, assures researcher Linda K. Massey, Ph.D., associate professor of human nutrition at Washington State, "If you drink 2 cups of coffee, remember to add an extra ⅓ cup of milk to your diet," she says.

Do I eat a high-protein diet? One study showed that protein pushes calcium out of the body. Young women eating a diet very high in protein (123 grams a day, the equivalent of between five and six three-ounce hamburgers) excreted almost twice as much calcium as women on a normal diet (46 grams of protein a day). This put the high-protein group in what the scientists called a "negative daily calcium balance"—they lost more calcium than they took in.

You could cut your calcium losses by eating less protein, says nutritionist Patricia Hausman, author of *The Calcium Bible* (Rawson Associates). She suggests you opt for foods like fruits, vegetables and grains. Another option might be to take a calcium supplement. (We'll tell you more about those options shortly.)

Am I stuck on salt? If so, you may be shortchanging your calcium stores. Experiments performed by Ailsa Goulding, Ph.D., senior research officer of the Department of Medicine at the University of Otago in New Zealand, believes that salt increases the amount of calcium lost through the kidneys. In one study, animals given salt supplements lost more calcium in their urine and had less of the mineral in their skeletons than those animals not receiving salt.

So shake the salt habit. To add zest without zapping your calcium supply, use herb-and-spice seasoning blends, herbs, onions or lemon juice.

Am I a fiber fanatic? There's something wrong with fiber—the same stuff that is said to *reduce* the risk of colon cancer by hurrying cancer-causers out of the bowels? Yes, according to Lindsay Allen, Ph.D., professor of nutritional science at the University of Connecticut in Storrs, fiber is a mixed blessing: It has a substance called phytate that binds with calcium so that it can't be fully absorbed. But getting a healthy daily dose of fiber—about 25 grams—doesn't mean you have to be a calcium cripple. It means getting about 125 more milligrams of calcium—the amount in less than ½ cup of milk. If you've already been diligent enough to assure your fiber intake, it should be easy to up your calcium a notch. Another suggestion: If you take a supplement to get your calcium, don't take it at the same time as a high-fiber meal.

Do I take medications? Certain drugs impair calcium absorption—antacids that contain aluminum, for example, and some types of antibiotics, laxatives and diuretics. Ask your doctor to make sure the medication you're taking isn't taking your calcium.

HOW TO GET MORE CALCIUM IN YOUR DIET

All these tips are for absorbing calcium—but to do that you have to get the mineral *into* your body. And that's as easy as pie—with a glass of milk.

"It's easier than you think to get this nutrient from ordinary foods," insists leading calcium researcher, Robert Recker, M.D., professor of

MAKING SENSE OF CALCIUM SUPPLEMENTS

There's a dazzling array of calcium supplements in a dozen shapes and sizes. Selecting the best among them really depends on your pocketbook and your personal needs. As one nutritionist put it, "For many people, there is no right source of supplemental calcium, only a right dose to take."

The whole idea is to choose a supplement that gives you the most concentrated calcium in the smallest number of pills and for the least amount of money. Unfortunately your multivitamin/mineral supplements do not qualify because they usually contain only a small amount of calcium.

For most people, then, the best buy is calcium carbonate tablets, which usually provide 40 percent calcium per pill. Using these, you need to take fewer tablets than you'd have to take if you chose another type of tablet containing a much smaller percentage of calcium.

The strike against most calcium carbonate supplements is that they are bulky; they look like a piece of chalk and often don't taste much better. Many people take certain brands of antacids as calcium supplements. Made of calcium carbonate, they are inexpensive and easy to take. But don't rely on antacids for more than 800 milligrams of calcium a day. Prolonged use of high doses may actually stimulate acid secretion and create "acid rebound." Other options include calcium gluconate, calcium lactate and calcium phosphate, which are available over the counter. But you may have to take more of these pills to get your calcium quota.

As already noted, there is a lot of calcium to pack into each pill, so you may prefer to crush your tablets and mix them with skim milk (a good way to boost absorption). The table on page 90, Calcium Supplements, provides the pros and cons of common calcium supplements.

medicine at Creighton University in Omaha, Nebraska. Still, he admits, it does take some planning.

For example, next time the waitress asks, "What will you have to drink?" make your answer, "Milk, please." Milk—especially low-fat or skim milk—is a great source of calcium (almost 300 milligrams per eight-ounce glass). What's more, it contains vitamin D, which helps calcium absorption.

Still, one glass of milk may be one glass too many, especially if you're lactose intolerant—you become bloated and gassy due to an inability to digest lactose, or milk sugar. If that's the case, you'd be better off getting your calcium from yogurt made from skim milk. It's got a respectable amount of calcium (452 milligrams per cup) and has been found to be well-tolerated and well-absorbed by those who are lactose intolerant. What's more, some researchers have found that *Lactobacillus acidophilus,* the friendly bacteria in home-made yogurt, may play a part in protecting against colon cancer (see chapter 72, Yogurt).

If you've been dodging dairy products because of their calorie content, consider this. It's possible to have skim milk on your cereal at breakfast, a cup of yogurt made from skim milk at lunch and a slice of Swiss cheese at dinner and come out with over 1,000 milligrams of calcium while staying close to 400 calories.

Foods from the cow aren't the only sources of calcium, however. Nondairy foods rich in calcium range from sardines and salmon (371 and 167 milligrams, respectively, in three ounces), to tofu (109 milligrams in three ounces) and broccoli (one stalk has 205 milligrams of calcium).

In fact, says Dr. Recker, if you take advantage of all the calcium sources, from soup stocks to nuts, "it's hard *not* to get your calcium quota." But to make extra-sure you do, here are several easy ways to boost the calcium content in your daily diet.

- Choose watercress instead of iceberg lettuce. A half cup of finely chopped watercress contains 20 milligrams of calcium—almost six times the amount contained in lettuce.
- Use dark green, leafy vegetables for salads. Turnip greens, mustard greens and kale contain fair amounts of calcium, and collards are an even better source. (Certain vegetables such as spinach, beet greens, rhubarb and Swiss chard also contain calcium, but their oxalic acid content prevents it from being absorbed.)
- Eat the soft bones of canned salmon and sardines. When cooking soups and stews containing hard bones, add an acid ingredient such as tomatoes, vinegar or lemon juice to leach the calcium from the bones and provide 125 milligrams of calcium in each cup. That's as much as you'll find in ⅔ cup of low-fat cottage cheese.
- Substitute blackstrap molasses for other sweeteners—a single tablespoon gives you 137 milligrams of calcium.
- Add nonfat dry milk to soups, puddings, sauces and even to skim milk. (One suggested ratio is ¼ cup dry milk to 1 cup liquid milk.)

CALCIUM SUPPLEMENTS

SUPPLEMENT	CALCIUM/TABLET (%)	CALCIUM/TABLET (mg)
Calcium carbonate Antacids† (Tums, Chooz, etc.)	40	168–340
Generic and name brands (Caltrate, Biocal, etc.)	40	140–667
Oyster shell (Os-Cal, etc.)	40	200–500
Calcium phosphate (dibasic and tribasic forms, i.e., Posture)	23–39	89–600
Calcium lactate	13	42–100
Calcium gluconate	9	45–63

*Dose needed to supply 1,000 mg of calcium daily.
†Antacids do not all contain calcium.

- Look to cheese as an excellent choice for calcium. The top five are hard Parmesan (336 milligrams per ounce), part-skim ricotta (337 milligrams per half cup), Gruyère (287 milligrams per ounce) and Romano (302 milligrams per ounce). Even cheddar provides 204 milligrams an ounce, and good old American is 174 an ounce. One tablespoon of grated Parmesan added to vegetables gives you 69 milligrams of calcium with about one-third fewer calories than a pat of butter.
- Snack on figs—27 milligrams of calcium each.

NO. TABLETS/ DAY*	PROS	CONS
3–6	Available as gum and flavored chewable or coated tablets.	Long-term use of large doses can produce acid rebound; take no more than 800 mg per day; some forms require a greater number of tablets than calcium carbonate generic and name brands.
2–8	May be least expensive; usually requires taking fewer tablets; offers wide range of doses.	Occasionally may cause constipation, gas, nausea, which may require taking with meals.
2–5	Same as above.	Same as above.
2–12	Available in fortified foods; does not cause gas distress.	Same as above.
10–24	Well tolerated; recommended for those who cannot tolerate calcium carbonate.	Requires a greater number of tablets than calcium carbonate.
16–23	Same as above.	Same as above.

THE FACTS ABOUT FORTIFIED FOODS

Calcium is cropping up in some pretty convenient places these days. Foods like milk, cottage cheese, bread, flour—even hamburger buns—are now fortified with it. And the following fact should delight dedicated soda drinkers: A low-cal cola containing calcium is presently being test marketed.

Is fortifying our favorite foods with calcium a good idea? "Definitely," says Dr. Allen. "The more places adults—particularly the elderly and postmenopausal women—can find calcium, the better."

Yet no one knows just how calcium may be absorbed from enriched bread, let alone soft drinks. This is why some experts feel you shouldn't depend on them as your primary source of calcium. "I'd rather see fortification of calcium limited to foods where calcium naturally occurs, like dairy products, for example," states Kurt J. Isselbacher, M.D., chief of the Gastrointestinal and Nutritional Unit at Massachusetts General Hospital, Boston. "That would reinforce the healthier food choice."

Dr. Recker would agree. "I'd be more inclined to depend on Mother Nature's chemistry to get my calcium than on foods fortified with a single nutrient," he says. "Calcium from food does not work in the body alone. Sticking it all by itself in other foods may distort the carefully designed absorption pattern."

Wherever you choose to get your calcium, the bottom line is to get it daily. "Calcium is a lifelong mineral," reminds Dr. Allen. "It's never too early to start getting it."

THE RIGHT TIME TO TAKE SUPPLEMENTS

There's evidence that calcium obtained from food is much better absorbed than calcium in pill form. Still, some experts feel it may be necessary to take supplements, especially if you have trouble sticking to a balanced diet. But *which* supplement you select matters less than *how* you take it.

One expert suggests you take calcium in small, divided doses—say two or three times during the day—rather than all at once. "If you overload, there's a chance that a good bit will be lost through body wastes," says Stanton Cohn, Ph.D., professor of medicine at the State University of New York at Stony Brook. Another doctor believes a calcium supplement is best absorbed if taken right before you go to sleep. (A compromise might be to take one of your divided doses at bedtime.)

However, your best bet may be mealtimes, says Dr. Recker. He explains that in his experiments with volunteers who had low acid production, he found that calcium supplements were easily absorbed when taken along with meals. "The evidence is stacked in favor of taking calcium with foods for optimum absorption," concludes, Dr. Recker.

One of the recommendations of the National Institutes of Health is that calcium supplementation should not exceed recommended levels because of the risk of kidney stones in susceptible individuals.

Fortunately, kidney stones are not all that common, and most of us are blessed with a built-in regulator that adjusts calcium absorption. "I'm more concerned with people getting too little calcium than too much," says Dr. Recker.

Still, if you have any history of kidney stones, don't take calcium supplements without your doctor's approval. And no one should exceed 1,500 milligrams a day without medical supervision.

CANCER PREVENTION PLAN: CALCIUM

- Try to consume 1,000 milligrams of calcium daily.
- Drink skim milk and use low-fat dairy products.
- Consider taking calcium supplements if your diet is inadequate.

CHAPTER 27
Coffee

Coffee's the beverage many people hate to love.

That's evident in the fact that so much time is spent talking about ways to cut down on Joe, java, tar or mocha. But people keep on drinking it. It became America's favorite beverage soon after the American Revolution and continued to sweep popularity polls until just recently, when soft drinks took a slight lead. Even though it's now in second place, coffee is an American ritual, served in a variety of ways: black, New York City "regular" (lots of milk and sugar), cappuccino, iced espresso, brewed from gourmet blends and stirred up from a lowly instant. There's even coffee candy that packs the flavor and caffeine of the real thing.

Why do people demand so many varieties and still fret about drinking too much coffee? Jittery nerves is one reason. Stained teeth is another. And fear that coffee may cause cancer is one of the most powerful reasons of all.

But while it's hard to dispute that *too much* coffee can make you edgy and turn your tooth enamel brown, the coffee-cancer link is very debatable.

You might not know this, however, and it's not because of ignorance. Rather, it's because there has been so much conflicting and sensational news about coffee. Even the scientific reports are conflicting. Several studies implicating coffee as a carcinogen have been released, with their frightening results blared on television news shows and bannered across front pages as though they were gospel. Often a study's findings hadn't been duplicated by other researchers, meaning that they may have been the result of a one-time quirk in the procedure.

One study linked coffee consumption to pancreatic cancer. Still others mention bladder cancer, lung cancer and cancer of the ovaries. During the same time period, other reports came out refuting some studies that associated coffee with ill health effects. But an informal poll shows that these studies weren't as widely publicized. Poll yourself: Have you heard anything good about coffee and health lately—or even anything that wasn't condemning it? Probably not. Yet the supposed dangers of coffee aren't as clear-cut as they've sometimes been made to seem. In fact, the link between coffee and cancer may not exist at all.

According to the National Cancer Institute in Bethesda, Maryland, there is *no* scientific proof that coffee leads to any kind of cancer. They aren't recommending that you go out and drink vats of coffee without fear of cancer, because, while no one has proven that coffee does lead to cancer, neither has anyone proven that it *doesn't.* But the National Cancer Institute doesn't include coffee on any of its lists of dietary restrictions intended to reduce the chance of getting cancer.

Still, it's clear that all the effects of coffee on cancer *aren't* clear. It's important to understand this controversy, so you can decide just what role you want coffee to play in your diet. Here are the facts—and the recommendations from the experts.

COFFEE AND BREAST CANCER

One of the most widely publicized controversies surrounds the role—or lack of it—that coffee has in breast cancer.

Some researchers have proposed that coffee increases the incidence of fibrocystic disease—where benign lumps form in the breasts—and that this disease leads to cancer. So the controversy over coffee and breast cancer involves two questions: Does drinking coffee increase a woman's chance of getting fibrocystic disease? And does fibrocystic disease increase a woman's chance of getting breast cancer?

IS DECAF SAFE?

Even decaffeinated coffee has been hit with charges that it may cause cancer. Obviously the worry isn't caffeine. Rather, it's the chemicals that are sometimes used to remove caffeine from coffee that have come under attack.

Among the several ways to decaffeinate coffee, one is to treat the green, unroasted coffee beans with the solvent methylene chloride. Some residue from this chemical remains even after the coffee has been roasted, but the Food and Drug Administration (FDA) has limited the amount.

A study by the National Toxicology Program (NTP) however, says these chemicals can cause cancer in rats. Predictably, the study caused quite an uproar. The roar should have been more of a rat's squeak, because the amount of decaf coffee the rats were forced to consume equaled 12 million cups a day in one group and 24 million in another—a little bit more than the average person drinks. The experiment was later deemed so inappropriate that the draft of the report was withdrawn.

Further studies on rats found no correlation between cancer and methylene chloride or decaffeinated coffee, even at rates equivalent to about 80 cups a day. "Hence," concludes Diane H. Morris, Ph.D., R.D. of the American Medical Association, "available scientific evidence suggests that methylene chloride is safe for use as a solvent in decaffeinating coffee." And, if you're *still* worried about methylene chloride, here's one more assurance from an expert: "The amount of the chemical is so minute that it's insignificant," says Manfred Kroger, Ph.D., professor of food science at Pennsylvania State University in State College.

Let's answer the second question first. "The new thinking about fibrocystic disease and breast cancer is that certain types of fibrocystic disease are risk factors. But these affect a relatively small number of women," says Lynn Rosenberg, Sc.D., assistant director of the Drug Epidemiology Unit, Brookline, Massachusetts.

Fibrocystic disease is defined as a condition in which there are palpable lumps (you can feel them) in the breast, usually associated with pain and tenderness. These fluctuate with the menstrual cycle and become progressively worse until menopause. If a woman wants to know if she has the common type of lumpy breasts or the rare type that may be associated with cancer, she'll have to consult with her doctor, says Dr. Rosenberg.

LUMPY BREASTS ARE NOT USUALLY A RISK FACTOR

But clearly, lumpy breasts need not be associated with cancer. In fact, one study published in the *New England Journal of Medicine* reports that fibrocystic disease was found in 58 percent of *non*cancerous breasts but in only 26 percent of cancerous breasts.

The possibility of a connection between coffee and fibrocystic disease is further diminished by a recent National Cancer Institute study. It examined the relationship between methylxanthine consumption and several types of benign breast disease. (Caffeine, theophylline and theobromine—found in coffee, tea, colas, etc.—are methylxanthines.) The study followed 1,569 women with benign breast disease and 1,846 "controls." Among those with various types of benign breast disease, 813 had fibrocystic disease. The researchers found no increased risk associated with methylxanthine intake and the fibrocystic disease cases.

What does this mean for women who are concerned about fibrocystic disease and breast cancer?

Gary Lyman, M.D., professor of medicine and director of the Division of Medical Oncology at the University of South Florida College of Medicine in Tampa, says, "There is no evidence that cutting back on coffee will cut your chances of breast cancer."

COFFEE AND PANCREATIC CANCER

Most people probably don't think too much about their pancreas; they're just content to let it hum happily along secreting hormones, particularly insulin. But it's a vital organ, and when the incidence of pancreatic cancer began rising in the 1950s and peaked in 1970, scientists were eager to find the cause. Coffee took a lot of the scientific heat at the time, though it seems to have deserved more of a lukewarm reception.

One study that evaluated the coffee and pancreatic cancer controversy was done by a team of Harvard doctors led by Brian MacMahon, M.D. They questioned 369 pancreatic cancer patients and 644 cancer-free people about how much coffee, tea, tobacco and alcohol they consumed. While the researchers stressed the fact that this connection needs further evaluation, the report concluded that "an unexpected association of pancreatic cancer with coffee consumption was evident."

This led to dramatic headlines like "Study Links Coffee Use to Pancreas Cancer." Considering that pancreatic cancer accounted for 22,532 deaths in 1983 in the United States, a headline like that is pretty scary.

But it wasn't long before a pot of controversy was brewing over the study. An editorial in the *Journal of the American Medical Association* summed up the problem: "The recent report that coffee may cause pancreatic cancer was presented in a pattern that has become distressingly familiar. The alleged carcinogen is a commonly used product. The report was given widespread publicity before the supporting evidence was available for appraisal by the scientific community, and the public received renewed fear and uncertainty about the cancerous hazards lurking in everyday life." The editorial continued to outline a series of possible biases and problems associated with the Harvard study and suggested that the study linking coffee to pancreatic cancer was a type of "fishing expedition" that also contradicted the results of earlier research.

LITTLE SUPPORT FOR A FRIGHTENING THEORY

In light of the MacMahon report, many other studies and examinations of research have been done. Most don't support the theory that coffee enhances a person's chance of getting pancreatic cancer. According to Patricia Hartge, Sc.D., an epidemiologist at the National Cancer Institute, "Pancreatic cancer isn't a dead issue. But right now the general impression is that MacMahon's findings have not been confirmed." Dr. Hartge is now involved with a study that is examining the effects of many substances, including coffee, on pancreatic cancer, but the results won't be available for a few years.

Meanwhile, the results of other tests are available. Researchers at the Boston Collaborative Drug Surveillance Program examined interviews with 93 pancreatic cancer patients done over a period of 13 years. The study concluded that coffee consumption had nothing to do with their cancer.

Researchers at the Scripps Clinic and Research Foundation in La Jolla, California, came to the same conclusion. They reviewed the charts of 91 pancreatic cancer patients seen between 1973 and 1980 and a group of 93 people who were at the clinic because of other cancers. Coffee was not implicated as a risk factor for pancreatic cancer.

A study by researchers at the Fred Hutchinson Cancer Research Center in Seattle, Washington, may provide a clue as to why coffee was implicated in the first place. Researchers there studied pancreatic cancer patients, and after adjusting their statistics for age, sex and cigarette smoking, found that there was no strong connection between coffee and the cancer, but there was a strong connection between cigarettes and the cancer.

According to Dr. Hartge, "The reason coffee keeps popping up in cancer studies is because the control groups aren't weighted for cigarettes. Heavy coffee drinkers are often heavy smokers. In fact, it's partly biological—people who smoke require more coffee to get the same amount of stimulation as people who don't smoke. And it's also partly sociological." While Dr. Hartge says coffee is so complex that it is hard to be certain exactly what effect it has on the body, she doesn't think it is to blame for pancreatic cancer.

COFFEE AND BLADDER CANCER

As if its reputation weren't bad enough, coffee has also been implicated in bladder cancer, lung cancer and cancer of the ovaries. As for ovarian cancer, "I can say very fairly that the link does not exist," says Dr. Hartge. She saves her harshest thoughts for a study that tried to link lung cancer to coffee. "That association is most likely false," she says.

As for bladder (and renal-cell) cancer, several studies have tried to establish coffee as a risk factor. But many of them have not made allowances for cigarette smoking, age and exposure on the job to dyes, chemicals and rubber products. Dr. Hartge and her associates at the National Cancer Institute compared about 3,000 people with bladder cancer to about 6,000 people without the disease, and they found no association between coffee and bladder cancer.

"While the issue of bladder cancer and coffee hasn't been completely resolved in some scientists' minds, my opinion is that there is no relationship between the two," says Dr. Hartge.

When all this information is taken into account, it seems that coffee might have developed a worse reputation than it rightly deserves—at least in terms of cancer. Barring future developments, moderate coffee consumption doesn't seem to be a risk factor for cancer.

28

Colorectal Examination

$\mathbf{T}$rue or False: Colorectal cancer, the second deadliest cancer, can largely be avoided, though doing so involves a complete change of diet and lifestyle and a willingness to practically live on the doctor's examining table undergoing excruciating, humiliating, disabling tests.

Trick question. The answer, of course, is both true *and* false. Yes, it's true that cancers of the colon and rectum, second only to lung cancer in terms of incidence for both men and women, can, for the most part, be prevented. What's false is that you have to turn your life upside down to accomplish it. In fact, all you need do is take a few simple precautions.

Unfortunately, many people are unaware of this fact. A survey conducted for the American Cancer Society revealed that people lack confidence in the effectiveness of detecting colon and rectal cancer early. They seem to feel they have some control over the health and fitness of other organs, such as the stomach, heart and lungs, but they often feel they have no control over the colon and rectum. Many people believe that by the time cancer is detected, it is already too late. In fact, more than 50 percent of people surveyed in a Gallup poll said they do not believe anything can be done to cure it.

These findings are particularly disturbing because statistics show that the cure rate for this form of cancer approaches 75 percent when cancers are found early. Furthermore, many cancerous tumors in the colon begin life as benign polyps sprouting like mushrooms in a cave. Routine cancer checkups will reveal these growths while they are still harmless and can easily be scraped away in a simple outpatient procedure, often right in the doctor's office. So these exams serve not only to catch cancer in its early stages before it does irreparable damage but also to prevent cancer from forming. Yet, surveys of Americans in the high-risk group for colorectal cancer (that includes everyone over 40) show that less than half have *ever* had the kind of checkup recommended for early detection.

HOW TO TAKE CONTROL

First, take a long, "lean" look at your diet. Studies indicate that you will greatly reduce your risk for colorectal cancer if you cut down on fats and eat a lot of fiber. Roughage is said to push everything through the plumbing faster, before it can sit around and fester. (The colon, a ropy, four- to five-foot long tube, is the last stop in the digestive tract that ends at the rectum.) Calcium and vitamin D also seem to offer some protection against the disease. For that reason, experts advise drinking skim milk each day. Regular exercise may be another effective preventive.

Second, be aware of the warning signals of colorectal cancer. Early warning signs include blood in the stool and a change in bowel habits, such as persistent constipation or diarrhea. Signs of a more advanced cancer include cramps or gnawing pain in the abdomen (as though your bowels were always uncomfortably full), gradual weight loss and loss of appetite, anemia and blood red or black stools. Check with your doctor immediately if you notice any one of these symptoms.

Third, keep in mind that precancerous and even downright malignant tumors may be growing down there in the depths without giving any warnings. And that's why you want to get regular checkups. Fortunately, doctors can now use miraculous new fiberoptics to peer into these nether regions and catch any marauders. More about that later. First, a simple test you can even do by yourself at home.

TAKE AN OCCULT BLOOD TEST

Fear not: Though the name of this procedure makes it sound like it's some weird supernatural rite, it is merely a test to detect hidden (occult) blood in the stool, which might indicate the presence of a tumor. The test, however, is far from perfect. First of all, not all tumors bleed, and even those that do often bleed only intermittently (not necessarily on the day you happen to be doing the test). To further complicate matters, many other problems can cause blood in the stool, most commonly hemorrhoids. In an attempt to render the results more accurate, many of these tests require two samples from three different

---

QUICK QUIZ

Colorectal cancer is expected to strike 140,000 Americans this year; approximately 60,000 are expected to die of the disease annually. Test your awareness of colorectal cancer with the same questions asked in a recent Gallup poll conducted for the American Cancer Society. Compare your answers with those given by the people who were surveyed (all of whom were in the high-risk group of people over 40).

Q: Have you heard of the stool blood test?
A: Yes/No (66 percent of those surveyed had.)

Q: Have you had a stool blood test?
A: Yes/No (39 percent of those surveyed had.)

Q: Have you heard of the digital rectal examination?
A: Yes/No (70 percent of those surveyed had.)

Q: Have you ever had a digital rectal examination?
A: Yes/No (54 percent of those surveyed had.)

Q: If you had a stool blood test and no blood was found, would you still need a procto or digital rectal examination?
A: Yes/No (40 percent of those surveyed said you would need further tests, 25 percent said you would not, and 35 percent said they didn't know.)

Q: Have you ever asked a doctor to examine your bowel, colon or rectum, and, if so, why did you ask for the examination?
A: Yes/No (24 percent of those surveyed said they *had* asked a doctor for such an exam; 14 percent because they were bothered

stools. The samples are mixed with a chemical solution that may turn a different color if blood is present.

If you do the test under a doctor's guidance, you will probably be asked to prepare a set of slides at home, which you will then return to your doctor for evaluation. (If President Reagan did it, so can you.) During the test period, you may also be directed to eat a high-fiber diet (roughage is thought to encourage a tumor to bleed), avoid such foods

by something, 11 percent because they wanted a checkup; some people gave both reasons. Seventy-six percent had never asked a doctor for such a test.)

Q: Have you heard about a new flexible scope or instrument that doctors can use for doing procto examinations, and, if so, would you prefer doctors to use it?
A: Yes/No (39 percent of those surveyed had heard of the new flexible instrument; 13 percent would prefer doctors to use it; 26 percent felt the doctor should decide; 61 percent had never heard of the sigmoidoscope.)

Q: Colorectal cancer is one of the most common types of cancer.
A: True/False (61 percent of those surveyed agreed, and they were correct.)

Q: Men and women are equally likely to get colorectal cancer.
A: True/False (45 percent of those surveyed agreed with this correct statement.)

Q: By the time most colorectal cancer is found, it's already in an advanced stage and not much can be done about it.
A: True/False (47 percent said false, and they were right.)

Q: If a person is tested for colorectal cancer, there's a good chance the person will be permanently handicapped.
A: True/False (60 percent disagreed with this patently false statement.)

as red meat and certain vegetables, not take more than four aspirins daily and avoid vitamin C and iron, which may give false results.

You can also test yourself with a variety of home kits now on the market. These work in different ways; the directions may tell you to throw a chemically impregnated paper into the toilet bowl after defecation, or place a small amount of stool on a paper, or use a specially prepared wipe.

The American Cancer Society firmly endorses fecal occult blood tests and advocates these annual screenings (testing of people who have no symptoms) for all Americans over 50. Many doctors remain unconvinced of the benefits of this kind of screening, however. In a three-part study, John W. Frank, M.D., of the University of Toronto's Department of Preventive Medicine and Biostatistics, Ontario, has found no clear-cut benefits to patients who, through testing for occult blood, have been found to have colorectal cancer. In contrast, there may be substantial risks and costs associated with the widespread use of this preventive maneuver. Dr. Frank examined results of various studies and found that only 40 to 50 percent of the people whose blood tests were positive (indicating that they had a tumor) actually had a growth. About 12 percent turned out to actually have cancer, while the rest had benign polyps.

Worse is the high percentage of false-negative test results: those people whose tests say they don't have cancer when they really *do*. They may gain a false sense of security and relax to such an extent that they fail to seek medical attention and will even ignore warning symptoms. Equally serious—and much more likely, according to Dr. Frank— are false-positive results (you don't have a tumor, but the test says you do). Every test that turns up blood in the stool is followed by examinations and even treatments that are expensive, invasive and, nine times out of ten, unnecessary, he maintains.

The problem of false results made headlines when President Reagan had an occult blood test as part of a routine physical exam. Two of his tests were negative, two positive. Doctors thought the positive results might have been misleading—perhaps caused by his diet—so they asked him to avoid certain foods and take another series of tests. This time, the six tests were negative, yet all along, a tumor was growing in his cecum, the first part of his large bowel.

President Reagan's case is a perfect example of why these tests are "not adequate for screening," says Charles G. Moertel, M.D., chairman of the Department of Oncology at the Mayo Clinic, Rochester, Minnesota. Dr. Moertel believes the results can be "confusing or even completely misleading." A spokesman for Memorial Sloan-Kettering Cancer Center, New York City, takes a brighter view. Quoted in the magazine *Science,* he noted that the President was later given further tests. "Look at the President. It's practically a miracle. He smeared his own stool [on the test slide] and he had a colonoscopy [the exam that later permitted doctors to glimpse the tumor]—never mind when he had it. A large polyp was found and he had appropriate surgery. His chances of survival are excellent. Yet he had no symptoms of colon cancer and ten years ago he would not have been diagnosed until he had symptoms."

This conflicting evidence should serve to warn us not to be overconfident about the results of fecal occult blood tests. If the first results are positive, there is no need to panic, since so many of the positive results turn out to be false alarms. You should, of course, immediately consult a physician. If the results are negative, you should not be falsely secure, but stay on guard for symptoms and follow recommended schedules for further cancer checkups.

CHECKUP CHECKLIST

The American Cancer Society recommends the following tests for early detection of colorectal cancer.

1. For people age 40 and over: annual digital rectal examination (examination of the rectum by a physician).
2. For people age 50 and over: annual test to detect hidden blood in the stool.
3. Also for people age 50 and over: annual proctosigmoidoscopy (examination of the lower colon by a physician using a special instrument). If the results of two consecutive annual exams are normal, this test can be administered every three to five years.

People at high risk are those with a close relative with colon cancer, those with past adenoma or colon cancer, those with a family history of familial polyposis (Gardner's syndrome) and those with ulcerative colitis. They should consult their doctor about test schedules.

LOOK INTO THE COLON

The American Cancer Society recommends that everyone over 40 have a digital rectal exam. This, to be perfectly blunt, means that the physician inserts a rubber-gloved finger into your rectum. It may be embarrassing but it is not in the least painful. The doctor can not only feel any imperfections in the walls of the rectum, but with male patients, he can also check out the prostate, another favorite site for cancer. The digital rectal exam should definitely not be neglected.

Studies show that colorectal cancers have, in recent years, migrated further up the colon, so the rectal exam is not enough. Fortunately, medical technology has kept pace and physicians are now actually able to peer up inside the rectum and lower (sigmoid) colon through a long, flexible, lighted glass tube called a flexible sigmoidoscope.

Neither colorectal cancer nor sigmoidoscopy is new to the medical field. In Colonial days, a minuteman with rectal problems was told to bend over, whereupon a rigid tube the size of a large cigar was inserted into the troubled area and a candle used for illumination. Over the centuries, the candle gave way to the oil lamp and electricity, but the basic instrument changed little.

The rigid scope, still sometimes used today, can (uncomfortably) inspect only six to seven inches past the anus; the new flexible sigmoidoscope is about two feet long and has a four-directional tip to examine the entire sigmoid portion of the colon. The tube has a lighted tip that illuminates the dark regions, and flexible bundles of glass-coated fibers within the tube transmit a magnified image back to the eye.

"It's like looking down a well-lit pipe. The clarity is astounding and you can see a growth the size of a pinhead," says B. F. Overholt, M.D., a gastroenterologist in Knoxville, Tennessee, and past president of the American Society for Gastrointestinal Endoscopy. (Endoscopy is the general term for looking inside the body; sigmoidoscopy refers specifically to examination of the rectum and the sigmoid colon.) Attachments can be added to make photographs or even movies, and accessories, such as laser beams, snare wires, scissors and forceps can be passed through channels in the tube. Through separate channels, water can be squirted in to wash the lens (or the bowel) and air can be puffed in to expand the bowel so the physician can see around corners.

Before the sigmoidoscopy, the patient is given an enema to clear out the area, then (usually right in the doctor's examining room) the patient lies on his left side with his knees bent (much more dignified than the draped-over-the-table-bottom-in-the-air posture required for the rigid scope exam). "It can be somewhat embarrassing and uncomfortable (the tube is about as wide as a pencil), but patients say the thought is worse than the experience itself," reassures Jerome Waye, M.D., a New York gastroenterologist and expert in colon diseases. "A routine exam takes five to ten minutes. Knowing what to expect eases the discomfort, and it's several minutes of inconvenience once every few years that may prevent major surgery or ultimately save your life."

The flexible sigmoidoscope has been shown to detect nearly three times the number of cancers and polyps than the rigid scope, and it can potentially ferret out 60 to 70 percent of cancers and polyps, according to Robert S. Sandler, M.D., assistant professor of medicine and clinical assistant professor of epidemiology at the University of North Carolina.

Polyps can be removed by placing a wire snare around the base of the polyp and applying an electrical current that does two things: It seals off any blood vessels that bleed, and it helps to remove the polyp, explains Dr. Sandler. Generally, polyps are not removed with a sigmoidoscope but with a colonoscope, a flexible tube of fiberoptic bundles. It is similar to the sigmoidoscope, but longer—long enough to reach the entire colon.

The sigmoidoscope isn't used for such procedures for a couple of reasons. First is the risk of explosion. The enema given for sigmoidoscopy has cleaned out only the bottom of the colon, and there may be gases higher up. The electric current used to help remove the polyp could ignite those gases. ("It is considered bad form to explode the patient," comments Dr. Sandler dryly.)

Another reason for a deeper look into the colon is that if polyps *are* seen with the flexible sigmoidoscope, there's a 30 to 50 percent chance of other polyps somewhere else in the colon. "So if we see a polyp with sigmoidoscopy, we send the patient home, prepare the whole colon so it's clean, examine the whole colon, then take out the polyp we saw and any others we see higher up," explains Dr. Sandler.

Though it's expensive (about $70 to $150 just for the exam), this new technique is exciting a good deal of interest both in the medical community and among ordinary folks who wouldn't have considered submitting their personal posteriors to the old rigid sigmoidoscope. More and more people are *asking* the family doctor about flexible sigmoidoscopy (put the accent on the "os" when you ask). And doctors are responding.

The flexible scopes are expensive and require training to operate. Rigid and flexible sigmoidoscopy is now part of the curriculum for a growing number of medical students. For practicing physicians and internists who have no experience with the flexible scopes, the American Society for Gastrointestinal Endoscopy and the American Academy of Family Physicians have launched a national teaching campaign, says Dr. Waye, who helped write the training manual.

One such training program in Rockford, Illinois, surprised organizers. "We've been offering this since 1982, but for the past two years we've seen a large increase in the number of physicians interested in retraining," says William Basking, M.D., a practicing gastroenterologist and part-time instructor at the University of Illinois College of Medicine, Rockford. "Doctors are usually reluctant to spend much time on preventive-type examinations, but if there is interest in the community, they'll take the time. The increase in the number of physicians we've trained tells me that communities are becoming more aware."

Robert Johnson, M.D., a Byron, Illinois, general practitioner, says the time and effort spent retraining is paying off for his patients. Although the exam is not routine for everyone in the waiting room, he recommends it to all patients over age 45. He's found that one of every five patients in the high-risk group unknowingly has polyps. Because of early detection, most of the growths are removed while in the benign stage and pose no further problems.

Don't sit up nights waiting for your doctor, however. Dr. Waye advises that once you reach the high-risk age, be suspicious and don't always think your doctor knows it all. One patient, for example, was in the risky age group and went to his doctor complaining of rectal bleeding. Hemorrhoids, the doctor diagnosed. The bleeding persisted, so he was referred to Dr. Waye, who found that the man's troubled hemorrhoids were sharing a lower tract with a large polyp.

"The moral is that anyone over age 50 who has colon complaints should automatically have a total examination, and don't assume that changes in bowel habits are always innocent," he says. "Many doctors don't look past the obvious and blame most rectal problems on hemorrhoids."

Another thing to keep in mind is your family history, which some busy doctors simply don't take adequate note of. The risk for any one of us developing colon cancer is about 5 percent, remarks Dr. Sandler. "Having a close relative with the disease increases the risk three times, to 15 percent, which is fairly substantial." (A case in point: President Reagan's brother also had colon cancer.)

Now, how do you delicately quiz your doctor to find out whether he has enough experience with colorectal cancer in general and flexible sigmoidoscopes in particular? Dr. Sandler's advice: "If a physician is reasonably deft, he can probably learn the technique if he does 15 or 20 procedures. A patient might ask his physician how he learned to do the procedure. If the physician says he read it in a book, that might not be adequate. Also, a patient might ask how often the physician does the procedure; if he does it only once or twice a year, he may not be getting enough practice to do it competently, but if he does several a week, you can be pretty sure he knows what he's doing." Don't be afraid to (diplomatically) question your doctor. After all, it's your body. "If a physician is uncomfortable answering these questions, maybe you should find a different physician," says Dr. Sandler.

THE FUTURE

Researchers are well aware that the perfect test (reliable yet noninvasive) has yet to be discovered. Some scientists believe future tests may use a type of antibodies known as monoclonals. These are designed-to-order in the laboratory and, when injected into the body, will go right to work locating tumors and, eventually, destroying them. Tumors of the colon secrete a characteristic substance called carcinoembryonic antigen (CEA), which attracts antibodies that are made against this substance. These specific antibodies make these tumors particularly good candidates for search-and-destroy missions. It is possible that one day, a specific antibody may be developed for use in a (reliable) fecal blood test.

David Goldenberg, Sc.D., M.D., president of the Center for Molecular Medicine and Immunology, Newark, New Jersey, has tested about 400 cancer patients with anticancer antibodies "labeled" with radioactive iodine. The radioactivity is like a beacon used to trace problem areas, says Dr. Goldenberg. The tests had a 90 percent accuracy rate for colorectal cancer, but because of the obvious dangers always present with radioactivity, this test cannot be used for routine screening. It is suitable only for patients with a history of cancer or a high suspicion of cancer.

Those of us who are as yet untouched by colon cancer will have to make do with what we've got—and what we've got is plenty! If the only thing that's keeping you from discussing all these tests with your doctor is embarrassment and a reluctance to talk about an unmentionable body part, be like the nun who had to teach sex education. She practiced the necessary vocabulary at top voice while she ran the vacuum cleaner. And what price embarrassment, anyway? The American Cancer Society has reported that if everyone over age 40 went for regular checkups and had precancerous intestinal polyps removed, 100,000 lives could be saved. Maybe one of them is yours.

CANCER PREVENTION PLAN: COLORECTAL CANCER

- Cut down on fat.
- Increase fiber consumption.
- Drink skim milk fortified with vitamin D daily.
- Exercise regularly.
- Know the early warning signs.
- Have regular medical checkups.

Copper

In the bank, copper is not nearly as valuable as gold or silver. In the body, though, this metal is precious—it's necessary for healthy tissue development and function. But where copper could really shine, say experts, may be in controlling (and possibly preventing) cancer.

Normally, a supply of copper is stored in your liver, which then releases it into your blood to meet metabolic needs. But certain conditions—infections, neoplasias (tumor formation)—require a large supply of copper.

"Elevated levels of copper in the blood could mean that cancer is present," says Maria Linder, Ph.D., professor of biochemistry at California State University in Fullerton. "A number of laboratory studies have shown that certain forms of copper slow the growth of tumors in a variety of animals and cell cultures," she reports.

That's why Dr. Linder thinks that getting your blood checked for copper is a smart way to screen for cancer, especially if you are at high risk (if, for instance, you smoke or have a family history of the disease). "Perhaps getting serum copper level checks for cancer could become as routine as getting cholesterol level checks for heart disease."

In addition to slowing a tumor's growth, copper also may prevent its formation, according to John R. J. Sorenson, Ph.D., professor of medicinal chemistry at the University of Arkansas. In one of Dr. Sorenson's experiments, more than half of the mice subjected to a lethal dose of radiation managed to survive. The reason? They had been given copper compounds, which served to shield them from the harmful rays.

What all this means, says Dr. Sorenson, is that copper could play an important role in preventing cancer in humans. He predicts that "it may be entirely possible for people to take a kind of copper supplement prior to getting an x-ray and be protected from its harmful effects."

MAKING YOUR COPPER COUNT

From a health standpoint, then, copper is a wise investment. You'll have to "invest" on a daily basis, however, because the body continually spends its copper—losing it primarily in the feces but also from the top layer of the skin, the toenails and fingernails and in sweat and urine.

No Recommended Dietary Allowance (RDA) has been set for copper, but it's been estimated that two to three milligrams is a safe and adequate daily intake. Unfortunately, three-fourths of all Americans may not be getting this needed amount, warns Dr. Sorenson. Be sure your diet contains foods rich in this mineral. Copper is found in navy beans, avocados, liver, crabmeat, nuts and seeds, whole wheat foods, apricots, bananas and chicken. Be sure to include plenty of whole foods, which have much more copper than overly processed foods. White flour, for example, has 60 percent less copper than whole wheat flour.

Another word of warning: If you take large doses of zinc or vitamin C, you could interfere with copper absorption, says Leslie M. Klevay, M.D., S.D. in Hyg., research medical officer of the Human Nutrition Research Center in Grand Forks, North Dakota.

Generally, you don't have to worry about getting too much copper from your food. Still, overdoses can happen when acidic food or drinks, such as vinegar, carbonated beverages or citrus juices, have been sitting in copper containers too long or if acidic water stands in copper pipes for a long period of time. However, the problem usually takes care of itself, because the vomiting and diarrhea caused by ingesting too much copper generally protect us from its more serious toxic effects.

CANCER PREVENTION PLAN: COPPER

- Consume copper on a daily basis by eating foods rich in this mineral, such as navy beans, avocados, liver, crabmeat, nuts and seeds, whole wheat foods, apricots, bananas and chicken.

Early Detection

Most of us don't try to find cancer in our bodies, or ask our doctors to. We've got our reasons, of course. The cancer detection tests are too costly, or they take too much time, or they're too uncomfortable. And the early warning signs are too tough to spot. Who wants to examine 500 moles every month to see if one has turned black? Who wants to search their breasts for a tiny lump that's probably just a cyst? And who wants to think about cancer, anyway? If you've got it, you'd rather not know. If you've got it, you're probably doomed.

These reasons are real—but they're not too realistic.

"If people paid attention to the early warning signals of cancer and followed the recommended schedules for cancer testing, we could save many, many lives," says Dexter L. Morris, Ph.D., M.D. at Duke University Medical Center in Durham, North Carolina. "When you catch cancers early—while tumors are small, before they spread and take root in nearby tissues—you can, in most cases, easily cure them or cut them out. And that is really a form of prevention—one people can and should be actively involved in."

The key to that involvement is confidence. Confidence that you can find a cancer if it's there. Confidence that detection tests can do the same, without subjecting you to a lot of needless pain and indignity. Confidence that if a cancer is found, it can be cured. And enough confidence to make detection tests a positive, easy part of your self-care health program.

Notice the words "self-care." Even though your doctor is involved, the main responsibility for cancer prevention is yours. "The patient is often able to notice cancer symptoms sooner than the doctor," says Dr. Morris. "Patients see themselves every day. The doctor may see them only once a year—if then—so the patient is much better able to notice a lump or bump, a change in stools, or signs like that.

"The patient should also be aware of recommended schedules for cancer detection tests. I would certainly question my physician about the various tests when I visited. A woman should keep track and have regular Pap smears, for example. And if you're a man or woman over 50, you might want to make sure you have a proctoscopy or other test for colon cancer. It's important for people to be aware of testing schedules, because if they are otherwise healthy and don't have any reason to visit a physician, they may miss the routine cancer screening and the chance to pick up something early.

"It is also important for people to be aware of whether or not they are in a high-risk group for certain cancers. Women whose mother or sister had breast cancer, for example, run a higher risk of getting breast cancer themselves and may want to get a mammogram earlier than is normally recommended and have more frequent tests."

NOTE THESE SCHEDULES

So, note the recommended schedules for testing, paying particular attention if you happen to fall into one of the high-risk groups. If you are due for a test sometime this year, mark it on your calendar. Also, be aware of the early warning signals; if you notice one of the signs, don't ignore it. Remember, they're called early warnings because they come early—in most cases in time for a cure. See your doctor immediately. Days count.

Finally, even if you are free of symptoms, you should shop around and find a doctor you can really work with. You might want to contact the American Society of Preventive Oncology to locate someone in your area who will understand the importance of taking a thorough and complete cancer-related history, including such factors as cancers in the family, past and present occupations, smoking habits and diet—someone who will be able to assess your personal risk level for various cancers and how best to schedule your regular cancer tests. Your physician should treat you as an active partner—you are working together to prevent cancer.

BREAST CANCER

Breast cancer will strike one in every ten women. Fortunately, if the tumor is found early and removed, most breast cancers can be cured.

Warning signs: Firm lump. Small changes in the nipple or discharge from the nipple.

Tests: *Monthly self-examination of breasts.* Have your doctor teach you the technique. So you'll remember, schedule your self-test for the same time each month—just after your period when you are in the bath (irregularities are easier to feel when fingers and breasts are wet). Self-tests are vital. It is the woman herself who discovers the telltale lump in 95 percent of all cases.

Mammography, or x-ray of the breasts. Since a tumor has to be at least one centimeter in diameter to be felt, we need a way to find the tumor earlier and mammography is the answer, says Leon Speroff, M.D., professor and chairman of the Department of Reproductive Biology at Case Western Reserve University School of Medicine in Cleveland, Ohio. Several large-scale studies have found that consistent screening with mammography greatly reduced breast cancer death rates. In Sweden, for example, 162,981 women were divided into two groups. One group received no tests, the other group had a mammogram every two to three years. After just seven years, the results show that the tested group had 31 percent fewer deaths and 25 percent fewer cases of advanced disease than did the untested group.

Many women are reluctant to expose themselves to a mammogram because they fear the effects of radiation. "With a modern-day mammogram," says Dr. Morris, "the amount of radiation you get is very small and the amount of risk of developing cancer from the radiation is extremely small. It is not dangerous. I would urge women to get the tests because they can greatly decrease their risk of dying from cancer."

Schedule: Doctors recommend a monthly breast self-exam starting at age 20. In addition, they recommend a physical examination of the breasts by a doctor every three years for women between the ages of 20 and 40, and every year after age 40. Also required is a baseline mammogram between the ages of 35 and 40 (with which future mammograms will be compared) and periodic mammograms thereafter until age 50, depending on the woman's x-ray results and risk factors. Having an annual mammogram after age 50 is recommended.

High-risk factors: Early onset of first menses. Late menopause. First child after age 35. Childlessness. Family history of breast cancer. Diet high in animal fat and low in fiber.

Breast cancer seems to be related to hormones. It is estimated that women who have a natural menopause at age 55 or older have twice the risk of developing breast cancer than women who had a natural menopause before age 45. Women who bear their first child after age 35 have three times the risk of the disease than do women who have their first child before age 18. If your mother or sister had breast cancer, studies show you have two or three times the risk of getting it as well.

CERVICAL CANCER

An estimated 8,000 women died of cervical cancer in 1985. A simple screening test will detect cancers early, and the cure rate is then close to 100 percent.

Warning signs: Abnormal vaginal bleeding between periods or after intercourse. Prolonged heavy bleeding during menstruation.

Tests: *The Pap smear.* This screening test involves gently scraping the cervix during a pelvic exam to remove cells from the surface. These cells are then smeared onto a glass slide and examined under a microscope. Abnormal or malignant cells can then be identified.

A cervical tampon. This do-it-yourself exam is currently being tested. Researchers say it is not intended to replace the Pap smear but simply to reach women who do not normally see a doctor regularly. A woman takes her own samples of cells and mails them in for evaluation.

Cervicography. This new test permits the physician to take a picture of the cervix to study later. This test is meant to supplement the Pap smear and increase the accuracy of diagnosis.

Schedule: Have a Pap smear annually for two years starting at age 20, or earlier if you are a sexually active teenager. Subsequently, schedule your exams every three years, more frequently if you fall into one of the high-risk groups. (The American College of Obstetricians and Gynecologists, however, suggests yearly examinations for all.)

High-risk factors: Sexual intercourse at an early age. Multiple sex partners. Many children.

COLORECTAL CANCER

In 1985, an estimated 138,000 Americans developed cancers of the colon or rectum and about 59,900 died of the disease. "Early detection holds great promise for improving the outcome of therapy for colorectal cancer and perhaps even preventing colorectal cancer through treatment of precancerous polyps," says Robert G. Norfleet, M.D., of the Marshfield Clinic in Marshfield, Wisconsin.

Warning signs: Blood in the stool. Feeling of being bloated. Change in bowel habits. Constipation. Diarrhea. Gas pains.

Tests: *Digital rectal examination.* The physician will insert a gloved finger into your rectum and be able to feel any rectal abnormalities. At the same time, he will be able to detect possibly cancerous growths of the prostate in male patients.

Fecal blood testing. This is a home test to detect hidden blood in the stools, which might indicate colorectal cancer. Your doctor will give you a kit, or you can simply buy one in a drugstore. The test kit will come with instructions on taking samples of stools (usually about six samples) and on preparing the samples so they may be examined. You will also be told to avoid certain foods that might falsify the results.

This test is far from 100 percent accurate. If your results do show blood, you should see your doctor immediately for further evaluation, but usually the blood doesn't mean cancer (it may mean you have hemorrhoids, though). Similarly, a negative test doesn't necessarily mean you don't have cancer; it may be that your tumor just wasn't bleeding on the days of the test. So no matter what the results, be sure to follow the recommendations for further tests.

Proctosigmoidoscopy. This test permits the doctor to examine the inside of your rectum and your colon through a glass tube lit by fiberoptics. The rigid sigmoidoscope views only the lower few inches of the colon. The flexible sigmoidoscope actually bends around corners, so it is much more comfortable, and it allows the physician to see the entire lower colon. Dr. Norfleet estimates that he and his colleagues detect about twice as many cancers and six times as many benign tumors with the flexible tube than they would with the rigid tube.

Schedule: Since 95 percent of colorectal cancers occur after age 40 and 98 percent after age 50, Dr. Norfleet recommends that people who are free of symptoms have a digital rectal exam annually beginning at age 40. Starting at age 50, people should have an annual fecal blood test. Following the recommendation of the American Cancer Society, Dr. Norfleet examines his patients with the flexible sigmoidoscope when they reach age 50, again at age 51 and then every three to five years thereafter as long as findings are normal and the patient remains free of symptoms.

People who fall in the high-risk groups should begin this schedule ten years earlier.

High-risk factors: Over age 40. Family history of colorectal cancer. Inflammatory bowel disease, especially ulcerative colitis. Past history of colorectal cancer or polyps. Familial polyposis. For women— history of breast cancer or cancer of the reproductive organs.

LARYNGEAL CANCER

This cancer is vary rare among non-smokers. It affects the larynx (Adam's apple) and, in advanced cases, can result in the loss of the voice. When caught early, however, 85 percent can be treated without surgery, thus saving the ability to speak.

Warning signs: Persistent hoarseness, soreness in the neck, feeling that you have a lump in your throat and difficulty swallowing.

Test: *Examination of larynx by a physician.* This cancer can easily be caught at a curable stage. A physician will simply examine the larynx with a mirror and if he sees anything suspicious, he will recommend a more complete examination.

Laryngoscopy. An examination in which the doctor looks at the larynx with a lighted tube.

Schedule: No set timetable recommended. See your physician if you notice any symptoms, particularly if you are in a high-risk group.

High-risk factors: Pipe, cigar and cigarette smoking. Excessive drinking of alcohol.

LUNG CANCER

Lung cancer is the leading cause of cancer deaths, claiming more than 100,000 lives a year. Ironically, this most deadly of cancers is also one of the most preventable.

Warning signs: Among high-risk group members: Chronic cough or hoarseness. Change in a cough, coughing up blood, pain or shortness of breath. Difficult to diagnose early, so see a doctor immediately.

Test: None specifically recommended. "Be sure to see your doctor if you notice any symptoms," urges Dr. Morris. "Lung cancer is not hopeless; if the lesion is small, they can cut it out and sometimes effect a cure."

Schedule: Lung cancer frequently will not show up in an x-ray until it is quite well developed, and studies show that routine testing for lung cancer in people who have no symptoms is not effective, even among smokers who have been exposed to asbestos.

High-risk factors: Smoking. Exposure to such products as asbestos, coal tar derivatives and radiation.

ORAL CANCER

Smoking, drinking and dental problems may lead to cancer of the oral cavity (tongue, gums, mucous lining). This form of cancer is most prevalent among older men.

Warning signs: Persistent red or white patches, usually painless. Be aware of any persistent lump, swelling or painful area and be sure to have it examined.

Test: *Screening.* Your dentist will examine your mouth during a regular checkup by looking for ulcers, sores or red areas. He will ask you to stick out your tongue so he can move it from side to side to look for lumps.

Schedule: See your dentist every six months.

High-risk factors: Chewing tobacco and snuff. Drinking alcohol and smoking.

PROSTATE CANCER

This is one of the leading causes of cancer death in men.

Warning signs: Weak or interrupted flow of urine. Inability to urinate or difficulty in starting urination. Need to urinate frequently (especially at night). Blood in the urine. Urine flow that is not easily stopped. Painful or burning urination. Continuing pain in lower back, pelvis or upper thighs. These symptoms may simply indicate prostate enlargement, but if you experience any of them, see your physician immediately.

Test: *Digital rectal exam.* The cure rate for prostate cancer is excellent, if it is caught early.

Schedule: Have an annual exam after age 50.

High-risk factors: A diet high in fats, according to some studies.

SKIN CANCER

The skin makes up approximately 15 percent of our body weight. It is exposed to the sun's ultraviolet rays, which are the primary cause of skin cancer. In fact, more than 90 percent of all skin cancers occur on body areas unprotected by clothing. Skin cancer is the most common form of cancer, but is easily detected because you can actually see it growing. The only danger is that it may grow slowly so that you become so used to it you don't even notice it anymore. Skin cancer is almost always curable. Catch it early.

Warning signs: Bumps and small sores. Any change in a scar or blemish or any new bump or sore that lasts for more than three weeks. Birthmarks or moles that get bigger or start to itch or bleed. See a physician.

Test: *Self-examination.* Undress and inspect your entire body in front of the mirror.

Schedule: Do an annual self-test.

High-risk factors: Frequent and prolonged exposure to the sun. Fair complexion.

STOMACH CANCER

Rates for stomach cancer have dropped, but more than 18,000 people still die of this disease every year. Almost everyone who gets stomach cancer dies of it, simply because it is not diagnosed in time.

CANCER PREVENTION PLAN: EARLY DETECTION

Breast Cancer

- Perform a monthly breast self-exam starting at age 20.
- Have a physical examination of the breasts by a doctor every three years between the ages of 20 and 40, and every year after age 40.
- Have a baseline mammogram (to which future mammograms will be compared) between ages 35 and 40 and mammograms periodically thereafter until age 50.
- Have an annual mammogram after age 50.

Cervical Cancer

- Have a Pap smear annually for two years starting at age 20, or earlier if you are a sexually active teenager.
- Have exams every three years, or more frequently if you fall into a high-risk group.

Colorectal Cancer

- Have a digital rectal exam annually beginning at age 40.
- Have an annual fecal blood test starting at age 50.
- Have an examination with a flexible sigmoidoscope at age 50, again at age 51 and then every three to five years thereafter.
- If you are in a high-risk group, you should begin this schedule ten years earlier.

Oral Cancer

- See your dentist every six months.
- Check your mouth and lips for smooth or scaly spots.
- Check your lips, neck and tongue for swelling or lumps.
- Recognize as warning signs any pain, burning, dryness, bleeding of unexplained origin, sores that do not heal within two weeks, or trouble speaking or swallowing.

Prostate Cancer

- Have a digital rectal exam after age 50.

Skin Cancer

- Perform an annual self-test by undressing and inspecting your entire body in front of a mirror.

Warning signs: Nausea. Gas. Burning pain after meals. A sensation of fullness. Loss of appetite. One reason stomach cancer is often not caught early is that the symptoms are just like those of ulcers or even plain indigestion. If the symptoms persist, see a cancer specialist.

Tests: None specifically recommended.

Schedule: No fixed timetable.

High-risk factors: A diet high in processed and preserved meats and smoked and salted foods and low in fresh fruits and vegetables.

UTERINE CANCER

This is the most common female reproductive cancer.

Warning signs: Irregular bleeding and, especially, bleeding after menopause.

Tests: *Cell sampling.* In order to detect this cancer, a physician must get a sample of the cells that line the uterus, either by scraping the lining or by injecting salt water into the uterus and then removing it and examining the cells present.

Schedule: Both test procedures are painful and expensive and are not recommended for women without symptoms, particularly since the symptoms appear early on in the disease.

High-risk factors: Occurs primarily in women after menopause. Overweight. History of relative infertility. Scientists now believe that it is probably caused by exposure to estrogen, either from failure to menstruate or from doses of estrogen prescribed for the symptoms of menopause.

VAGINAL CANCER

This was an extremely rare cancer until 1971, when it was discovered that daughters of women who had been treated with DES were susceptible to this cancer in adolescence and young adulthood.

Warning signs: Vaginal bleeding or discharge among DES daughters.

Test: *Pap Smear.* Thorough examination by your physician will help determine the presence of this cancer. The doctor takes a scraping from the cervix to test for cancerous cells.

Schedule: DES daughters should be examined annually beginning at age 14 or at onset of menstruation unless there is vaginal bleeding or discharge. These symptoms call for immediate evaluation.

High-risk factors: DES daughters.

Estrogen Replacement Therapy

Menopause heralds a new era of a woman's life. Many women rally to its call, welcoming it as a time of freedom from periods, pregnancy and family responsibilities and an opportunity to enjoy the good life.

Other women, though, are sidelined by unpleasant—even dangerous—conditions that occur when the body no longer produces sufficient estrogen. They may experience such drenching hot flashes they cannot sleep. Others have vaginal tissues so dry that sex is no longer pleasurable. In time, many of these women will have bones so brittle that even bumping their hips on a piece of furniture could prove fatal.

What could get many of these women back on the track is ERT, or estrogen replacement therapy, which, quite literally, gives back the hormone that keeps tissues and bones healthy and makes you more comfortable. And now there is some evidence that the new hormone therapy may even protect you from certain forms of cancer.

Unfortunately, many women have not heard the good news about the new ERT and remain reluctant to take it. No doubt they are recalling the flurry of reports that accused the old ERT of causing cancer.

121

Since 1975, at least 18 scientific studies have come out saying that women who took estrogen increased their risk of cancer of the endometrium, the lining of the uterus, by 2 to 15 times. One study reported that a woman's risk of endometrial cancer rose twentyfold after taking estrogen for 10 to 15 years. Another showed that even after women discontinued taking estrogen, the risk of endometrial cancer lingered.

These reports are not so suprising when you consider that, at that time, many women were virtually taking *megadoses* of estrogen because it was believed to be a kind of "eternal youth" pill. Little did they know it could cut their health short.

THE NEW ERT: SAFER, BETTER

But times have changed and so has ERT. Today's therapy carries less of a cancer risk, and a whole new batch of studies proves it.

What makes the current ERT different is a built-in safety feature: progestin. Researchers discovered that adding this synthetic version of the hormone progesterone can counteract the risk that comes with estrogen. You get the benefits of hormone replacement therapy but with little or none of the cancer risk.

It's only natural that these hormones work well together. After all, before menopause, your body produced them together. The estrogen grew endometrial tissue for possible implantation of a fertilized egg. Its sidekick progesterone further prepared the endometrium and made sure that the tissue wasn't overproduced so that it became troublesome. Progesterone causes the endometrium to slough off; it brings about your period. This counteracting effect of progesterone is one reason that endometrial cancer is rare before menopause.

Given as part of replacement therapy, progestin appears to work its same protective magic even after menopause. If you take estrogen without it, though, you run into the same cancer risk as did women a generation earlier.

"Estrogen itself does not cause cancer. It is not a carcinogen," explains Lila Nachtigall, M.D., associate professor of obstetrics and gynecology at the New York University School of Medicine and author of *Estrogen: The Facts Can Change Your Life*. "It can, however, cause endometrial hyperplasia, which is an excessive buildup or proliferation of the cells of the uterine lining. When sufficient progesterone is given each month along with a minimal dose of estrogen, there is no buildup of tissue that could lead to cancer."

THE PROTECTIVE POWER OF PROGESTIN

Progestin does its job so well, says Dr. Nachtigall, that if you take it in replacement therapy, you may be better protected from cancer of the endometrium than if you didn't take hormones at all.

To illustrate her point, Dr. Nachtigall cites her 1979 study, which was aimed at identifying the long-term effects of ERT. In it, she compared one group of women who took the estrogen/progesterone combination with another group of women who took no hormones. The results? "After ten years of therapy, we found a positive and protective effect when estrogens were combined with progesterone," she says. "In spite of the fact that higher dosages of hormones were used in the study than are normally taken by menopausal women today, there were no cases of endometrial cancer among the women treated with ERT."

Other researchers have reported similar findings. A 1980 study conducted by R. Don Gambrell, Jr., M.D., and his colleagues at the Medical College of Augusta, Georgia, demonstrated that the incidence of endometrial cancer among women who took estrogen with a progestogen was less than that of women who took no hormones at all. (A progestogen is any substance—natural or synthetic—that acts like progesterone.)

What's even more reassuring is that progestogen seems capable of reversing endometrial hyperplasia (established as a precancerous condition in some women), so that, in one study, the endometrium returned to normal in 94.5 percent of the cases. Other studies also seem to indicate that progestogens can prevent this abnormal overgrowth of the endometrium after estrogen treatment and reverse hyperplasia once it occurs.

Does this mean that ERT has been cleared of all charges of causing cancer? Not exactly, say experts. "We still do not know for sure just how or if estrogen or progestin affects the breasts," cautions Isaac Schiff, M.D., director of Reproductive Endocrinology Services, Brigham and Women's Hospital in Boston.

Admittedly, says Dr. Schiff, the studies have been confusing, to say the least. The early studies seemed to say that you were more than twice as likely to get breast cancer if you took estrogen than if you did not. Other studies involving certain subgroups of women, such as those with benign breast lumps, showed an increased risk the longer ERT was used. Still other research showed just the opposite results. One researcher went so far as to conclude that progesterone may even protect the breasts from breast cancer.

That may be going a little too far, says Dr. Schiff. "To say that progestins have a positive effect on the breasts seems a bit premature," he cautions. "There have been no long-term, careful studies on estrogen/progestin therapy and its role in breast cancer." At this point, he says, it's much safer to say that estrogen probably has no effect on the breasts. "That's where there is the most convincing evidence."

He's referring to studies like the one published by the Drug Epidemiology Unit at Boston College, in which researchers looked at more than 1,600 women with breast cancer and 1,600 without. Among the postmenopausal women, a mixture of estrogens did not appear to increase the risk of breast cancer, even when taken for many years or in the distant past. Researchers concluded that "the results of this study suggest that estrogens do not increase the risk of breast cancer."

Other experts prefer to remain somewhat cautious about the long-term effects of estrogen and progestin on the breasts—especially when it comes to certain subgroups of women. "It would appear that overall, ERT has no effect on the breasts," says Sadja Greenwood, M.D., assistant clinical professor of gynecology at the University of California Medical Center in San Francisco. "But we do know the risk rises with doses of hormones used and the length of time taken, and whether a woman is prone to breast cancer because of a family history, or she has a benign breast lump or she is overweight."

CANCER FEARS UNFOUNDED

Since breast cancer could take 25 years to manifest itself, we can't be sure if long-term use of the new ERT causes the disease until long-term studies are completed. Only then will we know whether an effect is genuinely lacking or only apparently lacking because there hasn't been enough time to see the real results. In the meantime, ERT is not recommended for women at high risk for breast cancer.

The rest of us should stop worrying, assures Dr. Nachtigall. "If you want to take estrogen for its benefits, ERT will probably not give you cancer and may even protect you in some ways if you are sure to take it in low doses and with progestin."

IS ERT FOR YOU?

The new ERT is not for everyone. It is not for women at high risk for cancer or heart disease. It is not for overweight women, who naturally have an elevated estrogen level. It's also not for women with lumpy breasts or uterine fibroids, since these conditions may be aggravated by estrogen.

Even if you don't have these conditions, though, you may not need or want to use ERT, reminds Dr. Nachtigall. Or your symptoms may be mild enough that you can get along fine on short-term doses of ERT.

Ms. F., for example, decided not to take hormones because her hot flashes were mild, she had a late menopause and, as a widow, she felt sexual functioning was not an issue for her. Mrs. J., on the other hand, took oral estrogen/progesterone for only about three years until her hot flashes and insomnia subsided. After that, she got along very well with the occasional use of vaginal estrogen cream which allowed for pain-free sexual intercourse.

Mrs. G., however, is a likely candidate for long-term ERT. She is a thin woman who had an early menopause, a family history of osteoporosis, vaginal soreness and sexual difficulties, not to mention horrendous hot flashes that kept her awake nights. Her problems, says Dr. Nachtigall, could be safely countered by ERT. "The point is," she says, "you should decide on ERT based on your symptoms, your history, risk factors and your personal needs."

But don't, adds Dr. Greenwood, fall into the same trap as women in earlier eras—ERT is not a magical menopause potion. It won't eliminate depression, although some women report feeling better (and some report feeling worse). And while estrogen sometimes makes the skin thicker, oilier and smoother, ERT cannot wipe out wrinkles and should never be taken for this reason. If you have a "leakage" problem due to a slackened urethra, you might want to try nondrug therapies like vaginal muscle exercises for incontinence.

ERT RELIEF

If you have any of the following maladies, you may want to consider estrogen replacement therapy.

Osteoporosis. It's been called the silent epidemic: "silent" because in its early stages, osteoporosis may have no symptoms, and "epidemic" because it affects one out of four postmenopausal women.

When estrogen is no longer produced to keep calcium in the bones, they can become brittle, porous and prone to fracture. At present, hip fractures caused by osteoporosis are believed to result in 50,000 deaths per year—greater than the annual number of deaths from breast and endometrial cancers combined.

At highest risk for brittle bones are thin white women with a family history of osteoporosis, early menopause or removal of ovaries, poor diet (low in calcium, high in caffeine, alcohol, protein and phosphate), women who are sedentary and/or who smoke.

According to a special panel convened by the National Institutes of Health, a highly effective method of curbing bone loss is ERT. In one California study, 245 long-term estrogen users were compared to 245 nonusers and followed for an average of 17.6 years. The researchers found that the osteoporotic fracture incidence in estrogen users was 53.7 percent lower than that of the controls, and the estrogen users showed less bone loss.

In order for ERT to work for those at high risk of developing osteoporosis, though, you need to take it when menopause occurs. What's more, if you stop ERT, the gains in bone density are rapidly lost.

Does that mean you need to take ERT for the rest of your life? Not necessarily, says Edmond F. Maes, Ph.D., Epidemiologic Studies

Branch, Division of Reproductive Health, Centers for Disease Control. "Bone loss occurs at an annual rate of 1 to 2 percent every year," he explains. "It may be possible to take ERT for only the first 10 years following menopause, which would sufficiently postpone bone loss so that severe problems wouldn't show up for another 10 or 15 years."

There is also growing evidence that much lower—and possibly safer—doses are able to halt bone loss. Half of what is now given (0.3 milligrams instead of 0.6 milligrams of estrogen), along with 1,500 milligrams of calcium supplementation and regular weight-bearing exercise such as walking may work in keeping brittle bones at bay.

Severe hot flashes. Nearly 80 percent of women experience hot flashes within the first year of menopause, and nearly 70 percent will have them for five years. Within two years, most hot flashes may lessen. If you do not find relief from measures such as dressing in layers, cutting back on caffeine and alcohol and exercising, you might try taking progestin only or a nonhormone drug called clonidine that suppresses the abnormal activity of blood vessels causing the hot flashes.

If that doesn't work, some doctors suggest trying a low dose of ERT. Remember, hot flashes will return once you stop ERT but can be reduced by gradually tapering off your dosage.

Vaginal soreness. When hormone levels drop, the cellular layer of the vaginal lining becomes thinner, drier and less elastic. And that can make sexual intercourse painful. Many women find effective relief by using lubricants such as vegetable or vitamin E oil, or water-soluble jellies, such as K-Y Lubricating Jelly. Regular sexual activity also helps reduce vaginal soreness.

If these methods are not successful, ask your doctor about using small doses of estrogen cream. It is inserted into the vagina with a measured applicator. The hormone is absorbed into the bloodstream and affects other parts of the body but exerts the major influence on tissues of the vagina, which is restored to a thicker, healthier condition.

Remember, the estrogen cream in high doses can be stronger than pills, as hormones from the cream enter the bloodstream directly and are not subject to the digestive process. However, lower doses of estrogen cream—less than an eighth of the length on the applicator—have been found to work as well. The risk of uterine cancer with such small doses is probably small, but to be on the safe side, doctors recommend using progestin for ten days after having used the cream for a few months, and taking progestin every six months thereafter.

THE PATCH POSSIBILITY

If you've been advised not to take ERT because of circulatory problems, liver disease or gallbladder problems, an estrogen patch might prove an effective solution. Called Estraderm, the round, bandagelike patch is worn on the stomach twice a week and delivers estrogen through the skin directly into the bloodstream; it therefore does not affect these conditions.

In addition, the estrogen remains in its purest form, estradiol, which is less likely than other forms to cause hyperplasia.

At this point, the patch has only been approved to treat hot flashes. However, the future looks promising for its use in the prevention of osteoporosis, says Dr. Nachtigall. "Preliminary studies lead us to believe it will be just as effective as oral estrogen for osteoporosis."

CANCER PREVENTION PLAN: ESTROGEN REPLACEMENT THERAPY

- If you are at high risk for breast cancer, if you have lumpy breasts or uterine fibroids, be aware that ERT is not recommended for women with these conditions.
- Take the lowest possible dose for the shortest possible time. Consider using creams or patches. Reevaluate your need for estrogen at least once every six months.
- Have your doctor prescribe progesterone.
- Watch for abnormal bleeding. Tell your doctor immediately if your bleeding is heavy or occurs at an unusual time.
- Don't quit ERT cold turkey. Gradually reduce your dosages so your endocrine system will not be shocked.
- Practice monthly breast self-exams.
- Make sure you get annual Pap smears, blood pressure and cholesterol checks.
- Monitor side effects.

C H A P T E R *32*

Exercise

Sure, you believed the scientists when they said exercise could help prevent heart disease and lower blood pressure and keep your weight down and make you feel less tense. That heart-pumping bicycle ride . . . that calorie-burning aerobics class . . . that brain-clearing brisk walk—it seemed obvious that exercise was good for your body. But prevent cancer? Stop a tumor? Any scientist who made *that* claim should have to spend an hour in a health club sweating the fantasy out of his system. And maybe you should be right there with him—preventing cancer. Because new studies show that scientists who say exercise may help prevent cancer are probably right.

The study of exercise's relationship to cancer is still in the early stages, so exercise recommendations aren't precise. No one knows enough to say, for example, that working out with weights to bring your heart up to 88 percent of its maximum 3.5 times a week will reduce your risk of cancer by 22.5 percent (and if anyone tries to give you such an equation, give them a look of suspicion). But several studies have forged a strong link between exercise in general and the prevention of various cancers, including colon, breast, and cancers of the female reproductive system.

STUDY: COLLEGE ATHLETES ARE PROTECTED

Perhaps the largest study of the relationship between cancer and exercise was done in 1985 by a team of researchers led by Rose E. Frisch, Ph.D., associate professor of population sciences at the Harvard School of Public Health in Boston. This study analyzed the responses 5,398 women graduates of eight colleges and two universities gave to a detailed questionnaire. The women who were tested had been at college sometime between 1925 and 1981, and ranged in age from 21 to 80. But perhaps the most important fact of the study was that about half (2,622) of the women were former college athletes.

To be counted as an athlete by the researchers, the women had to have played on a least one intramural or varsity sports team, including basketball, dance, field hockey, softball, tennis and volleyball and other energy-intensive sports, for one or more years, or earned a college letter. The team had to train at least twice a week during the college year. Women who didn't play on teams were included as athletes in the study if they regularly worked out by doing something like running two miles a day, five days per week.

According to the study, "A remarkable result was that the subjects who had participated in athletic activity while in college had a lower lifetime occurrence rate of cancers of the reproductive system (uterus, ovary, cervix and vagina) and breast cancer than their nonathletic classmates."

ESTROGEN MAY BE KEY TO PREVENTION

Dr. Frisch says no one knows exactly why exercise may protect against breast and female reproductive cancers. "But estrogen may play a key role," she says. "Exercise may lead to lower levels and less potent forms of this hormone in the body."

The connection between exercise and estrogen might center on weight, because overweight women tend to have higher estrogen levels. And since exercise helps people become leaner, that may be how it lowers their estrogen production. The women in the study who exercised were leaner in every age group than the women who didn't (see chapter 49, Obesity). All of the women had similar family histories of cancer, a similar number of pregnancies and similar smoking habits.

In another study, Dr. Frisch found that women who began training early also ate less fat, and this may be a clue to the favorable results of the exercisers in this study. Dietary fat can be a risk for cancer (see chapter 33, Fat).

Finally, the athletes in the study had later onset of menstruation and earlier menopause than the nonexercisers. Both of these traits put a women at lower risk for cancers of the breast and endometrium.

REGULAR EXERCISE IS IMPORTANT

Dr. Frisch is encouraged by the data and, while she says more studies have to be done, she also says, "This information suggests that exercise helps prevent cancer. The key seems to be regular, long-term exercise. This study suggests that young girls should start exercising early, participating in sports like basketball and track two times a week for several hours, or daily for shorter periods of time.

"We can't extend our data, which looked at exercise habits in college-aged women, to women who begin exercising later in life. But everything suggests that it wouldn't hurt for women to start exercising even in their twenties and thirties. Since the risk of cancer rises with age, young women have a long time to work at reducing their risk, and exercise should be part of their plan. Exercise is good for many things, including building up your bone strength."

SITTING IS AN OCCUPATIONAL HAZARD

While Dr. Frisch didn't study men, other studies did.

David H. Garabrant, M.D., of the University of Southern California School of Medicine in Los Angeles, led a study which found that men with sedentary jobs, including accountants, lawyers, musicians and bookkeepers, have a greater risk of colon cancer than men with more active jobs. And other studies have come up with similar results.

A team of researchers led by John E. Vena, Ph.D., of the Department of Social and Preventive Medicine at the School of Medicine, State University of New York, Buffalo, also found that men with sedentary jobs had a greater risk of colon cancer. Dr. Vena studied the occupational histories of 210 white males with colon cancer, 276 with rectal cancer and 1,431 without cancer who were admitted to a hospital in Buffalo between 1957 and 1965. He looked at the type of work the men in the study did and found a correlation between sedentary and light work and colon cancer. Sedentary was defined as never lifting more than 10 pounds, but occasionally lifting dockets, ledgers and small tools. A person in a sedentary job would usually sit, but sometimes would have to walk or stand. Light work was defined as never having to lift more than 20 pounds, but with frequent lifting of objects weighing up to 10 pounds. A person who does light work also would have to walk or stand frequently.

The study concluded that the risk of colon cancer went up in relation to the number of years a person spent working a sedentary or light job. And the greater the portion of a person's life that is spent working a sedentary or light job, the greater the risk for colon cancer. In fact, according to this study, people who have spent their entire lives doing light or sedentary work have twice the risk of colon cancer as people who always worked in more active types of jobs.

ACROSS-THE-BOARD BENEFITS

"The benefits of exercise on colon cancer appear in all age groups," says Dr. Vena. "We know very little about the exact mechanism of exercise and colon cancer, or the threshold level of exercise. So it's hard to say that a person should exercise this much to get this much protection. But the bottom line is that more exercise won't hurt, and there's a good chance it would help someone prevent colon cancer."

Dr. Vena says exercise might help reduce cancer risk by lowering a person's stress levels and thus boosting overall immunity. Or it might be that when people exercise they change other parts of their lifestyle, like eating a better diet. "Research shows that people increase their calorie intake when they exercise, and maybe they eat more carbohydrates, vegetables and fiber, which would help prevent cancer," says Dr. Vena.

Another possible explanation is that exercise lowers the amount of time it takes for food to pass through the colon and out of the body. This would reduce the contact the colon would have with carcinogens from a person's diet or environmental exposure.

But in the long run—or the long walk, if that's more your speed—it doesn't matter *why* exercise works to prevent cancer. What matters is that you actually exercise—at least three times a week, for a half hour or longer each time. Start slow and easy, and see your doctor first if you're over 30, overweight or become breathless even while inactive. But do get going. Cancer might be more likely to catch up with you if you just stand around.

CANCER PREVENTION PLAN: EXERCISE

- To help protect against breast and female reproductive cancers, exercise regularly.
- Young girls should start exercising early, two times a week for several hours or daily for shorter periods of time.
- To help prevent colon cancer, exercise at least three times a week for a half hour or longer each time.

33

Fat

If a tumor were a growing plant, fat would be its Miracle-Gro.

Just as a seed won't grow into a plant without fertilized soil, a cell won't grow into a tumor without the right environment. And fat may create that environment for some kinds of tumors.

"Probably, all of us have had some kind of 'initiating' event in our lifetime," says Leonard A. Cohen, Ph.D., who has researched fats and cancer at the American Health Foundation in Valhalla, New York. Such an event exposes cells to a damaging element—like x-rays or asbestos. The exposure changes the cell in a way that "programs" the cell to grow into a tumor. "Most women develop little lesions on the ducts of their breast, probably during puberty. About 95 percent of all men have little clusters of abnormal cells in their prostate by the time they're 70 years old. [These cells have been initiated.] Then the question is whether these cells will turn into a tumor or just sit there for the rest of their lives," he says. For an initiated cell to grow like Jack's beanstalk, it requires the right environment—one that promotes growth. "Fat is one of the chief promoting agents we've seen so far in breast cancer. It may also be a major factor in colon, pancreatic and prostate cancer."

We have little control over initiators. Initiation happens rapidly and is irreversible. But promotion—providing the proper growth environment—usually requires repeated exposure over a long period of time. And it is reversible, at least in its early stages, scientists believe.

HOW FAT PROMOTES BREAST CANCER

"Out of all the cancers, breast cancer shows the strongest association with fats," says Dr. Cohen.

In 1942, a scientist demonstrated that there's a probable link between breast cancer and fat in the diet. And the evidence for that link has been getting stronger ever since. Now more than 100 studies show that something's going on between dietary fat and cancer.

In a typical study, a group of researchers from Canada interviewed 577 women with breast cancer and 826 disease-free women, asking them how often they ate certain foods. They discovered that the more beef, pork and desserts a woman had eaten, the more likely she was to have breast cancer. Women who used butter or margarine in cooking or at the table also increased their risk. In fact, the women with the highest intake of animal fat had more than twice the risk of the women with the leanest diet.

Another study showed that a low-fat diet may actually prolong the lives of women who already have breast cancer. Researchers studied 953 women with breast cancer and discovered that the women's risk of death increased 1.4 times for every 1,000 grams of fat eaten per month (equivalent to about 2¼ tablespoons of butter per day). This connection between life expectancy and fat intake was especially strong for women with cancers that were spreading.

BLAME IT ON THE HORMONES

Scientists suspect that fat doesn't cause cancer directly—instead, it may use hormones to do the dirty work. Prolactin may be one of these hormones. Let's take a look at what it does in animals.

"When a bird is about to migrate, a lot of prolactin shoots out of the bird's pituitary gland," says Dr. Cohen. "The bird starts eating like crazy until 50 percent of its body is fat. Prolactin gives the bird a message to store fat. Until recently, scientists didn't believe prolactin and fat worked together in humans. We knew that prolactin 'tells' a new mother's breasts to start producing milk. But now we know it does other things too. What's more, we have a new way to detect prolactin levels, and we found that high-fat diets increase the biologically active form of prolactin in humans."

Too much of this prolactin may promote cancer. "Prolactin stimulates the breast to grow," says Dr. Cohen. "It's possible that it also can stimulate a tumor to grow."

Prolactin may not be the only middleman between fat and cancer. Estrogen also seems to be involved.

"Fat changes the activity of enzymes in the gut," says David P. Rose, M.D., Ph.D., chief of the Division of Nutrition and Endocrinology at the American Health Foundation. "The result is that people on a high-fat diet may reabsorb more estrogen than vegetarians. High estrogen levels in the blood may promote breast cancer."

And these are not the only body chemicals fat manipulates. Fat is also involved with prostaglandin levels. Prostaglandins are a group of hormonelike substances that have the ability to lower blood pressure, regulate body temperature and control inflammation. But don't think they're all good. Some prostaglandins can cause headaches and menstrual cramps. Other prostaglandins may cause cancer. The body actually converts essential fatty acids into a variety of prostaglandins with all sorts of biological effects.

"When we eat essential fatty acids, which are contained in vegetable oils, our liver and other organs process them until they turn into prostaglandins," says Dr. Cohen. "Too much vegetable fat may cause your body to overproduce certain types of prostaglandins at the expense of other types. And overproduction of certain types of prostaglandins seems to be associated with tumor growth, perhaps by inhibiting the immune response."

THE VULNERABLE PROSTATE

Since breast cancer is a woman's disease, are men off the hook, fat-wise? Not quite. Men's area of vulnerability is the prostate.

The prostate is a gland, about as big as a walnut, that surrounds the beginning of the urethra, just below the bladder. It's not essential for everyday health—its only known function is to produce the lubricating fluid that combines with sperm to make semen.

But for a second-class organ, it causes a lot of first-class problems. The American Cancer Society estimates that 26,100 men in the United States will die from prostate cancer each year, while another 90,000 will have it diagnosed.

Once again, fat seems to have some part in these statistics. Researchers from the University of Hawaii interviewed 4,657 adults to find out how often they ate 83 different foods and in what amounts. The results indicated that the more fat a man ate, the more chance he had of getting prostate cancer. A second study by the same researchers showed an increased risk only for men at the age of 70 and older.

Researchers at California's Loma Linda University found similar results. They studied male Seventh-Day Adventists, most of whom are vegetarians. Those vegetarians who ate a lot of fatty foods like cheese and eggs and those who did eat meat were 3.6 times more likely to have fatal prostate cancer than Adventists who stuck to a diet that included no animal products.

"The evidence so far on prostate cancer is very sketchy and strange," says Dr. Cohen. "The prostate is much more difficult to study in the laboratory, so much less is known about prostate cancer than breast cancer."

ANOTHER TARGET OF HORMONES

But scientists can guess how fat affects the prostate by comparing it to the breast. "Some scientists call the prostate 'the male breast,' " says Dr. Cohen. "The glands look similar in structure if you look at them under a microscope. Both have little spaces throughout, in which fluid accumulates. In the breast, it's milk and in the prostate, it's prostatic fluid."

They also seem to act alike when it comes to cancer and fat. Most countries that have a lot of breast cancer, for instance, also have a lot of prostate cancer.

And both the mammary and the prostate glands are affected by some of the same hormones. "The prostate and the breast are both target organs for estrogen, prolactin and prostaglandins," says Dr. Rose. "Prostate and breast cancer are both treated by manipulating hormones. And prostate cancer never occurs in men who are sterilized, just as breast cancer is uncommon in women who've had their ovaries removed. There's a whole list of similarities between these two glands. The thought is, probably hormones stimulate cancer cells in the prostate to become tumors, just as they do in the breast."

Of course, there are differences. "Prostate cancer tends to show up much later in age than breast cancer," points out Dr. Cohen. "Also, the prostate's always making prostatic fluid, while the breast makes milk only when the woman has a child. So we have to be careful about making parallels."

A RISK FACTOR FOR COLORECTAL CANCER

If breast cancer is for women and prostate cancer is for men, colorectal cancer is, for the most part, an equal opportunity killer. More than 100,000 new cases of colorectal cancer strike Americans each year—only lung cancer is more prevalent in this country.

When we track down the risk factors, we find that fat has struck again. Personal or family health history and age seem to play some part in who gets this disease. But because diet is the one factor that you have control over, say researchers from the American Institute for Cancer Research, it may be the most important one on the list.

Researchers in Greece studied a group of people to see whether people with colon cancer had eaten fattier foods than healthy people. And they found that those who ate the most meat (especially beef and lamb) and the least vegetables had eight times the risk of getting this form of cancer.

Other studies show significant, but more modest, results. A Canadian study of 1,425 people, for example, found that a high-fat diet more than doubled a person's risk of getting colon cancer.

"Even though some experiments show conflicting results, no one doubts that fat plays an important role in colon cancer," says Dr. Cohen. "The only good theory that explains how fats may cause cancer has to do with bile acids."

Bile is a greenish-yellow fluid that is manufactured in the liver, stored in the gallbladder and squirted through ducts into the intestine. Your body needs bile to digest fats, but too much fat may cause too much bile.

How would bile cause cancer? Right now, there is no answer to that question, only theories.

It could be that bile acids remove the mucous layer and the uppermost layer of cells from the intestine's lining. This damage needs to be repaired, so replacement cells are created at a more rapid rate. These growing cells are vulnerable to any cancer-causing chemical that may be lurking in food.

"Bile acids seem to increase the rate of cell turnover in the bowel," says Selwyn A. Broitman, Ph.D., professor of microbiology and pathology at the Boston University School of Medicine, who worked on the committee on diet, nutrition and cancer for the National Academy of Sciences. "Faster cell activity may make it easier for tumors to grow," he says.

According to another scenario, a high-fat diet encourages a type of bacteria in the large intestine which converts bile into secondary bile acids. Some experts theorize that this form of bile acid may help tumors grow.

Fat doesn't always have such devastating effects on the colon. In most countries where high-fat diets prevail, the frequency of colon cancer soars. But not in Finland. Finns eat about as much fat as the average American, but they have one-quarter the rate of colon cancer.

They get away with it because they eat about twice the fiber we do. Fiber may protect against colon cancer by diluting bile acid in the intestine. For more information, see chapter 34, Fiber.

FAT MAY HARM THE PANCREAS

Fat may cause a fuss in another digestive organ, too. We're talking about the pancreas, a digestive organ shaped like a bunch of grapes, which manufactures enzymes your body needs for digestion. "Some experiments on animals suggest that fat may cause pancreatic tumors to grow," says Dr. Cohen.

And recently, Swedish researchers conducted a study on fats and pancreatic cancer, which showed startling results. People who ate fried meat almost every day had five to ten times the risk of getting pancreatic cancer. Eating other fried foods and using margarine also increased the risk. The researchers concluded that fat consumption may be associated with pancreatic cancer.

How might fat affect this grape-cluster organ? Once again, by forcing the body to produce too much bile, scientists speculate. When your intestines are clogged up with too much fat and bile, some of the bile backs up into the pancreatic duct. But the bile is an unwelcome visitor—it irritates the tissue, and may promote a tumor.

IS AMERICA SHAPING UP?

America's track record on fat and cancer has been pretty dismal. The most common cancers in America, outside of those connected to smoking, are related to fat.

Such cancers aren't so common in other nations. North Americans have up to five times more breast cancer than people who live in Japan and other Asian nations, as well as most undeveloped nations. When these people move to the United States, their risk of getting breast cancer increases until it catches up with that of Americans. And the incidence of colon cancer follows the same pattern.

Once again, you can blame it all on fat. "In general, low-risk populations eat grains, vegetables, fish and low-fat meat," explains Dr. Cohen. "When their countries become more industrialized, or when they move to America, they often start eating foods which are higher in fat— processed cheese, milk and domesticated cattle, which have been fattened up."

Over the past few years, however, the popularity of red meat and dairy products has been waning, as the public becomes more aware of the harmful effects of fat. Livestock producers are responding to a fat-conscious America by reducing the fat content of meat animals.

And we're already starting to reap the benefits. "For the past two decades, women have been getting less colorectal cancer," says Dr. Broitman. "And the 1984 statistics show a continuing decline in colorectal cancer for women. Because of the decreasing meat fat intake,

I believe we'll see a greater reduction of colon cancer rates 20 years down the line."

TYPES OF FAT

Does it matter what type of fat you eat? If you're talking about heart disease, the answer is yes, but if you're discussing cancer, the answer is maybe.

Several studies with rodents have suggested that unsaturated fat could promote cancer more effectively than saturated fat. For a while, this finding startled doctors. They worried that the fat which might be good for preventing heart disease might be bad for preventing cancer. But scientists later found that if the fat content in food is high enough, it doesn't matter which type of fat it is.

Adding further to the confusion over types of fat, recent wrinkles in research show that some oils actually may protect against cancer. "People in Mediterranean countries such as Greece and Italy had lower breast and colon cancer rates than other Western countries, even though they ate about the same amount of fat," says Dr. Cohen. "The crucial difference was that they cooked with olive oil. But recently, they're starting to use different types of oils, and their breast and colon cancer rates are rising."

A few preliminary animal studies have also suggested that there might be something to this olive oil theory. Unlike corn oil, olive oil does not promote tumors in rats, and it might even protect against cancer.

Fish oil also may ward off cancer. A group of investigators at Rutgers University found that they were able to protect laboratory rats against breast cancer by feeding them fish oil. "Fish oil inhibited the growth of transplanted tumors, helped block development of chemically induced tumors and lowered levels of a biochemical indicator of cancer activity," they concluded. For more information about this development, see chapter 35, Fish Oil.

HOW ABOUT CHOLESTEROL?

Some time after the saturated fat conflict was cleared up, heart and cancer recommendations seemed to clash again over cholesterol.

"There was a mad panic in the National Institutes of Health when reports showed that people with colon cancer had low levels of cholesterol in their blood," says Dr. Rose. "They were afraid that we would have to choose between cancer and heart disease. But then they realized that cancer *causes* low blood cholesterol. A rapidly growing tumor may use large amounts of cholesterol from the blood to grow."

But even if cholesterol in the blood is off the hook, cancer-wise, there is a large body of evidence that cholesterol in our food *is* associated with colorectal cancer.

When researchers ask cancer patients what they have been eating, for instance, the answers seem to implicate cholesterol. A group of Canadian researchers compared 542 people who had bowel cancer with people who didn't have the cancer. They found out that the more cholesterol a person consumed, the greater his or her chances of getting colorectal cancer.

Other studies have shown conflicting results, but Dr. Broitman believes that positive results outweigh the negative. "I'd estimate that if you eat too much cholesterol, you increase your risk of developing bowel cancer significantly. Your risk may be anywhere from 1½ to 3 times greater."

Nobody knows for sure how cholesterol would do the work, but some scientists believe that high cholesterol intake leads to high levels of bile acids. And we've already mentioned that high bile levels seem to help tumors along.

HOW MUCH FAT IS TOO MUCH?

The evidence on fat has not escaped the notice of health organizations—virtually all of them recommend that Americans reduce their fat intake. The National Research Council recommends that to lower the risk of breast and colon cancer, people should pare down dietary fat to 30 percent of total calories. "Indeed," the Council admits, "the data could be used to justify an even greater reduction."

And some organizations and scientists *do* recommend a greater reduction. The American Health Foundation suggests no more than 20 to 25 percent of total calories should come from fat.

But who knows what 20 percent means? Few people, if any, would take the trouble to add up their daily caloric intake and calculate what percentage came from fat.

So we took the trouble for you. Take a look at the table, Fat Content of Foods, on page 140, which shows the percentage of calories from fat in various foods. It can help you select foods that are lower in fat.

The table shows, for instance, that a turkey breast has *one-fourth* the fat of a chicken breast. And whole milk, which contains 3.3 percent fat by volume, actually contains 48 percent of calories from fat. Skim milk has a mere 4 percent of calories from fat.

Sauces, dressings and gravies may add a dash of flavor to a meal, but they also can add a glob of fat. Canned chicken gravy contains 64 percent of calories from fat, while chicken breast only contains 20 per-

(continued on page 145)

FAT CONTENT OF FOODS

FOOD	PORTION	CALORIES	% OF CALORIES FROM FAT
DAIRY PRODUCTS			
Butter	1 tbsp.	102	99
Cheese			
Blue	1 oz.	100	72
Brie	1 oz.	95	73
Cheddar	1 oz.	114	72
Colby	1 oz.	112	71
Cottage, low-fat, 1%	½ cup	82	12
Cream	1 oz.	99	88
Feta	1 oz.	75	71
Mozzarella, part-skim	1 oz.	72	55
Muenster	1 oz.	104	72
Neufchâtel	1 oz.	74	79
Parmesan	1 tbsp.	23	57
Provolone	1 oz.	100	66
Ricotta, part-skim	½ cup	171	50
Swiss	1 oz.	107	64
Cream			
Half-and-half	1 tbsp.	20	76
Heavy whipping	1 tbsp.	52	94
Light, coffee or table	1 tbsp.	29	88
Milk			
Buttermilk	1 cup	99	19
Low-fat, 1%	1 cup	102	22
Skim	1 cup	86	4
Whole, 3.3% fat	1 cup	150	48
Yogurt			
Low-fat, fruit varieties	8 oz.	225	10
Low-fat, plain	8 oz.	144	21
FRUITS			
Apple	1	81	5
Avocado	1	324	80
Banana	1	105	4
Blueberries	½ cup	41	6
Cantaloupe	¼	47	7
Grapefruit	½	38	3
Grapes	10	15	4
Orange	1	62	2
Strawberries	¼ cup	11	10

FOOD	PORTION	CALORIES	% OF CALORIES FROM FAT
GRAINS			
Bran muffin	1	104	31
Bread			
French	1 slice	102	9
Italian	1 slice	83	2
Pumpernickel	1 slice	79	4
Raisin	1 slice	66	9
Whole wheat, firm			
crumb	1 slice	61	11
Cereal			
Cornflakes	1 cup	100	1
Oatmeal, cooked with			
no salt	½ cup	73	14
Crackers			
Cheese	10	52	37
Graham, plain	1 lg.	55	20
Oyster	10	33	25
Saltine	10	123	23
Whole wheat	10	161	29
Pancake, plain or			
buttermilk	1	164	27
Popcorn, plain	1 cup	23	11
Pretzel	1 rod	55	9
Rice			
Brown, long-grain,			
cooked	½ cup	116	4
White, long-grain,			
cooked	½ cup	112	1
Tofu, raw, regular	4 oz.	85	53
Wheat germ, toasted, plain	½ cup	216	23
MEATS			
Bacon	3 strips	109	77
Beef			
Bottom round roast,			
choice, no fat, braised	3 oz.	191	40
Broth	1 cup	16	30
Chuck steak, choice,			
braised	3 oz.	164	33
Corned, brisket,			
cured, boiled	3 oz.	213	68
Flank steak, choice,			
no fat, braised	3 oz.	208	51
Gravy	1 tbsp.	8	40
Ground, lean, broiled			
medium	3 oz.	231	61

(continued)

FAT CONTENT OF FOODS—*Continued*

FOOD	PORTION	CALORIES	% OF CALORIES FROM FAT
MEATS—*continued*			
Beef—*continued*			
Liver, fried	3 oz.	184	33
Porterhouse steak, choice, broiled	3 oz.	185	45
Rib roast, choice, no fat, roasted	3 oz.	209	53
Sirloin steak, choice, wedge-bone, no fat, broiled	3 oz.	180	39
T-bone, choice, no fat, broiled	3 oz.	182	44
Tenderloin, choice, broiled	3 oz.	176	42
Frankfurter, beef	1	142	82
Ham			
Chopped	3 oz.	195	68
Cured	3 oz.	140	42
Fresh pork, roasted	3 oz.	187	45
Lamb			
Chop, loin	3 oz.	160	36
Leg	3 oz.	158	34
Liverwurst	3 oz.	276	79
Pork			
Loin	3 oz.	208	51
Spareribs	3 oz.	338	69
Salami, hard pork	1 oz.	115	75
Sausage, Italian, cooked	3 oz.	274	72
Veal			
Boneless, for stew	3 oz.	200	49
Loin cut	3 oz.	199	52
NUTS			
Almonds, dried, unblanched	¼ cup	209	74
Peanut butter, no added salt	1 tbsp.	95	72
Peanuts, unroasted	¼ cup	207	73
Pecans, dried	¼ cup	180	85
Walnuts, English	¼ cup	193	81
POULTRY			
Chicken			
Breast, roasted	3 oz.	140	20

FOOD	PORTION	CALORIES	% OF CALORIES FROM FAT
Drumstick, roasted	3 oz.	147	30
Liver, simmered	3 oz.	133	31
Thigh, roasted	3 oz.	178	47
Wing, roasted	3 oz.	174	36
Broth, canned	1 cup	39	32
Gravy, canned	1 tbsp.	12	64
Duck, domesticated, roasted	3 oz.	171	50
Goose, domesticated, roasted	3 oz.	202	48
Turkey			
Breast, roasted	3 oz.	115	5
Leg, roasted	3 oz.	135	21
Gravy, canned	1 tbsp.	8	37

SALAD DRESSINGS

Blue cheese	1 tbsp.	77	92
French	1 tbsp.	67	84
Italian	1 tbsp.	69	91
Italian, low-calorie	1 tbsp.	16	84
Russian	1 tbsp.	76	91
Thousand island	1 tbsp.	59	84

SEAFOOD

Bluefish, baked with butter	3 oz.	137	30
Clams, cherrystone, raw	6	84	10
Cod, broiled with butter	3 oz.	144	28
Crab, king, steamed	3 oz.	79	18
Fishcakes, fried	5 bite-size	103	42
Flounder	3 oz.	171	37
Haddock, fried	3 oz.	140	35
Halibut, broiled with butter	3 oz.	145	37
Lobster, cooked	3 oz.	81	14
Mackerel, broiled with butter	3 oz.	200	60
Ocean perch, fried	3 oz.	193	53
Salmon, pink, canned	3 oz.	120	38
Sardines, in oil	3 oz.	172	49
Scallops, steamed	6	67	11
Shrimp, cooked	½ cup	21	9
Tuna			
in oil	3 oz.	245	38
in water	3 oz.	108	6

(continued)

FAT CONTENT OF FOODS—Continued

FOOD	PORTION	CALORIES	% OF CALORIES FROM FAT
VEGETABLES			
Alfalfa sprouts	1 tbsp.	1	17
Asparagus, cooked	4 spears	15	11
Broccoli, cooked	½ cup	23	8
Brussels sprouts, cooked	4	32	12
Carrots, cooked	½ cup	35	3
Cauliflower, cooked	½ cup	15	6
Celery, raw	1 stalk	6	7
Corn, cooked	½ cup	89	10
Cucumber, sliced	½ cup	7	8
Eggplant, cooked	½ cup	13	7
Lima beans	½ cup	104	2
Mushrooms, raw	4	20	13
Onions			
boiled	½ cup	29	5
raw	¼ cup	14	7
Peas, green, cooked	½ cup	67	2
Potatoes			
Baked with skin	1	220	.8
Broiled, without skin	1	116	1
French fried, frozen, heated in oven	10 strips	111	35
French fried, restaurant prepared	10 strips	158	46
Hash brown	½ cup	163	56
Mashed, with milk added	½ cup	81	6
Potato chips	10	105	56
Potato salad	½ cup	179	51
Squash			
Acorn, baked	½ cup	41	2
Zucchini, raw	½ cup	9	8

Table information adapted from the following sources:

Nutritive Value of American Foods in Common Units, Agriculture Handbook No. 456, by Catherine F. Adams (Washington, D.C.: Agricultural Research Service, U.S. Department of Agriculture, 1975).

Composition of Foods: Vegetables and Vegetable Products, Agriculture Handbook No. 8-11, by Nutrition Monitoring Division (Washington, D.C.: Human Nutrition Information Service, U.S. Department of Agriculture, 1984).

Composition of Foods: Dairy and Egg Products, Agriculture Handbook No. 8-1, by Consumer and Food Economics Institute (Washington, D.C.: Agricultural Research Service, U.S. Department of Agriculture, 1976).

Composition of Foods: Beef Products, Agriculture Handbook No. 8-13, by Nutrition Monitoring Division (Washington, D.C.: Human Nutrition Information Service, U.S. Department of Agriculture, 1986).

Composition of Foods: Fruits and Fruit Juices, Agriculture Handbook No. 8-9, by Consumer Nutrition Center (Washington, D.C.: Human Nutrition Information Service, U.S. Department of Agriculture, 1982).

Composition of Foods: Poultry Products, Agriculture Handbook No. 8-5, by Consumer and Food Economics Institute (Washington, D.C.: Science and Education Administration, U.S. Department of Agriculture, 1979).

Composition of Foods: Pork Products, Agriculture Handbook No. 8-10, by Consumer Nutrition Center (Washington, D.C.: Human Nutrition Information Service, U.S. Department of Agriculture, 1983).

Composition of Foods: Nut and Seed Products, Agriculture Handbook No. 8-12, by Nutrition Monitoring Division (Washington, D.C.: Human Nutrition Information Service, U.S. Department of Agriculture, 1984).

Composition of Foods: Fats and Oils, Agriculture Handbook No. 8-4, by Consumer and Food Economics Institute (Washington, D.C.: Science and Education Administration, U.S. Department of Agriculture, 1979).

Composition of Foods: Soups Sauces and Gravies, Agriculture Handbook No. 8-6, by Consumer and Food Economics Institute (Washington, D.C.: Science and Education Administration, U.S. Department of Agriculture, 1980).

Composition of Foods: Breakfast Cereals, Agriculture Handbook No. 8-8, by Consumer Nutrition Center (Washington, D.C.: Human Nutrition Information Service, U.S. Department of Agriculture, 1982).

Composition of Foods: Legumes and Legume Products, Agriculture Handbook No. 8-16, by Nutrition Monitoring Division (Washington, D.C.: Human Nutrition Information Service, U.S. Department of Agriculture, 1986).

Composition of Foods: Sausages and Luncheon Meats, Agriculture Handbook No. 8-7, by Consumer Nutrition Center (Washington, D.C.: Science and Education Administration, U.S. Department of Agriculture, 1980).

Composition of Foods, Agriculture Handbook No. 8, by Bernice K. Watt and Annabel L. Merrill (Washington, D.C.: Agricultural Research Service, U.S. Department of Agriculture, 1975).

cent of calories from fat. Butter has more fat than any food. And mayonnaise is' hardly better. In fact, the dab of mayonnaise on a fast-food 'superburger' contains nearly as much fat as the entire beef patty. So try to use less butter, mayonnaise, salad dressing and gravies, or use light versions of these foods. See the box, Rating the Cooking Methods, on page 170 for tips on low-fat cooking.

As for cholesterol reduction, the American Health Foundation recommends that you limit cholesterol to 200 milligrams a day. One egg yolk alone has about 272 milligrams of cholesterol, and more fat than a teaspoon of corn oil.

Not ready to give up your recipes that call for eggs? Then throw away the yolks. Use 1½ or 2 egg whites in place of each whole egg you need and, chances are, you won't be able to taste the difference. Check the table, Cholesterol Content of Popular Protein Foods, on page 146 for cholesterol content of other foods.

CHOLESTEROL CONTENT OF POPULAR PROTEIN FOODS

FOOD	PORTION (oz., except where indicated)	CHOLESTEROL (mg)
DAIRY PRODUCTS AND EGGS		
Cheese		
Cheddar	1	30
Cottage, low-fat, 1%	4	5
Cream	1	31
Feta	1	25
Mozzarella, part-skim	1	16
Neufchâtel	1	22
Ricotta, part-skim	4	35
Swiss	1	26
Egg whites, raw	3 lg.	0
Eggs, whole, raw	2 lg.	548
Milk		
Skim	8	4
Whole, 3.3% fat	8	33
Yogurt, low-fat, plain	6	11
MEATS, FRESH, RED (MOST TRIMMED OF FAT, COOKED MEDIUM)		
Beef		
Brisket, whole, braised	3.5	92
Ground, extra lean, broiled	3.5	83
Ground, regular, broiled	3.5	89
Flank, choice, broiled	3.5	70
Liver, braised	3.5	386
Round, full cut, choice, broiled	3.5	82
Sirloin steak, wedge-bone, choice, broiled	3.5	90
Lamb		
Chop loin, broiled	3.5	91
Leg, roasted	3.5	88
Pork		
Loin, roasted	3.5	90
Spareribs, not trimmed, braised	3.5	120
Veal		
Cutlet, medium fat, fried	3.5	127
Rib, roasted	3.5	127

FOOD	PORTION (oz., except where indicated)	CHOLESTEROL (mg)
MEATS, PROCESSED		
Bologna		
Beef and pork	2	32
Turkey	2	56
Canadian bacon, unheated	2	28
Chicken roll, light meat	2	28
Frankfurters		
Beef	2 franks	44
Turkey	2 franks	96
Ham		
Extra lean (5% fat)	2	26
Turkey, cured, thigh meat	2	. . .
Italian sausage, pork	3.5	77
NUTS AND BEANS		
Almond butter, plain	2 tbsp.	0
Kidney beans	1 cup	0
Lentils	1 cup	0
Peanut butter	2 tbsp.	0
Peanuts, dried or oil-roasted	1	0
Tofu	4	0
Walnuts, black or English	1	0
POULTRY		
Chicken		
With skin, roasted	3.5	88
Without skin, roasted	3.5	89
Turkey, light meat, without skin, roasted	3.5	69
SEAFOOD		
Clams	3.5	50
Cod	3.5	40
Flounder	3.5	58
Mackerel	3.5	79
Ocean perch	3.5	42
Salmon	3.5	70
Scallops	3.5	35
Shrimp, canned	3.5	150
Tuna, in water	3.5	56

(continued)

CHOLESTEROL CONTENT OF POPULAR PROTEIN FOODS— *Continued*

Table information adapted from the following sources:

Composition of Foods: Dairy and Egg Products, Agriculture Handbook No. 8-1, by Consumer and Food Economics Institute (Washington, D.C.: Agricultural Research Service, U.S. Department of Agriculture, 1976).

Composition of Foods, Agriculture Handbook No. 8, by Bernice K. Watt and Annabel L. Merrill (Washington, D.C.: Agricultural Research Service, U.S. Department of Agriculture, 1975).

Composition of Foods: Beef Products, Agriculture Handbook No., 8-13, by Nutrition Monitoring Division (Washington, D.C.: Human Nutrition Information Service, U.S. Department of Agriculture 1986).

Nutritive Value of Foods, Home and Garden Bulletin No. 72, by Susan E. Gebhardt and Ruth H. Matthews (Washington, D.C.: Human Nutrition Information Service, U.S. Department of Agriculture, 1986).

Bowes and Church's Food Values of Portion Commonly Used, 14th Ed., by Jean A. T. Pennington and Helen Nichols Church (Philadelphia: J. B. Lippincott, 1985).

Composition of Foods: Sausages and Luncheon Meats, Agriculture Handbook No. 8-7, by Consumer Nutrition Center (Washington, D.C.: Science and Education Administration, U.S. Department of Agriculture, 1980).

Composition of Foods: Nut and Seed Products, Agriculture Handbook No. 8-12, by Nutrition Monitoring Division (Washington, D.C.: Human Nutrition Information Service, US. Department of Agriculture, 1984).

Nutritive Value of American Foods in Common Units, Agriculture Handbook No. 456, by Catherine F. Adams (Washington, D.C.: Agricultural Research Service, U.S. Department of Agriculture, 1975).

"Provisional tables on the content of omega-3 fatty acids and other fat components of selected foods," by Frank N. Hepburn, Jacob Exler and John L. Weihrauch, *Journal of the American Dietetic Association* (June, 1986).

Composition of Foods: Pork Products, Agriculture Handbook No. 8-10, by Consumer Nutrition Center (Washington, D.C.: Human Nutrition Information Service, U.S. Department of Agriculture, 1983).

Composition of Foods: Legumes and Legume Products, Agriculture Handbook No. 8-16, by Nutrition Monitoring Division (Washington, D.C.: Human Nutrition Information Service, U.S. Department of Agriculture, 1986).

Composition of Foods: Poultry Products, Agriculture Handbook No. 8-5, by Consumer and Food Economics Institute (Washington, D.C.: Science and Education Administration, U.S. Department of Agriculture, 1979).

CANCER PREVENTION PLAN: FAT

- Pare down dietary fat to 20 to 30 percent of total calories.
- Cook with olive oil.
- Limit cholesterol. Eat no more than two to four egg yolks a week.

C H A P T E R 34
Fiber

Breakthrough advertising!"
"Innovative!" "Bold!" "Gutsy!" "Misleading!"

Such were the reactions when the Kellogg Company started publicizing the National Cancer Institute's (NCI) dietary recommendations in 1984. Where many cereal boxes feature send-in-your-boxtop prizes, the All-Bran box trumpets the news that a high-fiber diet "may help to prevent certain kinds of cancer." Some conservative medical researchers were unsettled by the sudden blare of Madison Avenue hype.

"The argument against the campaign was that John Q. Public might hear that ad and think, 'Oh, All-Bran prevents colon cancer, I'd better go get some,' instead of changing his overall diet," says Jon A. Story, Ph.D., who researches fiber and cancer in the Department of Foods and Nutrition at Purdue University, West Lafayette, Indiana. "But the information on the Kellogg's All-Bran box and in its ads is very carefully worded and is very accurate."

The public responded. The NCI received more than 60,000 calls on a toll-free information hotline that the Kellogg Company mentioned in their advertising. And All-Bran sales reportedly increased 41 percent.

But All-Bran is just a piece of the high-fiber pie. We are living, as one researcher puts it, in the era of the "fiber fuss." Not since Sylvester

Graham campaigned for the revival of whole wheat bread in the 1830s has there been so much energy and attention focused on the mainly undigestible portion of the foods we eat—the bran of grains, the pulp of fruit, the crunchy cell walls of vegetables and the squishiness of beans. In other words, the fiber.

Why all the fuss? Because evidence shows that fiber protects against a number of the chronic illnesses that plague us today, and possibly even colon cancer. And because the news about fiber is *good* news.

"We've been told to cut down on so many foods we like in order to prevent cancer," points out David Klurfeld, Ph.D., who researches fiber and cancer at the Wistar Institute in Philadelphia. "Finally, with fiber, we are told to eat more of something. And it's much more appealing to hear encouraging advice."

PROTECTION AGAINST COLON CANCER

The fiber fuss all started in 1974, when Denis P. Burkitt, a British doctor, visited Africa as a medical missionary. He noticed that people in Uganda ate plenty of fiber-rich foods such as ground nuts, sweet potatoes, yams and bananas. As a result, they took in 50 to 250 grams of fiber per day, as compared to an American's 3 to 5 grams per day. And they suffered much less colon cancer.

And Africans weren't the only ones who seemed to benefit from fiber, either. "There are a number of international comparisons, and they're probably the strongest evidence for the protective role of fiber," says Dr. Klurfeld. "In general, those countries where people eat a high-fiber diet have a much lower colon cancer rate than countries that have a low-fiber diet."

But fiber can protect you whether or not you live in a "high-risk" country. That's what Israeli researchers found when they asked hundreds of people how often they ate 243 different foods. The only significant difference between the diets of the 198 colon cancer patients and their healthy neighbors was how much fiber they ate. In fact, cancer patients ate 61 of the 73 fiber-rich foods less often than their neighbors.

Researchers from the Kaiser-Permanente Medical Care Program in Oakland, California, found similar results when they investigated the rising colon cancer rates in black people. A woman went door-to-door, asking 99 black colorectal patients and 280 black cancer-free people to describe their eating habits. The results? Cancer patients ate less fiber foods such as oatmeal, bran cereal, cornbread, beans, fruits and vegetables.

But what about that other "f" word—fat? Study after study has proven that dietary fat is a major cause of colon cancer (see chapter 33, Fat.) Since a high-fiber diet is usually low in fat, could it be that fiber itself has nothing do to with preventing cancer?

Probably not. In fact, a high-fiber diet may even counteract the harmful effects of fat. Finns in Kuopio, for example, eat as much fat as the Danes in Copenhagen, but they have only one-third the rate of cancer.

"At first, researchers were confused by this finding, because a high-fat diet is usually associated with colon cancer in international studies," says Leonard A. Cohen, Ph.D., of the American Health Foundation in Valhalla, New York. "Then they noticed that most Finns eat this funny porridge at every meal. You can tell this cereal is rich in fiber because it goes right through them. If you don't mind my being indelicate here, they produce enormous amounts of stool." To be precise, the Finns ate an average of 31 grams of fiber each day—almost twice the amount of the Danes, who took in 17 grams a day.

Here, the United States Department of Health and Human Services announced that if Americans ate less fat and more fiber, cases of colon cancer could fall by 30 percent, saving about 20,000 lives each year. Researchers at the National Cancer Institute are even more optimistic. They have estimated that if everybody ate 20 to 30 grams of fiber a day, a 50 percent reduction in colon cancer would be possible.

THE FIVE FACES OF FIBER

Until the late 1960s, some experts announced that fiber was bad, because it resisted digestion and thus "irritated" the intestine. But now we know fiber is good. In fact, in the intervening years, science has learned a great deal about fiber and the way it works in the body. And even though there is still much to learn, what is known is fascinating.

We know, for example, fiber isn't just "roughage." In fact, fiber isn't even just one substance, but many different kinds of substances. "We can't think of fiber as one big type of food—like starch, for example," explains Dr. Story. "Even though there are variations in kinds of starch, they all behave similarly when we eat them. They all get digested. But you can't generalize about fiber, because the types are so varied."

"Indeed, fiber is just a generic term," says Dr. Klurfeld. "There are different classifications under that label. There is crude vs. dietary fiber, as well as soluble [it dissolves] vs. insoluble fiber." And these broad classifications are broken down into even smaller categories: cellulose, pectin, hemicellulose, lignin and gums.

Although fiber's overall role as a protective factor in colon cancer appears well established, the particular role of each type of fiber is still being investigated. Each type's anticancer power is described by fiber researchers in careful, cautious terms. Clearly they are on the threshold of a breakthrough, but afraid to claim too much too soon. Here is a summary of what is known and what is theorized about the different fiber types.

Cellulose. This type of fiber, which is the most prevalent, probably comes closest to the old notions of what fiber ought to be. It is indeed fibrous, softens the stool and shows up in all the expected places—fruits, vegetables, bran, whole-meal bread and beans.

But it does more than the old notions suggest. It increases the bulk of intestinal waste and eases it quickly through the colon. All of which means that it prevents constipation—we're 100 percent sure of that, says Dr. Klurfeld.

But many investigators say these actions may do more. They may dilute and flush cancer-causing toxins out of the intestinal tract before they can do much damage.

Your body itself secretes potential carcinogens into the intestine every day. These are bile acids. As you may recall from the chapter on fat, eating a lot of fat increases bile acids in the colon. And abnormally high levels of these acids may promote tumors.

"Cellulose dilutes bile acids in the intestine," says Dr. Klurfeld. "That's one of the ways in which fiber is thought to protect against colon cancer—by diluting intestinal contents such as bile acids that may irritate colon walls and set up conditions for cancer. So fiber probably counteracts the effect of dietary fat."

Research continues, and Dr. Story is confident the theory will stand. "I'm convinced that fiber prevents colon cancer, mainly because of the bile acid connection," he says. "There's *so* much evidence showing that bile acid concentration determines colon cancer susceptibility, and I *know* that dietary fiber affects bile acid concentration."

Pectin. That very same substance that sets your homemade jelly also appears to counteract bile acids in the intestinal tract and therefore may offer protection from colon cancer. "Pectin-rich fruits may have a protective effect against colon cancer, but those same fruits are also rich in vitamins," says Dr. Klurfeld, implying that the benefits that come from eating fruit may be as much the result of their vitamin content as their pectin content.

Hemicellulose. "This type of fiber seems protective, too," says Dr. Klurfeld. "The mechanisms haven't been investigated enough to know *how* it works, but we know that hemicellulose is fermented significantly in the intestine. One theory is that the fermentation products are substances thought to prevent the development of tumors. And while there is fairly good laboratory data to suggest this, I'd say we're at least five years away from proving it."

Lignin. "It represents a minority of total dietary fiber. And it appears to be protective against colon cancer in rats," says Dr. Klurfeld.

Still, lignin is something of a mystery fiber. "No popular hypothesis explains how lignin protects. It doesn't increase fecal volume very much, and it doesn't dilute bile acids very much. It's the only fiber that's not a carbohydrate. Lignin is a very weird-looking chemical—a very large molecule which appears to go right through you, untouched by your intestines and the bacteria that live in them."

Gums. These are the sticky fibers you eat every day without even realizing it. You usually encounter them as plant-derived thickening agents in everything from ketchup to store-bought cookies.

But investigators have discovered that gums can do far more than give "body" to condiments. They've found that guar gum, oat gum and others can lower cholesterol significantly. And they've shown that a few gums can even help people with diabetes to handle blood sugar better.

Do they prevent cancer? Possibly. "We've tested a number of gums and found that they behave similarly to pectin," says Dr. Klurfeld. "But we've had conflicting results—sometimes they seem to protect, and sometimes they don't. There's no consensus yet."

Even though scientists are still hot on the trail, testing what each type of fiber does, they all agree that you should eat all types.

"That's what I argue for all the time," says Dr. Story. "There's no question that the average American doesn't get enough dietary fiber. And since different fibers have different effects, you should cover all bases by eating a mix of foods."

See the table, Finding the Fiber You Need, on page 154 for more sources of the kinds of fiber you need.

HOW TO GET YOUR FAIR SHARE

The National Cancer Institute recommends Americans double their current intake of fiber, which is considered to be approximately 11 grams a day, to a minimum of 20 grams a day, with a maximum of 35 grams a day. "This intake can be easily obtained from eating two to three servings of fruits and vegetables each day, plus substituting some whole grain products for refined bakery products," says Elaine Lanza, Ph.D., of the Division of Cancer Prevention and Control, NCI.

Eating plenty of fruits, vegetables and grains does more than just increase fiber. You'll end up eating fewer refined foods that are high in fat, sodium and sugar, thereby doing yourself double and triple favors.

The advice seems simple enough, but when you're in the supermarket trying to make fiber-smart choices, it may seem pretty complicated. So consult the table, Fiber Content of Some Common Foods, on page 155 to see how much fiber you're really getting. And try to abide by the following guidelines.

RECOGNIZING FIBER-RICH BREADS

Refined flour. It sounds classy. But refining flour removes the bran and the germ portion of each grain—in other words, most of the fiber. White rice and pasta have also been subjected to refining—brown rice and whole wheat pasta have more fiber.

FINDING THE FIBER YOU NEED

FIBER TYPE	FOOD SOURCE
Cellulose	Apples
	Bran and whole grain cereals
	Brazil nuts
	Brussels sprouts
	Carrots
	Lima beans
	Peanuts
	Pears
	Peas
	Rhubarb
	Whole wheat flour
Pectin	Apples
	Bananas
	Beets
	Carrots
	Okra
	Oranges
	Potatoes
Hemicellulose	Apples
	Bananas
	Beets
	Bran and whole grain cereals
	Green beans
	Radishes
	Sweet corn
Lignin	Bran and whole grain cereals
	Brazil nuts
	Cabbage
	Peaches
	Peanuts
	Pears
	Peas
	Strawberries
	Tomatoes
Gums/Mucilages	Dried beans
	Oat bran
	Oatmeal

Why do they take out the fiber? "In food processing lingo, it gives food a better 'mouthfeel,' " explains Dr. Klurfeld. "I think the popularity of white bread is a holdover from a century ago, when the poor people could only afford coarse, dark bread, and eating white bread was a mark of affluence. But now we know whole grain breads are healthier."

FIBER CONTENT OF SOME COMMON FOODS

FOOD	PORTION	FIBER (g)
BREADS AND CEREALS		
Bran muffin	1	2.5
French bread	1 slice	1.0
Oatmeal	½ cup	1.3
Pumpernickel bread	1 slice	2.4
Whole wheat bread	1 slice	2.2
FRUITS AND VEGETABLES		
Alfalfa sprouts	1 tbsp.	0.1
Apple, raw with skin	1	2.8
Applesauce, canned, unsweetened	½ cup	1.0
Apricots, raw	3	1.4
Apricots, dried	½ cup	15.6
Avocado	1	4.7
Banana	1	1.6
Brussels sprouts, cooked	4	1.2
Cauliflower, cooked	½ cup	1.0
Dates, chopped	¼ cup	2.3
Figs, dried	¼ cup	8.0
Papaya	½	1.4
Peas, cooked	½ cup	3.0
Potato, baked with skin	1	3.7
Potato, boiled without skin	1	1.4
Prunes, dried, uncooked	½ cup	13.0
Raisins, seedless	¼ cup	2.8
Raspberries	¼ cup	1.4
Rice, brown, long-grain, cooked	½ cup	5.4
Rice, white, long-grain, cooked	½ cup	2.2
Spinach, raw	1 cup	1.8
Squash, acorn, baked	½ cup	1.5
Strawberries	¼ cup	0.7
NUTS AND LEGUMES		
Almonds, dried, unblanched	¼ cup	1.7
Lima beans	½ cup	3.6
Peanuts, unroasted	¼ cup	3.4
Pinto beans	½ cup	4.8
Soybeans, green	½ cup	2.5

But when faced with a large selection of breads, making a high-fiber selection can be tricky. "Wheat bread," for instance, isn't necessarily high in fiber. "Whole wheat" is the one with fiber.

Beware of breads that list "powdered cellulose" in the ingredients. "Powdered cellulose is added to bread to increase fiber content and decrease calories," says Dr. Klurfeld. "I refer to it facetiously as 'sawdust,' because it's made from trees. Actually, by the time it's all processed, it's similar to the cellulose that would come from a carrot or an apple. But we're becoming more and more convinced that once fiber is ground up and powdered, it doesn't work as well as when it's in the original form. It turns out that powdered cellulose actually *increases* cancer in laboratory animals. The risk is small, but it's better to eat bread with beneficial fiber in it."

CHOOSING A CEREAL

One cereal promises "high fiber." The next promises "more fiber." Yet another claims to have "more fiber than any other cereal!" Should you read every label in search of the true winner?

Not necessarily, says Dr. Story. "I'm not sure which cereal is the winner in the fiber horse race right now," he says. "But in my opinion, 13 grams a serving is too much, because you sacrifice taste almost completely. Also, if you're an average American and you eat about 10 grams of fiber a day, one serving of such a cereal would double your intake. You should double your intake, but not just with cereal. It's better to divide your extra fiber into several different sources of food."

So what should you do? "It's easy to get more fiber in cereal by switching from Fruit Loops to bran flakes, granola or something," says Dr. Story. "And if you eat a wheat bran cereal one day, eat an oat cereal the next day. You hedge your bets if you get some of each fiber."

POPPING FIBER PILLS

"The data that shows the effectiveness of fiber is based on a diet and a lifestyle, not on taking a bunch of fiber pills," says Dr. Klurfeld. "A bad diet with a bunch of pills is still a bad diet. I'd rather see people change their diets and eat fresh fruits and vegetables and whole grain products, because a diet based on high-fiber foods is usually a healthy diet overall. Eating fiber-rich food generally gives you less fat and more vitamins and minerals."

"Personally, I would rather eat fiber-rich food than have to eat a fiber bar at every meal to get my fiber," says Dr. Story. "It's a lot more fun to have broccoli and asparagus and whole wheat bread and bran muffins."

But maybe you have trouble eating high-fiber foods. In that case, a fiber supplement is better than no fiber at all, according to Dr. Klurfeld. Ask your doctor which supplement provides the types of fiber you're lacking. Or try sneaking a few sprinkles of wheat bran on your food. Bran, the flaky remnant of grains, is one of the world's richest sources of dietary fiber. It contains several types of fiber, including cellulose, hemicellulose and pectin. And wheat bran seems to be the most effective fiber against colon cancer.

WHAT ABOUT SIDE EFFECTS?

Let's say you're inspired by this chapter. You immediately start eating more fruits and vegetables, bran muffins, oatmeal and beans. How do you think your body will respond?

That's right, with intestinal distress. If the bacteria in your intestine have been weaned on white bread, they cannot completely break down whole wheat. The fermentation products of fiber build up, causing bloating and flatulence. What's more, the minerals you've eaten may bind to the undigested fiber, so the intestine can't absorb them.

These problems can be avoided, however, if you increase fiber gradually, says Dr. Klurfeld. A gradual change in diet gives the right bacteria a chance to appear. And your risk of colon cancer a chance to disappear.

CANCER PREVENTION PLAN: FIBER

- Increase your intake of fiber to a minimum of 20 grams a day, with a maximum of 35 grams. (A bowl of high-fiber cereal, for example, has about 10 grams.)
- Eat plenty of fruits, vegetables and whole grains.
- If you have trouble eating high-fiber foods, try a fiber supplement.
- To avoid unpleasant side effects, increase fiber gradually.

Fish Oil

It has been quite some time since we heard any *good* news about fat in our diets. In fact, those of us whose mouths water at the very sound of a good hearty sizzle from the frying pan have been downright gloomy lately, faced with statistics on the correlation between a high-fat diet and the increased risk for heart disease and certain types of cancer (see chapter 33, Fat). The evidence has piled up as, in country after country, researchers studied local diets and tabulated the corresponding disease rates. It wasn't until they had practically reached the North Pole that they found a group of people who failed to fit the fatal formula.

Greenland Eskimos. Their diets consisted of tremendous amounts of high-fat fish and other fatty marine animals such as seals and whales, yet their arteries were clear and their cancer rates low. How could anyone who dined nightly on blubber *not* show an increased susceptibility to heart disease and the breast, colon and pancreatic cancers researchers had come to associate with fatty diets? The scientists were puzzled.

They noted also that Japanese fishermen and their families in remote coastal villages ate a great deal of fish and remained relatively free of cancer and atherosclerosis. When these peoples migrated into regions that offered them a Western diet, their rates of cancer and heart disease increased. Might there be something protective in the fish itself?

WHY FISH FATS ARE DIFFERENT

In the laboratory, scientists found that fish oils are polyunsaturated like vegetable oils, but there is one structural difference. Marine oils are built of omega-3 long-chain fatty acids, particularly those known as eicosapentaenoic acid (EPA) and docosahexaenoic acid (DHA).

The building blocks of vegetable oils, on the other hand, are known as omega-6 fatty acids, particularly arachidonic acid (AA). These very same omega-6 fatty acids have been implicated in the body's production of chemicals called prostaglandins. Certain kinds of prostaglandins are thought to incite the formation of tumor cells, foster tumor-cell proliferation and lead to suppressed immune response. Omega-3's in fish oil interfere with that process, according to William Cave, Jr., M.D., associate professor of medicine and oncology at the University of Rochester School of Medicine, New York.

Dr. Cave and others have been examining just how the fishy omega-3 fatty acids are influencing tumor development. "Our feeling is that the omega-3 fatty acids get substituted into the membrane of these cells and compete with the omega-6 fatty acids, which are one of the precursors of prostaglandin synthesis," explains Dr. Cave. Once they are in the cell, omega-3's grab on to and somehow neutralize the enzyme that the omega-6 fatty acids need to produce prostaglandins. "No one knows quite how it all works," says Dr. Cave. "Understanding the process is the aim of our research."

Dr. Cave and his associates studied mammary tumors in animals and found that diets containing 20 percent fish oil produced a reduction in tumor incidence and delayed the onset of chemically induced tumors. This finding contrasted sharply with the enhanced tumor development and the speedy onset of tumors in animals fed an equivalent amount of vegetable oil. (Of course, this represents a very high-fat diet for a laboratory animal—about four times the normal intake, says Dr. Cave.) "No one is suggesting you swear off vegetable oils, though these results indicate that there are important differences in the biological effects among these different families of fat (saturated versus polyunsaturated; omega-3 versus omega-6)," says Dr. Cave.

Similar results have been reported by researchers studying colon cancer at the American Health Foundation and by professor Rashida

Karmali, Ph.D., and others in experiments on breast cancer at Rutgers University in New Brunswick, New Jersey. At Memorial Sloan-Kettering Cancer Center in New York City, Michael Osborne, M.D., began a study of the effects of fish oil on women who have a family history of cancer or who have had a biopsy showing precancerous changes.

THE RESEARCH CONTINUES

The research community seems cautiously excited about the whole field of fish oils. According to one study, an increased dietary intake of marine oils, particularly those rich in EPA, may reduce the risk of coronary artery disease in patients on a mixed diet. Others are concentrating on the possible effects of fish oils on rheumatoid arthritis, psoriasis and even migraine headaches. And in 1986, the National Cancer Institute issued a formal invitation for scientists to submit plans for further study into the effects of omega-3 fatty acids on tumor development.

We must recognize, however, that promising as it may sound, all of this research is still in preliminary stages. No one is even thinking of prescribing daily doses of fish or fish oil for cancer. "This research is very important to do," says Dr. Osborne, speaking of his own work at Memorial Sloan-Kettering. "The fish oil looks very interesting, but until we finish up our work, there is no evidence that it prevents cancer in humans. It's simply too early to say that."

In the meantime, Dr. Karmali suggests that substituting salmon or mackerel for beef or pork might be your best bet for cancer protection. And Dr. Cave adds, "It is all very intriguing. I would like to encourage people to stay interested in the concept because it's through their interest and support that we're going to find an answer. There does seem to be some hope that by better understanding how this phenomenon occurs, we may be able to uncover ways of improving our chances against cancer." And that's the best news we've heard all day.

CANCER PREVENTION PLAN: FISH OIL

- Substitute salmon or mackerel for beef or pork to increase the amount of fish oil in the diet and lower the amount of saturated fat.

Food Additives

Hackettstown, N.J.: "Red-colored "M&M's" chocolate candies are back, much to the delight of their fans . . . "

Perhaps you remember reading this news item, which made national headlines in 1987. The M&M/Mars Company announced in January of that year that they would once again be coating their chocolate candies in crimson—after giving the tint a ten-year sabbatical.

If you can remember as far back as 1976, you may recall why they originally decided to can the color. Public anxiety over cancer risks from food additives—particularly over Red 2—ran high. The company was not using Red 2 in its product (it has used Red 3 and Red 40); but just to eliminate any confusion, Mars executives decided to "remove ourselves from the controversy."

Does the triumphant return of the red M&M signal a shift in public attitudes toward food additives? "I believe so," says Mars company spokesman Hans Fiuczynski. "We did a lot of research, and I believe the attitude has toned down. There was a fair amount of concern, arising out of confusion."

It's hardly any wonder that consumers were concerned and confused—not just about food dyes, but about any number of substances being added to foods.

Cyclamates. Red 4. Butter Yellow. Violet 1. All were subjects of intense debate over whether they caused cancer—and all were eventually banned. Today, we still read occasional headlines about food additives, and carcinogenicity is one worry. Scientists are also investigating allergic reactions to some additives like sulfites, Yellow 5, and monosodium glutamate. A related issue is the *unintentional* food contamination that may be carcinogenic, such as contamination with pesticides and animal drug residues (see chapter 53, Pesticides in Food).

Given what we know today, scientists agree that most food additives probably do not pose a significant cancer risk. Nitrites and nitrates and saccharin are the source of the greatest ongoing concern (see chapter 48, Nitrites and Nitrates). Nonetheless, food additives are at the center of a controversy among scientists, legislators, regulators, and the courts over the question of whether it's acceptable to have even very small amounts of carcinogens in our foods.

WHAT ARE FOOD ADDITIVES?

Since ancient times, people have added chemicals to food to make it look or keep better. Salt and spices were used to preserve meat and fish. Plant extracts were used for coloring. Today, some 2,800 substances are intentionally added to foods: colors, flavors, antioxidants (to prevent products from becoming rancid), humectants (to keep products moist), emulsifiers (to prevent oil and water from separating, as in peanut butter), stabilizers (to improve consistency) and more.

Food processors say that without additives, much of the food in our supermarkets would be unattractive and unpalatable and would not keep. Our modern, pressured lifestyles seem to demand convenience foods, a breed of products that wouldn't stay fresh or be easy to prepare—and of course be bright and colorful—without additives.

"We've got a culture now in which the food supply is dependent on food additives," says Peter Goldman, M.D., professor of health sciences in nutrition and director of the Division of Biological Sciences in Public Health at the Harvard School of Public Health, Boston. "I don't think people recognize how many colorings are in food. That nice white vanilla ice cream has several colorants in it. So even when you think, 'Oh that's a natural food,' it may really contain a color to make it look natural." The colorings are used, Dr. Goldman adds, because consumers demand them. "I'm like everybody else—if I pick oranges out of the bin, I don't like to see brown spots on them—and they're often *orange* because of colorings."

ASSESSING THE RISKS

Most scientists agree that, in general, cancer risk from food additives should not be a major concern.

"Food additives are probably a limited cancer risk, in the sense that they are systemically tested on animals. I think it's widely recognized that there are quite a number of *natural* compounds found in common foods that can be carcinogenic," Dr. Goldman says. "In that sense, we have at least the assurance today that food additives have had some kind of testing, whereas old-fashioned natural products have just been accepted on faith.

"On the other hand," adds Dr. Goldman, "unpredictable things happen." He notes that some drugs believed to be safe have caused unexpected side effects. "It seems possible that this is a model for what could happen with food additives—that there could be rare, occasional [problems]."

Cancer epidemiologists Richard Doll and Richard Peto concur with the "probably safe" verdict. "Because of the uncertainty regarding the position of nitrites and the possibility that other additives might have unsuspected effects, we have not excluded food additives as a source of risk, but have attributed them a token proportion of less than 1 percent [of cancer deaths]," they say in their report, *The Causes of Cancer.*

Says Sidney Weinhouse, Ph.D., Professor Emeritus of biochemistry at the Fels Institute of the Temple University School of Medicine, Philadelphia and advisor to the American Cancer Society on diet and nutrition: "I don't think it's ever been shown that there's a really serious danger in food additives on the market today."

With those assurances, it may surprise you to learn that there are known or suspected carcinogens being added to food. And that's where the controversy begins.

To understand the debate, some legislative history is in order. Back in 1958, like today, the U.S. Congress was concerned about cancer risks. The way they saw it, food additives, and especially colorings, serve little nutritional purpose and therefore should be strictly regulated. So, they passed the Delaney Clause to be included in the Food Additives Amendment. The Delaney Clause said that additives should not be permitted in food if the additive is found to induce cancer in humans or animals.

The scientific theory behind the Delaney Clause is that no safe threshold can be established for cancer-causing agents. In other words, because scientists didn't know where the line was between a safe dose and a cancer-inducing dose, the regulators decided the safest bet would be to ban carcinogens entirely.

Today the problem remains: Scientists *still* don't know if there's such thing as a "safe dose" of a carcinogen. What's changed is partly science, and partly politics.

New methods of analyzing chemicals now allow detection of carcinogens in quantities as low as parts per trillion—a million times smaller than could be traced in 1958. Some scientists assert that it is unreasonable to ban such infinitesimal amounts.

It's also been discovered that some foods *naturally* contain larger amounts of more potent carcinogens than man-made food additives contain. Natural carcinogens include aflatoxins (made by mold which can grow on peanuts and other stored foods) and polycyclic hydrocarbons, which are produced when meat or fish is broiled or smoked. For more information on polycyclic hydrocarbons and smoked foods, see chapter 37, Food Preparation and Cooking, and chapter 23, Barbecued Foods.

THE DOCTRINE OF DE MINIMUS

For these and other reasons, the Food and Drug Administration (FDA), which regulates the use of additives, has decided that "striving for absolute safety makes no sense." They no longer seek to interpret the Delaney Clause literally. Instead, they have decided to apply a legal doctrine called *de minimus.* This doctrine allows for known and suspected carcinogens that pose very little risk to be added to food. "*De minimus* literally means that the law does not concern itself with trifles," FDA Commissioner of food and drugs, Frank Young, M.D., Ph.D., explains.

"*De minimus,* in the way we use it, connotes safety," adds Commissioner Young. "What we have done is to set a reasonable standard of safety that poses virtually no human health risk.

"In applying the *de minimus* concept and in setting other safety standards, FDA has been guided by the figure of 'one in a million,' " says Commissioner Young. "It is not an actual risk—we do not expect one out of every million people to get cancer if they consume foods which may contain carcinogenic substances. Rather, it is a mathematical risk based on scientific assumptions used in risk assessment . . . When FDA uses the risk level of one in one million, it is confident that the risk to humans is virtually nonexistent."

A LOOK AT SOME ADDITIVES

Let's take a look at some of these food additives. One that's brewed up quite a storm is methylene chloride, a solvent that the U.S. Consumer Products Safety Commission (CPSC) says poses "one of the highest cancer risks ever calculated for a consumer product." Some companies used it to decaffeinate coffee. The FDA asserts that it is far from dangerous in the very small amounts that remain in coffee. "The residue of methylene chloride left in coffee following the decaffeinating process posed a risk so small as to be virtually no risk at all," says commissioner Young.

Another additive is butylated hydroxytoluene (BHT). Admittedly, this one is a real puzzler. It's an antioxidant that is added to foods that contain oil—everything from chewing gum to potato chips and enriched rice—or to their packaging, to prevent rancidity. BHT is not believed to be carcinogenic by itself, but it has been reported to promote lung tumors in mice. On the other hand, the use of BHT may contribute to the decline in mortality from stomach cancer.

The FDA also permits the use of about 26 food colorings for general use in food—including, yes, a red dye—in spite of evidence that it may be an animal carcinogen or that it may be contaminated with traces of known animal carcinogens.

FDA spokesman Emil Corwin explains. "Red 3 is still under investigation, because of evidence it causes thyroid [cancers] in laboratory animals. Another food coloring, Yellow 5, may contain carcinogenic impurities, which were detected in various batches at very low levels, or not at all.

"And with Yellow 6, there has been some concern regarding adrenal medullary lesions and kidney lesions but the results have not been found to be biologically significant." He adds that Yellow 6 as a "whole entity" has not been shown to cause the cancers, but that it contains very small amounts of six carcinogenic impurities. At the maximum concentrations for the impurities allowed by the FDA, the potential risk is estimated to be less than three in ten million, Corwin says.

At this writing, the FDA has permanently listed Yellow 5 and Red 3 as acceptable for use in food. However, Red 3 was permanently listed for food use before the FDA received data showing that it caused thyroid tumors. The FDA is reassessing its status in light of these data. Yellow 6 remains on the "provisional list" until the FDA responds to objections regarding the final order that would have permanently listed the color additive for use in food, drugs and cosmetics.

DELANEY DEBATED

Some members of the scientific community support the FDA's new approach. "The Delaney Clause was written almost 30 years ago, when it was hoped that we could eliminate all carcinogens from the diet," notes Elizabeth Weisburger, Ph.D., D.Sc., assistant director for chemical carcinogenesis, Division of Cancer Etiology, National Cancer Institute.

"Now we're finding that's impossible. The analytic capabilities have increased so significantly—we can now measure parts per trillion, when 20 years ago we thought parts per million were really great."

Noting that so many natural carcinogens have been found in foods, she adds, "The aim of the Delaney Clause, to prevent additional carcinogens from being added to foods, was a very fine idea, but when it comes down to practice, it seems we're surrounded by [natural] carcinogens."

Dr. Goldman says that the debate is really over values and politics rather than science. "There is no doubt that the Delaney amendment makes life easier, in the sense that it's pretty much black and white. The moment you have evidence that anything is carcinogenic, it cannot be deliberately added to food," he says.

"When you get rid of the Delaney amendment, you have to make a very careful evaluation of risks and benefits. And there you have a problem because you have value judgments." Ultimately, says Dr. Goldman, we all have to make these value judgments ourselves.

"Color dyes are a good example of risk/benefit judgments. I personally shrink away from pink frostings and green candies—I emphasize *personally*. These are my value judgments. I find it difficult to make decisions for other people."

HOW TO AVOID FOOD ADDITIVES

If you're concerned about food additives, the good news is that they're fairly easy to avoid. Federal regulations require labels to list whether artificial colors and additives are used in products.

The bad news is that most colors are not required to be listed by name. However, one controversial color—Yellow 5 (alias tartrazine)—is required by rule to be listed on the label, because it is also an allergen for some people.

Remember, too, that avoiding food isn't the most effective way to help prevent cancer. In fact, adding certain foods to your diet—high in fiber, low in fat—can be one way to protect yourself.

CANCER PREVENTION PLAN: FOOD ADDITIVES
- Read food product labels carefully.
- Avoid additives when possible.

C H A P T E R 37

Food Preparation and Cooking

In the struggle against cancer, our pantry becomes our arsenal; our fruits, vegetables and grains become our weapons. These are the foods rich in fiber and the anticancer nutrients like vitamin C, beta-carotene and selenium that may help counteract cell breakdown or defend us from fat.

If we aren't careful, though, we can disarm our food allies without ever knowing it. How? By peeling our potatoes, for example, we strip them of fiber. By boiling them, we drain them of vitamin C. Worse, we may even do things that unintentionally turn our food allies into food enemies.

"What adds the element of danger is how we prepare foods," writes Donald R. Germann, M.D., clinical professor of radiology at the University of Missouri School of Medicine in Kansas City and author of *The Anti-Cancer Diet* (Wyden Books).

Take the Japanese diet, for example. Japanese people eat plenty of vegetables and fish—two food groups which supposedly protect against cancer. Yet, says Dr. Germann, the Japanese have a higher rate of stomach cancer than we have here. "This has led researchers to suspect that there was something about the manner of preparation of these two food items . . . that makes eating them an additional cancer risk factor."

Sure enough, it was discovered that the salt used in pickling brine for the vegetables and for processing salt fish contains nitrites, which "[are] at least partially responsible for the high rate of stomach cancer among the Japanese.

"The point is not that salt promotes cancer . . . nor that fish is a bad food," he explains. Rather, "what we do with our food before we eat it may be as important as the food itself."

But let's look at our own eating habits for a moment. How many of us, without giving it a second thought, add dressing to a salad? Or slather a baked potato with sour cream? "When you bury your peas in butter," says Paul Lachance, Ph.D., professor of nutrition and food science at Rutgers University in New Brunswick, New Jersey, "you may counteract any anticancer effects."

The idea, then, is to retain as many healthful nutrients in your food as you can, without adding harmful substances. Given these best possible conditions, what you eat can help defend you against disease.

PICKING THE PEAK NUTRIENTS

Step one is to recruit the best foods available, those packed with the most vitamins and minerals. The first place to look is in the garden. Why? Because fresh-off-the-vine foods are the least tampered with and therefore have the most nutrition.

In other words, if you pluck an orange from your backyard tree and eat it, you're probably getting every bit of nutrition that orange has to offer. If you squeeze the juice from that orange, you'll reduce the vitamin C somewhat, simply because it will have been exposed to oxygen. Even so, that juice is better than orange juice that has been sitting in a carton. While the cartons don't leak, they do breathe, causing vitamin C loss. The store-bought juice has up to 30 percent less vitamin C than fresh-squeezed.

Unfortunately, gathering our foods fresh from the garden is not possible for many of us. That's because we don't have a garden or we can't shop at the farmer's stand out of season or we live in regions where year-round garden produce is as unlikely as an iceball in Hades.

What, then, is the best substitute for fresh produce? Here's where frozen foods come in. Believe it or not, the foods frozen into those hard-as-rock blocks are the next best thing to fresh. "Farmers grow crops especially for frozen food companies," explains Dr. Lachance. Because of that special arrangement, produce can be frozen within a few hours of picking. "The nutrients are preserved before the shock of handling can lower their nutritive value."

Still, there are some vegetables—like tomatoes and lettuce—that have such delicate tissues they can't be frozen. For these foods, advises Dr. Lachance, your best bet is to buy them "market fresh" and store them in the refrigerator. "Chilling will slow down the degeneration of the nutrients," he says.

Canned fruits and vegetables should be your choice only in a pinch. They usually have about two to three times less vitamin B and C than when fresh—particularly since we discard the water they are packed in.

As for boxed foods, such as instant potatoes, keep them around only for can't-get-to-the-store emergencies. If you're snowbound, eating them will fill you up, but not with as many nutrients—they may have very few.

THE CARE AND HANDLING OF NUTRIENTS

So far so good. You've selected the best kinds of food for an anti-cancer diet. The next step is selecting the best way to handle them and to cook them, so their nutrients will work for you. The key to preserving vitamins, explains Dr. Lachance, is to keep them away from their enemies—heat, air and, for some, water.

The most vulnerable vitamin and the one that deteriorates most rapidly when exposed to its enemies is vitamin C, also known as ascorbic acid. A food high in this vitamin will lose its nutritional edge if it is cooked—particularly if it's boiled, which exposes it to both heat and water. Vegetables high in vitamin C—like potatoes, broccoli, cabbage or spinach, to name a few—should be cooked briefly and, where possible, whole and in covered dishes.

Luckily for us, most of the foods that are high in vitamin C—citrus fruits, strawberries, melons in season—don't need cooking. These mostly need protection from the air and from warm temperatures. A half of a grapefruit or wedge of cantaloupe needs only to be tightly covered in plastic wrap and stored in the refrigerator to keep its vitamin C levels relatively high for brief periods.

Vitamin C is not alone in its vulnerability. Take the B-complex vitamins like thiamine and riboflavin, for instance. Heating meat in water—as in soup or stew—can slowly destroy the thiamine, which is heat sensitive. Exposing milk to light can rob it of riboflavin and the added vitamin A. That's why it should be stored in cartons in the dark part of the refrigerator.

Other vitamins, the so-called fat-soluble type, are somewhat less susceptible to environmental damage. Yet even these lose potency when exposed to heat. Beta-carotene, a source of vitamin A, is one of these fat-soluble vitamins. Foods containing tocopherols are a source of

(continued on page 172)

RATING THE COOKING METHODS

There are many ways to skin a chicken—and even more ways to cook it. Among the many choices in any cook's arsenal, some rate healthier than others. Here's a rundown of some of the common ways of preparing food in the home kitchen.

Good Choices

Pressure Cooking. In comparative studies, pressure cooking beat out boiling and steaming in preserving the most vitamins and minerals. Why? Because it's quick, it uses a lower heat setting and a minimum of water, and you don't add fat. It's especially good for vegetables, dry beans, grains, meats, potatoes and soup.

Steaming. This is a good way to spare nutrients in vegetables and fish. In one study, asparagus lost 78 percent of vitamin C when boiled but only 43 percent when steamed.

Baking/Roasting. This method is ideal for fish, squash, potatoes and loaves. It also rates high for beef, pork, veal, poultry and roasts.

Braising. Also known as stewing, this method is best for the tougher cuts of meat and also for fish. When stewed, fish—an excellent source of selenium—loses only 15 percent of this nutrient, about half the amount it would lose if fried. Braised food is cooked in liquid in a closed container. The longer you cook it, the more fat will seep into the liquid. You can then chill and skim off the fat.

Poaching. It's good for lots more than cooking eggs in those cute little cups. Poach firm-fleshed fish or boned chicken in three parts water and one part lemon juice, seasoned with vegetables and herbs. Poaching has become so popular that a new kind of cookware has been invented just for that purpose. These are glass pots with special ridges on the bottom which capture the liquid in the food so very little added water is necessary.

Microwaving. Homemakers rave about microwave ovens—and nutritionists have joined in. Reportedly, microwave cooking preserves more vitamin C than either pressure cooking or boiling. This method works because it's fast, uses very little (if any) water, and doesn't require using problem ingredients like fat.

In fact, U.S. Department of Agriculture studies found that microwaving actually can reduce a food's fat content. Take a hamburger, for example. Microwaving cooks it from the inside out, so there's no firmly cooked surface to hold the fat in. And for reheated frozen leftovers, tests showed that potatoes, beef, carrots and peas had very little nutritional loss.

According to the Food and Drug Administration (FDA), you should not worry about microwaves leaking and causing harm if the oven door is not damaged and if the oven shuts off when you open it. Contact the appliance manufacturer or state health department if you suspect leakage.

Fair Choices

Slow Cooking/Crock Pots. Crock pots are a handy way to have your dinner cook all day while you are away. What's more, you get good results with a lean-but-tough cut of meat. And you have the opportunity to throw in lots of *whole* vegetables. Vitamins and minerals are retained—but so is the fat. Take care of that problem by chilling the stew, skimming off the fat and reheating before serving.

Stir-Frying/Sautéing. The best thing about briskly frying up bits of meat and vegetables is that it's quick and seals in soluble nutrients as well as flavor and color. What can make this method even better is using less than a tablespoon of oil or, better yet, none at all. Try steam-frying using stock, broth—even herb tea—in place of oil.

Poor Choices

Boiling. Good for pasta; not so good for veggies because water leaches out vitamins and minerals. If you do decide to boil, keep the skins on food, and use boilable plastic bags. Make sure your pots have tight-fitting lids and don't plop foods into the water until you've brought it to a rolling boil. Remember to save the liquid.

Frying. This is the least desirable of all cooking methods because it adds fat. Another problem with frying—especially the frying done at restaurants—is that the oil may have been over a very hot flame for a very long time. And that can cause polyunsaturated oil to break down, forming potential cancer-causing by-products. If you must fry foods, keep the heat low. Don't use the fat over, and don't use oil if it begins to smoke.

Toasting/Browning. If you torch your food, the resulting burnt material may be mutagenic, say experts. What's more, toasting can drain your bread of thiamine. So go "light" on browning. If you want your bread or bun warm, steam or microwave it.

Charbroiling. The surfaces of food cooked this way may be exposed to high temperatures. When cooking meat and other protein foods over flames, the fat that drips into the fire causes smoke to rise and deposit potentially harmful substances on your food. You can safeguard your grilled food by wrapping it in foil and keeping it away from the flame.

vitamin E. Green vegetables are a significant source of yet another fat-soluble vitamin, vitamin K. High heat can turn this nutrient from warrior to wimp.

To simplify the matter, says Dr. Lachance, just aim to preserve vitamin C. "If you are careful to prevent deterioration of ascorbic acid, you are bound to preserve the other nutrients as well."

DO'S AND DON'TS OF NUTRIENT CONSERVATION

It's easier than you may think to keep the environment from robbing nutrients of their strength. Here's how:

Don't drown your food. You'll retain more vitamin C and other vitamins that leach when you cook vegetables without added water. The more water you use, the fewer vitamins you retain.

If you plan to boil your vegetables, add just enough water to cover them, or better still, steam them. Cabbage, which keeps its vitamin C better than many foods, loses about 10 percent of its vitamin C when cooked in just enough water to keep it from burning. Drown it, though, and it relinquishes five times that amount.

Do keep foods in one piece. The more you cut cells, the more you expose them to air or water and the more nutrients are lost. Whole baked sweet potatoes retain 89 percent of their ascorbic acid. Cut in half, they keep only 31 percent.

Try cabbage wedges instead of cole slaw—the finely cut pieces have less vitamin C. Remember, if you french-cut your green beans, you'll increase the loss of vitamin C. Cutting carrots crosswise results in greater loss of vitamin C than cutting them half across the middle and then in half again vertically.

If you must cut your fruits and veggies, make sure your paring knife is super sharp. A dull blade could cause bruising and result in increased nutrient losses.

Don't allow sliced food to stand. Berries lose much of their vitamin C within hours if they are cut, mashed or hulled. Cucumbers lose nearly a quarter of their vitamin C when they're sliced, but they lose a third if those slices are left standing for an hour. After three hours, almost half the vitamin C has vanished. Resist buying precut vegetables like tossed salad and don't shell peas, cut beans or peel vegetables until just before you cook them.

Do use all parts of the plant. Collard greens, kale and broccoli have more vitamin A in their leaves, stalks and flower buds than in the stem. The outer leaves of lettuce have more calcium, iron and vitamin A. Simply scrub them well and add these rarely used parts to soups and stews.

Do freeze leftovers. Freezing leftover vegetables in their cooking liquid will preserve more vitamin C than merely refrigerating them.

Even after a whole year in the freezer, your leftover lima beans will retain 90 percent of their original nutrients. Remember to serve foods immediately upon thawing and don't thaw meats in water or room temperature—you'll melt away a lot of nutrients.

Do save cooking liquids. Keep a special container in your freezer and add to it all leftover vegetables and their nutrient-dense liquids until it's filled. Then add it to soups and stews.

FLAVOR WITHOUT THE FAT

What's toast without butter, pizza without mozzarella, asparagus without hollandaise? Healthy, that's what. They're healthy because they're not loaded with fat.

Fat is definitely one substance that is not in the anticancer camp. In fact, it is probably *the* enemy, having been implicated in the development of cancer in the breasts, prostate and colon (see chapter 33, Fat). Too much fat, it is believed, may upset the body's hormonal balance and increase hormone production. Others say that fat triggers the production of bile acid by-products, substances that attempt to break down the fat but which may promote cancer.

It is less important to understand how fat works, experts suggest, than to eat less of it. It should make up only about a fourth of your calories. For starters, you can choose leaner cuts of meat and trim away all excess fat from all meat, including roasts, steaks and chops, and remove the skins of poultry before cooking. Careful preparation can cut the fat content significantly. When you cook meats, don't fry them. A Swedish study revealed that fried and grilled meats have been associated with an increased risk of cancer of the pancreas. Instead, place them on a raised broiler pan in the oven so the excess fat will drip away into the lower pan.

You can defat soups, stocks and stews by refrigerating them for a few hours, then lifting off all the congealed fat that has formed on the top. Reheat the dish and serve. While some nutrients may be sacrificed in the process, the benefits of defatting override the losses.

What about flavor, you ask? Is it indeed possible to prepare and cook foods that are sumptuous and succulent without being saddled with extra fat? The answer is an emphatic *yes*, if you know a few tricks.

- Instead of using oil to make marinades and sauces, you can use stocks and juices.
- When you reheat meat, place it on a lettuce leaf on the bottom of a pie plate and cover it with another lettuce leaf. Add a splash of water, bake at 350°F until the meat is heated through, and you'll have a moist, flavorful dish without having added fat.

- Instead of using margarine to season your peas and carrots, try lemon juice, garlic, onions and delicate herbs like basil, parsley, or thyme.
- Invest in a set of nonstick cookware so you can bake, sauté and even pan-fry without a drop of oil.
- Saute with a bit of broth or stock rather than oil or butter.
- Learn to sauté vegetables with mushrooms—they produce a generous amount of liquid.
- Steam rather than sauté with butter or oil. You'd be surprised how sweet chopped onions can taste!
- Alter your recipes that call for cream, butter or other high-fat dairy products. You can make your pizza with part-skim mozzarella, for example. A soft dairy cheese called Neufchâtel can replace cream cheese in your recipes and give you almost 50 percent less fat. Often, low-fat yogurt can replace light cream in sauces.

Are you getting the idea? By now, you should be well on your way to learning how to slash your fat intake without sacrificing flavor.

**CANCER PREVENTION PLAN:
FOOD PREPARATION AND COOKING**

- Use fresh fruits and vegetables whenever possible, substituting frozen food when necessary.
- Steam rather than boil.
- Keep foods whole throughout storage and cooking.
- Freeze leftovers.
- Trim away excess fat from meats and remove chicken skin.
- Don't fry food.
- Defat soups and stews by refrigerating them and then lifting off the fat layer.
- When possible, use fat substitutes; sauté in stock, for example, instead of butter.
- Use skim milk or low-fat dairy products.
- Eat whole grains and other whole foods.
- Eat smoked foods as occasional treats or appetizers, not as frequent main courses.
- When choosing smoked foods as a snack, select those that are labeled "smoke-flavored."

FIBER TO FORTIFY YOUR MENU

If fat is your foe in the anticancer struggle, fiber is your friend. Certain fibers are believed to bind up excess fat and escort it from your body (see chapter 34, Fiber).

"Include a combination of fiber in your diet and keep it in its coarsest form," says Peter Van Soest, Ph.D., a professor at Cornell University, Ithaca, New York. Make it a habit to include wheat germ in your meat loaf as well as your muffins. Add seeds to your salads and legumes to your stews. Try using buckwheat, brown rice, bulgur, stone-ground wheat and oat bran, which, according to Dr. Van Soest, are better than, say, whole wheat flour, because they are in a coarser form.

Fruit

If scientists were trying to synthesize a a food that prevents cancer, what ingredients do you think they would choose? Probably the first thing they'd put in the test tube would be fiber. Then they'd add a dash of vitamin A, plus a heaping spoonful of vitamin C, for their protective value. Of course, this food would also have to be low in fat.

Sounds healthy, but maybe not so tasty? Imagine if it could taste tart and sweet, and even *look* colorful.

Well, this food exists, and it's better than anything any mortal has cooked up. It's provided in dozens of delicious forms by Mother Nature. One of the best foods that prevents cancer, of course, is fruit.

FRUITFUL RESEARCH

Studies have shown that people who eat more fruit are better protected against cancer. One persuasive example was a decade-long study of one million Japanese, which found that the lung cancer death rate of cigarette smokers can be affected by diet. Those who ate fruit or drank fruit juice five to seven days a week had a lower death rate than that of cigarette smokers who ate fruit or drank fruit juice zero to two days a week.

That study also found that smokers who dined on fruit three or four days a week were 25 percent more likely to die from cancer than more frequent fruit-eaters. The smokers who avoided fruit completely or ate it only one or two days a week were 75 percent more likely to succumb to the disease.

Interestingly, this study also showed that consumption of green salads, or of vitamin pills that might contain vitamin A and C, had little or no protective value against lung cancer deaths. The researchers concluded that "frequently taking multivitamin pills cannot substitute for eating fruit or drinking fruit juice."

In another study, a team of scientists from the National Cancer Institute in Bethesda, Maryland, discovered that women who eat foods containing beta-carotene are less likely to develop mouth or throat cancer. A study of a group of women who had these types of cancer and a control group of women who did not have cancer showed that those who ate 21 or more servings of fresh fruits and vegetables a week cut their risk in half. The researchers reported that those who ate moderate amounts of fresh produce—11 to 20 servings a week—reduced their chances by about 35 percent.

More evidence of the protective effects of fruit comes from a study of colon cancer death rates in the "fruit belt"—the parts of the country where two-thirds of the families have citrus trees in their backyard. In Florida, Southern California and Arizona, the incidence of bowel cancer is one-half the national average, *even though many residents of these areas formerly lived in higher-risk northeastern and midwestern states.*

A group of Florida researchers, working with the American Cancer Society, studied the colon cancer rates and prevalence of citrus trees. They hypothesized that the easy availability of the fruit may be what's protecting the Sun Belters. They speculated that the *combination* of anticancer ingredients in fruit work together to ward off the disease.

Just what are those ingredients? Some of fruit's cancer-prevention components can be spelled out precisely—from A to F.

FRUITS ON THE "A" LIST

The government's National Research Council says that eating foods rich in vitamin A is an important way to reduce the risk of developing certain kinds of cancer. Vitamin A boosts the body's natural immunity. Laboratory animals fed vitamin A show a marked ability to suppress the development of cancer. Fruit is one good source of this all-important vitamin.

What's more, there's a naturally occurring pigment that's plentiful in fruits and vegetables that may be especially important in protecting against cancer. Beta-carotene, which gives many fruits and vegetables their green or orange-yellow hue, converts to vitamin A once inside the body. Researchers aren't certain whether it's the beta-carotene or the vitamin A that has the protective effect against cancer. "We're not sure, but we suspect it's the beta-carotene," says Fred Khachik, Ph.D., from the U.S. Department of Agriculture's Human Nutrition Research Service in Beltsville, Maryland. "We can say, however, that there's definitely a relationship between foods with beta-carotene and cancer prevention."

One theory about why beta-carotene is so effective is that it apparently protects cells from free radicals, the by-products of fat metabolism that can turn a healthy cell cancerous.

To help you pick the best fruits for vitamin A, see the table, The Best of the Bunch, on page 181.

BIOFLAVONOIDS ON THE "B" LIST

Additional cancer-fighting substances in nearly all fresh fruits—especially citrus fruits—are the jack-of-all-trades nutrients known as bioflavonoids. Bioflavonoids appear to increase the anticancer activity of certain enzymes found in our skin, lungs, gastrointestinal tract and liver. These enzymes metabolize foreign compounds, according to leading bioflavonoid researcher Ralph C. Robbins, Ph.D., of the Food Science and Human Nutrition Department, Institute of Food and Agricultural Sciences at the University of Florida in Gainesville. The enzymes also help convert fat-soluble carcinogens to water-soluble form, so they can be safely excreted from the body. Citrus fruit bioflavonoids may be especially effective in this regard. Bioflavonoids may also protect the body from the cancer-causing effects of air pollutants such as benzo(a)pyrene. Finally, bioflavonoids increase the body's absorption of another important cancer-protector—vitamin C.

FRUITS ON THE "C" LIST

Vitamin C has been lauded for any number of health benefits. From stress relief to allergy relief, from reducing the severity of the common cold to clearing up bladder infections—vitamin C has been shown to be a protector and a healer.

So it should hardly be surprising that this beneficial substance, which does some of its "magic" by boosting the immune system, also appears to provide protection against cancer. Studies show that people with cancer are likely to have a severe depletion of vitamin C (see chapter 67, Vitamin C). Gastric cancer seems to be associated with a lower intake of vitamin C in the diet, and similar patterns have been found with esophageal cancer, colorectal cancer and bladder cancer. There are even indications that vitamin C can reduce the toxic or carcinogenic impact that more that 50 pollutants in air, water and food may have on our bodies. One example of a carcinogen that vitamin C may protect us against is nitrosamines, cancer-causing agents that form when common food additives called nitrites interact with body chemicals (see chapter 48, Nitrites and Nitrates). Vitamin C apparently combines with nitrites in the stomach to hinder their transformation into carcinogens.

Fruit, of course, is one of the very best food sources of vitamin C. Some scientists say that just one orange eaten before a meal can contain enough vitamin C to neutralize potentially cancer-causing nitrites. (The orange should be eaten just before meals, so it's waiting in the stomach.) That's one immediate incentive to eat fruits at every meal!

An important fact to remember when you're stocking up on fruits and fruit juices is that the shelf-life of vitamin C is shorter than you might think. Light and warm temperatures can deplete vitamin C levels. In order to get maximum vitamin C from your fruits, keep the following hints in mind:

- Buy the freshest fruits you can find. Shop at farmers' markets or supermarkets on days when you know the produce is fresh.
- Refrigerate fruit promptly when you get home, and don't let it sit around long before eating. Even a day or two in the refrigerator can rob a fruit of precious nutrients. Fruits can lose half their vitamin C after two or three days in the refrigerator, and they lose it even more quickly if stored at room temperature.
- If you can't get fresh fruit, buy frozen. It's second best to fresh in terms of retaining nutrients. However, long periods of freezing can destroy vitamin C. Canned fruits come in third, nutrient wise. The heat and water involved in canning deplete vitamins C and A.
- Cutting fruit and exposing the cut surfaces to the air causes oxidation, which destroys certain nutrients, especially vitamin C. So don't cut fruits before storing them. If you're making fruit salads, cut the fruit up immediately before serving. It's better to make small amounts at a time rather than to keep large amounts in the fridge for a week. When you do cut up the fruit, make large pieces. That minimizes nutrient losses.
- If oranges are your thing, keep in mind that seasons make a difference in vitamin C content. Oranges grown from November to January (mostly Hamlin oranges) and from January to

March (mostly Pineapple oranges) contain more vitamin C
than oranges grown from April to July (mostly Valencia oranges). One study showed that a six-ounce glass of juice
from June and July oranges barely contained the Recommended Dietary Allowance for vitamin C.

For the best fruit sources of vitamin C, consult the accompanying
table, The Best of the Bunch.

EAT FRUIT FOR THE BIG "F"

Perhaps you already know that the American Cancer Society and
the National Cancer Institute want you to add more fiber to your diet.
Maybe you've even bought yourself a box of bran, vowing to sprinkle it
onto your granola at breakfast, soup at lunch and spaghetti sauce at
dinner. But like a lot of people, you may find yourself falling short of
that noble but not necessarily appetizing goal.

If so, we have some very good news for you. You don't have to go
on "The Squirrel Diet" to get all the fiber you need for protection from
colon cancer (not to mention the other possible health benefits of fiber,
like control of heart disease, diabetic conditions and obesity). Delicious, natural fruit is one of the best fiber sources around—and, in
some cases, *a better source of fiber than bran!* Raspberries, for example, contain more fiber than bran.

How does fruit fiber fight cancer? Certain forms of fiber increase
the bulk of intestinal waste and ease it through the colon. This means
the well-known benefit of warding off constipation. But investigators
also say that these actions may dilute and flush cancer-causing toxins
out of the intestinal tract. That means significant protection against colon cancer.

There are five different kinds of fiber (cellulose, pectin, hemicellulose, lignin and gums/mucilages). Cellulose and hemicellulose have
this constipation-relieving effect. "Fruit fiber" actually means different
kinds of fiber—usually pectin, but also cellulose and lignin—with other
types mixed in, too. By eating a lot of fruit, you will guarantee that you
get a variety of all the cancer-fighting forms of fiber.

The best fruit sources of fiber are listed in the accompanying table,
The Best of the Bunch.

IS JUICE JUST AS GOOD?

Can you get the all the cancer protection benefits of fruit from your
morning glass of orange juice, instead of eating "the whole thing?"
Well, as noted above, the study of one million Japanese showed that
frequent consumption of fruit juice, as well as fruit, seemed to have a
protective effect. However, depending on the form, season and storage

THE BEST OF THE BUNCH

VITAMIN A

FRUIT	PORTION	VITAMIN A (IU)
Cantaloupe	¼ med.	4,304
Papaya	½ med.	3,061
Apricots, fresh	3 med.	2,769
Watermelon	10″ × 1″ slice	1,762
Avocado	1 med.	1,230
Nectarine	1 med.	1,001
Prunes, dried, cooked	5	835
Tangerine	1 med.	773
Peach	1 med.	465

VITAMIN C

FRUIT	PORTION	VITAMIN C (mg)
Orange juice, fresh squeezed	1 cup	124
Grapefruit juice, fresh squeezed	1 cup	94
Papaya	½	94
Orange	1	70
Cantaloupe	¼ med.	56
Strawberries	½ cup	42
Grapefruit	½ med.	41

FIBER

FRUIT	PORTION	FIBER (g)
Apricots, dried, uncooked	½ cup	15.5
Prunes, dried, uncooked	½ cup	13.0
Figs, dried	¼ cup	8.0
Avocado	1	4.7
Pear	1	4.1
Blackberries	½ cup	3.3
Nectarine	1	3.3
Raisins, seedless	¼ cup	2.8
Dates, chopped	¼ cup	2.3
Blueberries	½ cup	2.2
Cranberries, whole	½ cup	2.0
Tangerine	1	1.8
Apple	1	1.7
Banana	1	1.6
Plums	3	1.5
Papaya	½	1.4
Raspberries	¼ cup	1.4

of the fruit juice, it may have significantly fewer cancer-fighting nutrients, especially vitamin C. And frequently, juice contains less fiber than the fruit itself, since it doesn't contain as much pulp, skin, pith and so forth—the indigestible components that make up fiber.

If you don't want to trade your morning O.J. or grapefruit juice for a fruit eaten out of hand, at least consider the following when choosing a fruit juice.

- As you might expect, the citrus juice that you squeeze at home is *usually* the next-best thing to eating the whole fruit. While the fresh juice obviously has less fiber, it may have more vitamin C than a whole fruit, because you would be drinking the juice of several oranges to make a cup. One cup of fresh-squeezed orange juice contains about 120 milligrams of vitamin C. A medium orange might contain about half that much.
- In general, fresh-squeezed orange juice contains a little more total vitamin C than frozen or processed orange juice. It's best to drink juice you squeeze yourself, because it has been stored in the best container of all—the fruit's natural peel—instead of wax-coated paper cartons or glass, which allow depletion of vitamin C.
- Frozen juice is second best, in terms of vitamin C. However, in the spring and summer, frozen juice may contain even more vitamin C than fresh oranges. That's because, as noted above, the natural vitamin C content of oranges varies according to the type of orange you buy and the season. In the spring and summer, vitamin C content of oranges drops. Frozen orange juice, on the other hand, is made from a blend of different kinds of oranges, and the cans it's packed in protect vitamin C levels better than other forms of packing, so the vitamin C level stays fairly high.
- The container counts. Polystyrene bottles and wax-coated paper cartons are the worst for preserving vitamin C, because they are not airtight and allow light in. Both oxygen and light contribute to the decay of vitamin C. Airtight glass jars are a little better. Enamel-lined cans and tin cans are better still. The best containers are frozen concentrate cans—second only to the natural skin of the fruit!
- Pay attention to storage conditions. Even if the juice is sealed in an airtight can, keeping the can in a warm room encourages loss of vitamin C. So keep your cans of citrus juice in the refrigerator if possible; if not, keep them in as cool a place as you can.

HARVEST FRUITS EVERY SEASON

Just because it's winter and your watermelon supply has dried up doesn't mean you have to go without important nutrients from fruit that protect you from cancer. Make a point of enjoying fresh fruits at their peak. Look for fruits at their seasonal finest.

- In the fall, who can go without munching on crisp, fiber- and vitamin C-rich apples? Healthy harvests also include grape-fruits, grapes, guavas, kiwi fruits, oranges, peaches, pears and vitamin A-laden persimmons.
- Brighten your winter with harvests of grapefruits, guavas, kum-quats, oranges and pears.
- When spring comes, you can enjoy melons, oranges, peaches, lemons and limes at their peak.
- And in the summer, indulge yourself with the veritable cornu-copia of fruits on the market like apricots, grapes, kiwi fruits, mangoes, melons, nectarines, peaches and especially berries (often great sources of vitamin C and fiber), including straw-berries, blueberries, blackberries, boysenberries, loganberries and raspberries.

PESTICIDES AND THE APPEAL OF PEELING

Yes, Mother Nature made fruit an important food that protects us from cancer. That was the good news.

Now for a little bad news. Unfortunately, human beings have found it necessary to mess around with nature's fine gift.

Some 50,000 pesticide products are registered, including insecti-cides, fungicides, rodenticides, fumigants and more, according to the Environmental Protection Agency (EPA). Not to mention the colorings, petroleum-based waxes and oils that make that fruit you see on the supermarket shelf look gorgeous, shiny and flawless. These finishes, like a facelift, can even make fruit look fresher and younger than it really is.

Unfortunately, we cannot assume that all these chemicals are safe (see chapter 53, Pesticides in Food). The EPA admits that hundreds of substances have not yet been adequately tested for carcinogenicity. Fur-thermore, the EPA does "risk/benefit" analyses of known carcinogens, and they do permit carcinogens to be used on food crops when they feel the health risk is small and the necessity for the chemical is great.

If that kind of policy-making makes you a little queasy, by all means, peel away. You probably have more to gain by peeling than nutrients to lose. Peeling will remove many of the residues of chemicals that are applied to the exterior of fruit. It will also remove a small amount of nutrients and varying amounts of fiber. For example, one cup of unpeeled raw apples contains 59 International Units of vitamin A and 6.2 milligrams of vitamin C. The same amount of peeled apples contains 48 International Units of vitamin A and 4.4 milligrams of vitamin C. Peaches and pears also lose small amounts of these nutrients when peeled.

In apples, peaches and pears, an important fiber component of the skin, pectin, is lost if you peel. But for thin-skinned fruits like peaches, there really isn't that much of a loss. And although the thicker skins of apples and pears are rich in pectin, their fleshy parts are equally rich, so fiber loss is relatively small.

Peeling isn't the perfect solution—it won't strip away all the chemicals. Some are "systemic" and get into the flesh of the fruit—there's not much you can do about them.

There is also a way of washing fruit that removes excess chemicals. "Simply washing fruits and vegetables with water is not an effective way of removing pesticide residues," says the Carcinogen Information Program (CIP) in St. Louis. Instead, says the CIP, you can wash produce in water to which you've added a small amount of dishwashing liquid. The alkalinity of the detergent helps remove more chemicals. Follow that bath with a clear-water rinse to remove detergent residues. Scrubbing the fruit with a vegetable brush also helps.

Another way to avoid the problem, of course, is to seek out outlets of organically grown produce.

CANCER PREVENTION PLAN: FRUIT

- Eat fruit and drink fruit juice daily.
- Buy the freshest fruits you can find.
- Refrigerate fruit promptly.
- If you can't get fresh fruit, buy frozen.
- Limit cutting fruit and exposing cut surfaces to the air.
- To remove surface chemicals, wash fruit in water to which you've added a small amount of dishwashing liquid, then rinse thoroughly.

C H A P T E R **39**

Hair Dyes

Hate that gray? Why *not* exchange that silver for gold? Some 30 million women in the United States have, choosing to dye rather than live wearing the crown of aging. Others, equally chagrined at what they see in the mirror, squelch their urge to dye their hair, worrying that coloring products cause health problems. Even cancer.

What's the root of this worry? Well, back in the 1930s, researchers discovered that hair dyes could cause severe skin allergies in some people. In the late 1970s, they found that dye caused cancer in lab animals. Mice and rats were fed huge quantities of ingredients found in hair dyes such as so-called coal-tar dyes. Some of the rodents developed cancer.

It's true that feeding massive doses of dye to rats is a far cry from humans who shampoo it onto their hair once a month—it doesn't mean they'll get cancer that way. Even so, one hair dye manufacturer decided to remove the chemical in question and replace it with another dye that had similar properties.

As it stands today, some of the newer chemicals in hair dyes have not been tested for their cancer-causing properties. Yet experts are less concerned about the danger of humans absorbing them. Why? Because recent evidence shows that humans absorb a lot less hair dye through their scalps than previously feared.

"When scientists analyzed urine excreted from humans who dyed their hair, only a trace of dye could be detected," reports Patricia Engasser, M.D., associate clinical professor of dermatology at the University of California Medical Center in San Francisco. "This new evidence shows that scalp penetration of hair dye chemicals is actually much smaller than some previous animal studies had shown."

If you want more reassurance about the safety of hair dyes, consider this. Most epidemiological studies have looked at the hair-dyeing habits of cancer patients, and none has shown a definite link.

In one study conducted by the American Health Foundation, scientists compared 401 people who had breast cancer with 625 people who didn't. They considered possible factors relating to the use of hair dye among these two groups, including whether the dye was permanent or semipermanent, what shades were used, how often and for how long the dye was used. The results? No matter how they examined their data, the researchers could not find any increase in the odds of getting breast cancer among hair dye users—even among women who had been using the stuff for 20 years or more.

TAKE THE DOUBT OUT OF DYEING

If you still have doubts about the safety of dyeing, here are some precautions that help reduce whatever dangers may remain.

- Read directions carefully and follow them to the letter. Look to see if the preparations contain coal-tar supplements (4-methoxy-m-phylenediamine, known as 4-MMPD or 4-MMPDS). Some experts have suggested that you avoid these chemicals if you are pregnant or are trying to get pregnant.
- Wear gloves when applying dye.
- Don't leave dye on your head longer than necessary, and use the product as infrequently as possible.
- Consider frosting or streaking your hair, a process where coloring is not applied directly to the scalp.

C H A P T E R 40
Heredity

If you found out you had inherited a genetic predisposition to cancer, it might seem reasonable to live it up. To indulge in "nasty" habits! To smoke, drink and eat chocolate by the boxful! After all, you're going to get cancer anyway. Right?

Wrong.

"Most people perceive heredity as doom and gloom—if you have it in your genes, it's going to happen," says Sandra Wolman, M.D., associate professor of pathology at the New York University School of Medicine in New York City. "But this is not necessarily true with cancer—in most cases, the hereditary element involves a predisposition, which may or may not be realized depending on your behavior and environmental influences. Knowing you have an increased risk should *increase* your motivation to lead a healthy lifestyle and to cooperate with your doctor."

A few rare forms of cancer are considered to be completely hereditary. Among these are eye cancer in children (retinoblastoma) and a type of colon cancer that develops from genetically caused polyps.

In most cases, however, cancer develops from an interaction between genetic susceptibility and environmental and lifestyle factors. But to understand how that happens, we first have to understand genes.

DNA: THE CELLULAR BRAIN

Imagine a baby gurgling and playing in his crib. He knows nothing about politics, geography, biology—in fact, he hardly knows anything at all. However, this baby's genes already "know" that he will be tall and "know" that he will be bald by age 50.

That information—and much more—is stored in his genes, the basic carriers of traits from mom, dad and past generations. And the essence of a gene is its DNA, a chemical mind, an intelligence in the very center of each cell that instructs the body how to work.

But when that mind goes crazy, when DNA is even slightly damaged, the cells no longer have coherent orders to obey. They are out of control. They destroy instead of build. They are diseased cells. They are cancer.

DNA can be damaged in a variety of ways. Nuclear radiation can do it. So can certain chemicals. But DNA can also start off somewhat damaged (or mutated) when a parent with a mutated, cancer-prone gene passes it to his or her child. That child now has an increased risk of cancer—the same environmental insults that all of us receive, but usually repulse, are more likely to scramble his already weakened genes.

But that's not the only way a parent can bequeath cancer. Some inherited disorders decrease the rate of genetic repair. In a condition known as xeroderma pigmentosum, for instance, the mechanisms that fix environmentally induced damage to DNA in skin cells do not function well. So a person with this malady is more likely to develop skin cancer from exposure to the sun's DNA-damaging ultraviolet rays or to medications that work by altering DNA.

Other genetic syndromes—with tongue-twisting names such as ataxia telangiectasia and Fanconi's anemia—can cause cancer by encouraging mutation. These conditions cause chromosomes (strands of genes) to break easily in the presence of carcinogens, thus increasing the possibility of an abnormal recombination.

An immune deficiency can also be inherited, and some scientists postulate that an inadequate immune system allows cancer cells to reproduce unchecked, developing into tumors.

ARE YOU PREDISPOSED TO CANCER?

If your mother had cancer, that doesn't necessarily mean you'll get it, too. But it does mean that your risk may be higher than that of someone without cancer in their family.

"The actual risk depends on a number of factors, including the type of cancer and the number of affected relatives," says John J. Mulvihill, M.D., chief of clinical genetics at the National Cancer Institute in Bethesda, Maryland. "But a generalization could be made that if a first-degree relative (a sibling, parent or offspring) has cancer, you have about 3 times the chance of getting that same type of cancer. A woman is at a much higher risk if her mother and sister had breast cancer under the age of 40. This woman is 40 times more likely than her peers to get breast cancer in her early thirties."

GENETIC ENGINEERS:
CAN THEY BUILD A BRIDGE OVER CANCER?

Tremendous advances have been made on the genetic engineering frontier this past decade. This is good news for dwarf mice, and it may even be good news for families with high rates of cancer.

Scientists can now pluck a gene for a specific trait from one creature and transplant it into the cell of another. This cell should then follow the instructions coded in that gene.

The first successful application of this technology involved the aforementioned dwarf mice. Researchers injected a growth hormone gene into the fertilized egg of a mouse who was deficient in this hormone. Without the shot, the rodent would have grown up to be a midget. With the shot, the mouse overproduced growth hormones and grew to twice the normal size. The deficiency was overcompensated for, but this experiment did demonstrate that a particular genetic disease can be cured, at least in laboratory animals.

"This knowledge will probably one day be applied to benefit people with a high risk for hereditary cancer," writes Henry T. Lynch, M.D., professor and chairman, Department of Preventive Medicine at the Creighton University School of Medicine in Omaha, Nebraska, in *The American Cancer Society's Complete Book of Cancer* (Doubleday)."For example, if we could isolate cancer-resistant genes and transplant them into human cells that are deficient in them, we could conceivably prevent the influence of the cancer-prone genes and produce a higher degree of resistance to cancer-causing agents.

"In fact, plans to do just that are on the drawing boards of a number of genetic engineering laboratories throughout the world."

ADVICE FOR HIGH-RISK INDIVIDUALS

If all this talk of family cancer makes you suspect that you inherited a large cancer risk, you might consider genetic counseling. Medical geneticists (and some oncologists, or cancer specialists) can estimate your risk, based on family history. The information might indicate that you should be using some of the following measures for yourself, your family and future generations.

Limit exposures to known risks. Many people know that certain activities might cause cancer, but they decide that the pleasure is worth the risk.

"To illustrate, sunlight is the commonest known cause of cancer in the U.S., but most people look forward to sun exposure and congratulate each other on a healthy tan," points out Dr. Mulvihill. "However, the parents of a child with xeroderma pigmentosum [a condition that predisposes to skin cancer] who died of melanoma were told to protect their affected infant twin boys from ultraviolet light. They did so—and prevented cancer. In the same way, a person with a family history of lung cancer should be more motivated to give up smoking."

So if a genetic counselor tells you that you are particularly sensitive to a certain substance, steer clear of it.

KNOW THE SIGNS OF HEREDITARY CANCER

Any cancer can have a genetic component—but some types of hereditary cancer announce themselves in obvious ways. Here are the major signs:

Early onset. Hereditary cancers often hit a person at a young age. The theory behind this observation is that the cells were mutated before the person was born, giving the predisposed person a head start in the cancer process. What constitutes an early age depends on what type of cancer it is. In general, however, cancer that occurs before the age of 30 could well be hereditary.

Multiple sites. Hereditary cancer usually strikes more than once. It may hit more than one organ or a pair of organs (such as both kidneys), or it may cause several lesions to develop in the same organ.

Atypical of gender. Cancer that seems to transcend the sex barriers might also have the genes to blame. Breast cancer in a man or lung cancer in a nonsmoking woman are examples of types of cancer affecting the atypical sex.

If there's a high incidence of cancer in your family, you should examine any possible risk factors, advises Dr. Wolman. Do you come from a family of hard drinkers? Heavy smokers? High-fat eaters? If you've got the same habits, you should consider changing them.

Practice surveillance. If you can't stop cancer from developing, at least you can catch it in its early stages, before it is totally out of control. If you have a high risk for a particular type of cancer, don't ignore it. Find out the early warning signs and see a doctor for regular early-detection checkups.

Obtain prenatal diagnosis. A pregnant woman with a risk for a rare genetic cancer (such as xeroderma pigmentosum, retinoblastoma or Fanconi's anemia) can have a prenatal test to determine if the baby will inherit the disease. Knowing the risk will alert the doctor so that the disease can be detected and treated early. Most patients with retinoblastoma, for instance, can undergo radiation treatment before the age of 2. This is possible if the tumor is spotted early and removal of the eye is not necessary.

People who have survived retinoblastoma or Wilms' tumor may even decide not to start a family because of the excessively high risk they'd pass to their child. Here, too, a genetic counselor can advise prospective parents.

Consider prophylactic surgery. A drastic step is to remove the organ at risk for cancer before the cancer has a chance to develop. This is recommended only for people with a very large risk. People with familial polyposis, for instance, typically have more than 100 polyps in the colon by the time they're 20 years old. If they live to be 70, nearly everybody with this trait will contract cancer. Because of this risk, most people with this gene have their colon removed by the time they're 20 years old.

CANCER PREVENTION PLAN: HEREDITY

- If you have a family history of cancer, consider genetic counseling to estimate your risk, based on family history.
- Limit exposures to known risks.
- Learn the early warning signs and see a doctor for regular early-detection checkups.
- People who have hereditary cancer should inform family members so they, too, can take preventive measures.
- Consider prophylactic surgery when necessary.

Use genetic registers. People who have hereditary cancer should inform their family members so they, too, can take the preventive measures just discussed. Along the same line, inform your doctor of any blood relatives who have had cancer and ask if he or she uses a genetic register. Some doctors are starting to use these registers to keep track of hereditary cancer, for both diagnostic and research purposes. With such a record, a doctor should be able to better serve a future family member who gets the disease.

Remember, cancer genes aren't a death sentence—they're a loud announcement to take charge of your health and reduce the risk. And that could be a blessing in disguise.

Immune System

You may not have had any symptoms. You may not have had a diagnosis. There may not have been any x-rays. But somewhere deep inside you a toxic chemical, shaft of radiation or deadly virus altered, interrupted, modified or otherwise messed up the intricate "grow/don't grow" codes sent from one part of a cell to another. And yesterday you got cancer.

The cancer might have been in your liver, where that bout of hepatitis B you had last spring left some virus cells to set the stage for your destruction. Or it might have been on your cheek where the summer sun burned your skin. It might even have been on your lip, where the toxic chemicals from that pipe or cigarette you used to smoke were concentrated.

Scary, isn't it? But if yesterday you had cancer, today you don't. Today you woke up in the morning, the sun was shining, you stretched and your cancer was gone. You never even knew you had it, did you?

Sound like a fantasy? A pipe dream? Someone's idea of science fiction? According to researchers across the country, it's not. It's not because every one of us, scientists say, gets cancer. And the difference between those of us who get sick and die and those of us who get well and live is the immune system—that intricate defense network of lymph nodes, suppressors, helpers, killers and antibodies that can destroy an embryonic cancer before you're even aware of it. Before, perhaps, it even takes hold. It can, scientists say, prevent cancer.

"Your immune system is the major defense system of your body," explains Terry Phillips, D.Sc., director of the immunogenetics and immunochemistry lab at George Washington University Medical Center in Washington, D.C. Any foreign substance—whether it's an ordinary winter virus or an exotic occupational carcinogen—can only cause death or destruction, quite literally, over the dead body of your immune system. And if that sounds like war, adds Dr. Phillips, well, the metaphor is unavoidable.

AN ARMY-NAVY GAME

Your body's defense system actually begins in the bone marrow, Dr. Phillips explains. Special cells called "stem cells" break out of the marrow and travel either to the thymus gland in your chest or the bursa area in your intestines. Cells that pass through the thymus are referred to as T-cells—for "thymus-derived"—while cells that pass through the bursa are B-cells—"bursa-derived."

Both sets of cells are like the chiefs of staff for your body's army and navy. The T-cells head your land-based or cellular forces, while the B-cells control your body's waterways—that intricate system of arteries, veins and capillaries that permeates every microscopic piece of tissue in your body—and the equally complex system of lymph nodes, glands and fluids.

But just as an army divides its land-based forces into more manageable divisions, so your body divides its cellular forces into specialized teams: T-helpers, which call up the troops, and T-suppressors, which send the troops back to the barracks when their job is done, act as a committee and direct battlefield operations. Together they decide how many soldiers, called T-effectors, and their commandos, called T-killers, are necessary to repel an invader.

The B-cells, on the other hand, don't believe you need a bureaucracy to fight a war. They concentrate their efforts on producing a single elite warrior, the antibody—arguably your body's ultimate weapon.

It all adds up to a defense system with a variety of tactical weapons at its disposal, explains Dr. Phillips. The immune system can kill an invader with either T-killer soldiers or a warrior antibody, as its committee deems appropriate.

But how does the committee know when your body is under attack? How does it know when a virus invades or a cancer starts to grow?

That information, says Dr. Phillips, comes from a scouting party made up of white cells called macrophages. Macrophages constantly patrol your body carrying a molecular checklist—a list of what the body has determined from the time you were born as making up "self." And as they patrol, they use what amount to little fingers to conduct a body search, feeling every cell they meet. When something in a cell doesn't match their "this is self" checklist, the macrophages zap out a powerful chemical to destroy it.

But the macrophages are only patrols, not battalions. So when they're in danger of being overwhelmed—a single viral invader, for example, can multiply to 10,000 within a seven-hour period—they pull off a piece of the virus and take it back to the T-cell committee as an appeal for reinforcements.

That's when your T-cell committee calls in the navy. Or, in this case, the B-cells, your body's equivalent. The B-cells confer with the committee of T-cells, says Dr. Phillips, and decide how many antibodies the B-cells should make. Then the antibodies, which look more like little molecular lobsters than warriors, flood into your bloodstream, whip in and out among the cells and hunt the invader down.

The invader, of course, doesn't have a chance. Or at least not much. The antibodies' "claws" grab the enemy in a bear hug while their tails wave madly to bring in a whole cluster of enzymes, called complement, that leech onto the invader and drill holes in it.

Not even Rambo could withstand these puncture wounds. And— whether cancer cell or virus—neither can your body's invader. The primitive life force of the "not-self" cell is sucked out of the holes, and the few bits of immunological debris that may remain are gobbled up by the macrophage patrol. End of virus. End of cancer. End of whatever your body defines as "not-self."

But what would happen if your body's immune system were weak when an invader attacked? Well, says Dr. Phillips, then you might be in trouble. "Those are excellent times for cancers, if they're not (yet) being detected, to suddenly start to grow."

Look at the people who have acquired immune deficiency syndrome (AIDS), for example. One-third of these severely immuno-suppressed people develop a cancer called Kaposi's sarcoma. Also, people who are given drugs to suppress the immune system—in preparation for organ transplants, for example—have a threefold increase in various cancers. Perhaps it's not coincidental.

FEEDING THE TROOPS

That's why it's important to keep your immune system strong, says Dr. Phillips. "Then the first time your body sees any [cellular] changes, any little deviations from the checklist—Zap! They're gone."

But *how* do we keep our immune system strong?

VACCINATE YOURSELF AGAINST CANCER

How would you like to show up at your doctor's office one morning and get a vaccination against cancer? Well, immunologists share that dream. And reality is catching up. Because, of the four major viruses thought to trigger changes in cells that can set the stage for cancer—hepatitis B, Epstein-Barr, human papilloma virus and adult T-cell leukemia—there's already a vaccine for one, the hepatitis B virus, which can cause liver cancer.

How does a vaccine work? Basically, scientists say, they take a little of the virus you don't want to infect you and inject an inactive or weakened amount of it into your body. Your immune system reacts and produces antibody warriors to fight the virus. Cells that "remember" the virus are also produced, and in the event of a viral attack in the future, you are impervious to attack. You're immune.

Scientists are not only working on vaccines that make you immune to the viruses implicated in cancer production. They're also working on making you immune to cancer itself. At the Bionetics Research, Inc. facility in Rockville, Maryland, for example, Michael G. Hanna, Jr., Ph.D., has developed a vaccine that may prevent the recurrence of colon cancer. And at New York University Medical Center's Kaplan Cancer Center, Jean-Claude Bystryn, M.D., is developing a vaccine against melanoma.

Both vaccines already seem to work in the lab. Here's hoping they'll be just as effective in people.

"The immune system doesn't work well in anybody who's malnourished," says Dr. Phillips. You need to provide it with enough proteins, sugars and fats to make the antibodies, macrophages and T-killers that range throughout your body. And that's not as simple as it sounds, because your body has a food allocation system with more guidelines than a federal food bank.

Your brain, for example, is always fed first. Maybe the the brain figures that it's the most important since it's in charge of your body. Or maybe, since it is in charge, it's just pulling rank. Who knows? What we do know is that all the major organ systems get fed second and the immune system, if there's any food left, gets its share last.

Does this mean that if you go without breakfast your immune system doesn't get its Wheaties either? That's right, folks. And the resulting immune system famine can shut down your body's defenses.

But vitamins and minerals play almost as significant a part in immune function as how much, and whether or not, you eat. Vitamin C, for example, is believed by some scientists to help the thymus make T-cells and stimulate macrophages to kill bacteria. Vitamin A helps produce T-cells, while vitamin E is believed to speed up T-cell reaction time. The B vitamins may affect all aspects of the immune system, scientists suspect, and may be particularly useful in keeping the thymus on its toes. Vitamin D may be responsible for keeping the macrophages patrolling throughout your body. (See chapters 65 through 70, which discuss individual nutrients, for a complete discussion of your body's specific needs.)

The effect of minerals on your immune system is less well understood, although that there *is* an effect is undeniable. The right amount of a particular mineral such as zinc, for example, appears to regulate T-cells and help create enzymes—maybe even the ones that punch holes in an invading cancer or virus. Too much zinc (or too little) is believed to suppress your immune function.

As for supplements, to take or not to take, that is the question. "You may want to talk to your physician about it," suggests Dr. Phillips. "Otherwise as long as you're eating a reasonable diet, one of those standard one-a-day type vitamins is sufficient" to keep your immune system at maximum efficiency.

GETTING SOME REST AND RELAXATION

Another way to keep your immune system strong is to avoid excessive amounts of stress, says Dr. Phillips. That's because when you're bombarded with overwhelming problems—your workload is too much, your bank balance is too low, your husband has just run off with his secretary—the brain saturates your body with chemicals that can literally shut down your immune system. And a shutdown is the perfect time for any unidentified cancer to multiply.

"When I personally get really worked up, I'll go for a ten-minute walk," says Dr. Phillips. "I can feel myself calming down."

And one study showed that the immune system also perks ups when you calm down. At Albright College in Reading, Pennsylvania, for example, college students were randomly assigned to one of four 20-minute relaxation methods—the relaxation response pioneered by Harvard's Herbert Benson; guided visualization; massage; or lying quietly with eyes closed. Antibodies in the students' saliva were measured both before and after they relaxed. The result? The antibody level in each student shot up. In a control group that did not practice any relaxation techniques, the antibody level remained the same.

And why not also try writing? Or even laughing? A recent study at Southern Methodist University, Dallas, Texas, by psychologist James W. Pennebaker, Ph.D., found that writing about painful personal problems—and how you feel about them—not only reduces stress but may bolster the immune system as well. In his study, 25 college students were asked to write their thoughts on unimportant topics, spending 20 minutes a day for four days at the task. Another group of 25 students wrote for the same time period but described their feelings about problem situations that they hadn't been able to resolve.

Blood samples taken just before and just after the experiment, as well as six weeks later, showed that students who wrote out their troubling feelings had an increased T-cell response. Those who recorded thoughts on trivial subjects showed no such improvement in their immune system. Six weeks after the initial bloodletting, the "confiding" student-writers still had stronger immune defenses.

"I would guess that the kind of stress that makes you feel highly anxious or under an outside threat—especially if you feel hopeless or helpless—would lower the function of your immune system," says Dr. Pennebaker. And crying out our guts to a diary is one way to relieve it. But, adds Dr. Pennebaker, we can also learn to avoid the things or people that threaten us.

But if walking, relaxing or writing isn't your thing, how about laughter? "We're not quite to the stage where we can say a laugh a day will keep the doctor away," says Katherine Baker, Ph.D., a biologist and researcher at Millersville University of Pennsylvania. "But we do know that if you're sitting in an office under pressure and you get upset about it, your immune function will go down." Approach the situation with humor, she adds, and your immune function will go up.

How does she know? Because following the lead of Kathleen Dillon, Ph.D., a psychologist at Western New England College in Springfield, Massachusetts, Dr. Baker conducted a study that measured the concentration of antibodies in a group of ten students. The researchers showed the students two videotapes: one funny, "Richard Pryor Live," and one boring, an educational tape on anxiety. Then they measured the students' level of a particular antibody. The results were enlightening: While the students' antibody levels remained the same both before and after viewing the educational tape, they shot up after watching Richard Pryor.

Their results have not yet been duplicated by other studies, cautions Dr. Dillon, "but I think some exciting things are happening." Their next study on the immune system, she adds, will be to determine whether or not other positive emotional states, such as love, have the same effect as laughter. Is it possible, for example, to boost your immune system with a kiss?

But aside from weakening the immune system itself, says Dr. Terry Phillips, the major problem with excessive stress is that it usually interferes with your sleep. In fact, the way to tell the difference between stress that gives you an edge—keeping you sharp in your job, for example—and stress that suppresses your immune system—*distress*—is whether or not it interferes with your sleep. *Anything* that prevents sleep, says Dr. Phillips, is distress.

"Sleep is like the mechanic's shop for the immune system," he explains. "During sleep all your other body functions tend to shut down. Then your food materials—your building blocks—can be used by the immune system. The immune system can get out, get around, it can work a little better. It's like coming into the gas station after the rush hour."

MARCHING ORDERS

Another way to rev up your immune system, he says, is exercise. Exercise speeds up the blood flow throughout your body—increasing the response time of antibodies as they zip around with it—and also raises your body temperature. Since a slightly elevated body temperature during illness—triggered, scientists feel, by a brain-to-body messenger called endogenous pyrogen or interleukin-1—is generally believed to improve macrophages' munching, some scientists believe that the artificially elevated temperature caused by exercise may do the same thing.

Moreover, exercise seems to stimulate your body's production of beta endorphins, substances that—in labs at the National Institutes of Health, at least—latch onto your T-killer cells and increase their ability to destroy invaders by an average of 63 percent.

How much excerise is good? How much exercise is bad? Some scientists feel that investigations into exercise and the immune system are too preliminary to make a judgment. But Dr. Phillips disagrees. "There's a time when you stop exercising and you get that wonderful sort of euphoric feeling," he says. "And then there's a time when you finish something and it was a real strain—a time when you say, 'Oh my God!' " That's the difference, he says, between good and bad, between enough and too much, between stimulating the immune system and suppressing it.

ADDITIONAL IMMUNE-POWER TIPS

Suppressing the immune system is not hard to do. Especially inadvertently. That's because chemicals in everyday kinds of things such as alcohol, tobacco smoke—even antihistamines—can slow down or even halt immune function, as can constant physical irritations—false teeth that don't fit, tobacco pipes resting on a lip—and occupational exposures to radiation or toxic chemicals.

Viral infections—even those "harmless" seasonal sneezers you get every winter—can also do their share of damage. If a cancer starts to grow while the attention of your T-cell committee is even partially elsewhere, cautions Dr. Phillips, it's more likely to gain a foothold.

So the moral of this story is to practice good hygiene. "I've almost given up hand-shaking," chuckles Dr. Phillips. Hand to hand contact is one of the major ways we transmit viruses.

One controversial method that *may* boost your immune system to overcome all invaders, however, is psychoimaging—an experimental technique used by clinical psychologists to treat cancer. It involves picturing a weak tumor being obliterated by cells of the immune system, and it may indeed contribute to the regression of malignant tumors (see chapter 78, Mind/Body Healing). The question is, can it work in a preventive way? Can we literally *program* our immune system to bring it up to maximum killing efficiency? Can, as in this case, a psychoimage a day keep the cancer away?

"I'm not yet ready to make that jump; there are, as yet, no data that bear directly on this question," says Robert Ader, Ph.D., a leading researcher in the field and director of behavioral and psychosocial medicine at the University of Rochester School of Medicine and Dentistry, New York. But the question is intriguing, since, as he says, "We do know that you can condition changes in your immune system."

But whether or not we can use our minds to program a cancer-targeting antibody will have to wait until immunology has evolved further out of the Paleolithic era. In the meantime, says Dr. Phillips, our hope is that people who eat right, sleep well, exercise moderately, reduce excessive stress and avoid cancer-causing agents and immunosupressive drugs will be able to zip their immune system up to maximum capability and zap any insidious little cancers that mutate along the way. *Before* they know they're around.

CANCER PREVENTION PLAN: IMMUNE SYSTEM

- Make sure your diet is high in the B vitamins and vitamins C and A.
- Get sufficient vitamin D.
- Avoid excessive amounts of stress.
- Exercise regularly.
- Avoid tobacco smoke.

CHAPTER 42
Indoor Pollution

Would you ever invite a manufacturing plant to locate its smokestack in your backyard? To spew dark clouds into the air that your family breathes?

Of course not. But whether your neighborhood looks like an industrial zone or the Garden of Eden, the air *inside* your home may actually be *more* dangerously polluted than the air outside.

Scientists now know that the products we keep around the house—paints, cleansers, solvents, aerosol sprays—along with chemicals emitted by building materials and furnishings, plus certain personal activities, like smoking—can expose us to surprisingly high levels of worrisome chemicals. Some of these substances are established cancer threats.

Man-made products are not entirely to blame. Mother Nature is playing a villainous role in this scenario by pumping in a carcinogen that may be the worst threat of all: Radon.

What's made things even worse is our efforts at energy conservation. Sure, we sealed in the heat when we dutifully weather-stripped, caulked and insulated our homes—but we also sealed in the bad air. Scientists even have names for the phenomenon: "building-related illness" or "sick building syndrome." Symptoms of building-related illness may include throat, nose and eye irritation, fatigue, headaches, nausea and skin rashes. In the long term, more serious problems may develop, including heart, kidney or liver damage—and cancer.

Unfortunately, some of the known cancer risks in the indoor environment are invisible and odorless. That's why it's so important to be alert to the problem.

ASBESTOS

Once hailed as a versatile insulating material, asbestos—a mineral fiber derived from rocks—has been implicated in asbestosis (a progressive and disabling lung disease), lung cancer, stomach cancer and mesothelioma (a rare cancer of chest and abdominal membranes), as well as cancers of the esophagus, colon, rectum and other sites. The evidence that asbestos is a human carcinogen is strong.

What makes asbestos so lethal? It's composed of tiny, indestructible fibers. If these fibers—which are too small to be seen—become airborne, they can be inhaled, and that's when they wreak havoc. Health damage may not appear for 20 to 40 years.

The people most at risk of developing asbestos-related cancer are those who worked with large amounts of it, such as those in the shipbuilding industry, asbestos mining and automotive brake lining repair.

Asbestos was widely used in commercial buildings until recently. But it also was used in products made for private homes. Asbestos can be found, for example, in heat and acoustic insulation, roofing and flooring materials, fireproofing materials, ceiling panels, carpet underlays, artificial fireplaces, patching and spackling compounds, and more. It's also in some older appliances—no doubt you remember checking your hairdryer and, perhaps, buying a new one, in the 1970s.

The Environmental Protection Agency (EPA) estimates that 20 percent of buildings contain asbestos, which can be released if disturbed. The health consequences of this long-term, lower-level exposure to asbestos are uncertain.

Asbestos has been banned from pipe coverings, patching compounds, hairdryers and some other uses, and the EPA is considering the elimination of asbestos from all consumer products by the mid-1990s. The government is particularly concerned about asbestos in schools and has undertaken a major initiative to clean up the problem.

DANGER! HANDLE WITH CARE

If you do suspect that there is asbestos in your home, do not, repeat, *do not* attempt to remove it yourself! If the asbestos is intact and undamaged, removal can be more dangerous than leaving it in place, and should be done only as a last resort. If it is removed without proper precautions, you could cause yourself, or your family, serious health damage.

British doctors recently reported to the medical journal *Lancet* a case of a 28-year-old-man who died of mesothelioma. Five years earlier, he had knocked down a wall while renovating his house, without wearing a face mask. Over a 72-hour period he was heavily exposed to asbestos dust.

A sobering story. But there's no need to panic: It's encouraging to remember that most people exposed to small amounts of asbestos don't develop any related health problems.

There is a healthy way to go about dealing with asbestos. If you suspect there's asbestos in your home (or office), the first thing to do is consult an experienced plumber, building contractor, heating contractor or other building professional who can make a reasonable judgment if it really is asbestos, based on visual inspection or on knowledge of the products used.

If the verdict is yes, the next decision is whether to leave the asbestos in place, remove it, or seal it in. This decision will depend on the condition of the material containing asbestos.

But sometimes simply eyeballing the material is not enough. The only certain way to determine if the material is releasing asbestos fibers is to have it analyzed by a process called polarized light microscopy, at a testing laboratory. Contact your state health agency or a reliable, certified testing company to take a sample for analysis.

As noted, most asbestos-containing materials should be left alone. That's because asbestos is usually combined with a binding material so the fibers are not released into the air.

So, for example, if you find the patching compound or textured paints used on your walls *do* contain asbestos, but the material is in good condition, the best thing you can do is leave it alone. Scraping or sanding will release asbestos fibers. If, however, the material is damaged, the asbestos may become airborne, able to be inhaled—and dangerous.

Options for dealing with asbestos that poses a hazard include encapsulation or removal.

Encapsulation involves sealing asbestos-containing materials. Wide protective duct tape, for example, can be wrapped around asbestos insulation that surrounds pipes. Asbestos floor tiles can be covered with other flooring materials. (This procedure is effective only for undamaged substances which contain asbestos, not for soft or crumbly materials.)

Asbestos removal is a more expensive, hazardous procedure. Be sure that the contractor you hire is a certified, qualified and reliable asbestos abatement contractor. If you insist on doing it yourself, the EPA can provide detailed guidelines for safe asbestos control. If an older home is being renovated, be especially careful to follow EPA guidelines.

And, if you believe that you may have been exposed to any amount of loose asbestos, no matter how long ago, you should consult your physician immediately, according to the American Lung Association. Smokers, especially, beware: Asbestos and cigarette smoking together produce more lung cancer than either factor alone.

For help, contact your EPA Regional Asbestos Coordinator. There are also some toll-free numbers that you can call for information and assistance.

- For names of laboratories qualified to test and analyze asbestos samples, call the EPA at 1-800-334-8571, ext. 6741.
- For guidance, documents and technical assistance, call the EPA at (202) 554-1404.
- For information on asbestos in consumer products or homes, call the Consumer Product Safety Commission at 1-800-638-2772.

FORMALDEHYDE

Mobile homes were one of the first concerns. Because mobile homes are small, airtight, and built with plenty of formaldehyde-laden plywood, health officials worried about the high levels of this strong chemical that could build up indoors.

So formaldehyde levels in mobile home materials were restricted—but scientists, regulators and health officials are still concerned about formaldehyde in home and office air.

There are more sources of formaldehyde around you than you might suspect. These include plywood and particleboard; textiles such as those used in furniture, drapes and carpets; a certain kind of insulation called urea-formaldehyde foam insulation (UFFI); and even cigarettes and poorly vented gas stoves and heaters.

Often, you can tell it's there: Formaldehyde is a pungent-smelling chemical that is known to cause eye, nose and throat irritation, coughing, skin rashes, headaches, dizziness, nausea, vomiting and nosebleeds.

And it may also pose a cancer risk. "The animal evidence is absolutely clear-cut," says Aaron Blair, Ph.D., chief of the occupational studies section at the National Cancer Institute in Bethesda, Maryland. "Formaldehyde is a carcinogen without a doubt.

"For humans, the epidemiological evidence is not as clear," he adds. Dr. Blair directed the largest study to date of occupational exposure to formaldehyde. The study, released in 1986, found no overall link between formaldehyde and most cancers among 26,000 workers in industries where formaldehyde was produced and used.

However, the study did find higher-than-expected rates of cancers at certain sites in the upper throat, Dr. Blair notes.

His conclusion: "This study makes it plausible that formaldehyde plays a role in formation of this tumor [of the upper throat]. I would not come out and say it's definitely proven, but it might be prudent to assume it as a carcinogen."

The EPA is working under the same assumption. "We've classified it . . . as a probable human carcinogen," says Richard Hefter, project manager for formaldehyde risk assessment at the EPA in Washington, D.C. "That classification is one step—albeit a large step—below the materials for which there is definitive evidence, like asbestos and vinyl chloride."

CLEANING IT OUT

If you've noticed a pungent odor around the home or office, or are experiencing health problems like headaches or a scratchy throat, the first thing you should do is test the air for formaldehyde concentration levels. Detection devices are relatively inexpensive—about $30—or you can ask your local health department or a private testing company to perform the analysis.

If it is determined that there are excess concentrations of formaldehyde in the home, there are a number of different steps you can take.

Remove the source. Paneling, furniture, or carpeting can easily be removed and replaced with materials that are low in formaldehyde, such as low-formaldehyde particleboard and exterior grade plywood (which releases less formaldehyde than interior grades). You may have to contact the manufacturer to determine if their products contain formaldehyde. However, some significant sources of formaldehyde are trickier or more expensive to remove, like particleboard subflooring or urea-formaldehyde foam insulation.

Treat the source. Emission from particleboard subflooring can be blocked: The upper surface can be treated with varnish or paint to stop vapors from entering the home. Similarly, vapors from UFFI can be reduced by covering walls with vapor-barrier paint or vinyl wallpaper, or by sealing cracks in the walls.

Ventilate or purify the air. "When people started to make their homes tighter, formaldehyde levels increased in some cases," says Richard Hefter. Simply opening your windows a crack at night is a good idea. Or you can use a forced ventilation system that will bring in fresh air, diluting formaldehyde levels—although you'll lose heat. Air-to-air heat exchange ventilation systems are a better alternative. They bring fresh air in, but recover heat from exhaust air. Chemical air filter systems can also reduce formaldehyde levels, although they can be costly and require constant monitoring.

Along with keeping the air fresh, it's also important to keep it dry. The more humid the air is, the more formaldehyde is released. Dehumidification during humid seasons can relieve the problem.

For more information on formaldehyde reduction, you can contact your regional EPA office or the Consumer Product Safety Commission at 1-800-638-2772.

RADON

Back in 1984, a worker at the Limerick nuclear power plant in eastern Pennsylvania began setting off radiation detectors on his way *into* work.

This little mystery triggered national alarm after it was discovered that he was picking up radiation not from the nuclear power plant but from his *home*. An odorless, colorless radioactive gas called radon was seeping in from a natural low-grade uranium formation under the soil that his house was built upon. That geologic formation, the "Reading Prong," was found to extend through parts of Pennsylvania and into New York and New Jersey.

Since then, radon in homes has become a major national concern.

And no wonder. Scientists have long known that uranium miners suffer inordinately high rates of cancer, caused by years of exposure to radon gas. Based on exposure information, scientists now estimate that radon gas may be causing 10,000 to 30,000 cases of cancer a year. It's generally agreed that *radon is the leading cause of lung cancer among nonsmokers,* responsible for more cases than either outdoor air pollution or asbestos.

Over a million homes may be affected by radon. Bernard Cohen, Ph.D., a physics professor at the University of Pittsburgh, says virtually every state has areas of radon contamination that could pose a health threat. Regions of concern include the "Reading Prong," in the Northeast; in the West, areas with large deposits with uranium ore; and in Florida, reclaimed phosphate mining land that has been developed for homes. Trouble spots have also been identified in Canada, Europe and other areas of the world.

HOW DOES RADON GET IN?

Radium, the precursor of radon, is found in small amounts in most soil. It's highly concentrated in uranium and phosphate deposits, and at somewhat lower concentrations in granite and shale.

These materials give off radon gas. Normally, the gas escapes through fissures in the earth and dissipates harmlessly in the atmosphere. Unless a house gets in the way. Then the radon seeps in through cracks in a home's foundation, sump pumps, drains and the like. It can even diffuse through solid concrete walls.

The house bottles up the radon. Concentrations ten times higher than outdoor levels are not unusual.

In the house, the radon gas continues to decay, mostly into radioactive particles, which attach themselves to dust and smoke. These particles can be inhaled; they lodge in the lungs and upper respiratory tract, and continue to emit radiation.

Radon has a relatively short "half-life" of 3.8 days, meaning the radiation decays rapidly. So you wouldn't run much risk from cancer if you spent a week, or even a year, in a house with moderate radon contamination. But if you lived in such a house for 20 years or more, you might well increase your chances of getting cancer—and there are virtually no short-term symptoms to warn of trouble. Cancer might not show up for two or three decades.

IDENTIFYING THE PROBLEM

Is your home a radon trap?

That depends, first of all, on where you live. You've probably read in the newspaper if your area has a radon problem. But even if your neighbor has a radon problem, you may not. Levels may vary from house to house, or street to street. The home of the nuclear engineer who triggered the first alarm had radon concentrations 1,000 times higher than normal; levels in the home of a neighbor, 100 feet away, were found to be safe.

Levels in the home depend on the amount of radon coming from the earth below your house, the rate at which it enters the home, and the rate at which ventilation exhausts it from the home.

Houses that have flunked radon tests do have some things in common, however.

- Airtight homes have higher indoor radon levels than leaky ones.
- Single-level houses test higher than multilevel ones.
- Clay soil beneath a house more effectively blocks radon from entering the home than sandy soil does.
- Buildings with slab-on-grade construction collect more radon than those with basements or crawlspaces.

Energy efficiency aggravates the radon problem. Without adequate ventilation, radon will stay inside a house longer, and at high concentrations. Simply caulking and weather-stripping can increase levels of radioactivity by 20 percent.

TESTING TIPS

If you've heard of a radon risk in your area, you should get your home tested. Both public agencies and private laboratories can test for radon. To understand the results of your radon test, you need to know that radiation levels are measured in picocuries per liter (pCi/l). One pCi/l represents the decay of about two radon atoms in a quart of air.

What levels of radon require remedial action? That depends whom you ask. The National Council on Radiation Protection says anything below 8 pCi/l is safe; Florida's EPA recommends fixing any house with levels above 6 pCi/l. The U.S. EPA says any house with levels greater than 4 pCi/l should be repaired. And the American Society of Heating, Refrigeration and Air Conditioning Engineers says levels above 2 pCi/l is unsafe.

Julie Overbaugh, Ph.D., of the Harvard School of Public Health in Boston, says that based on an average risk estimate from past studies, the probability of getting cancer in a 4 pCi/l house is 1 in 32.

RADON REMEDIES

If unhealthy levels of radon have been detected in your home, there are plenty of things you can do to remedy the problem—although it will cost you. The average price of radon repairs ranges from $600 to $5,000—and, in extraordinary cases, can go much higher.

The simplest remedy is to block the pathways that the radioactive gas is following into your home. Cracks and crevices in the basement should be plugged with a concrete silicone sealant, such as those made by UGL and GE (they're available in most home centers). Floor drains can also be radon entry points, and they should be plugged if the basement doesn't take in water.

Opening a window in the basement is a temporary cure. The ventilation will dilute airborne radon. Air-to-air heat exchangers are a more permanent solution; they'll ventilate the house without causing major heating or cooling losses.

RADON IN WATER

Another source of radon in the home is well water. Most municipal water supplies are safe, because the radon disperses before the water reaches the home. But if the rock under a well is high in radon, some of the gas will be picked up by the water.

Drinking radon-contaminated water isn't the only problem: As the water splashes out of faucets, showers and washing machines inside the house, up to half the dissolved radon is released into the air—where, again, it can be inhaled.

That's why it's especially important to keep shower and laundry areas well ventilated and, in the bathroom, use the exhaust fans while running water. Jerry Lowry, Ph.D., professor of environmental engineering at the University of Maine, recommends purifying water with an activated carbon filter that treats the whole water supply, not just drinking water, and costs about $700 to $800. Two pamphlets, "Radon in Water and Air," and "Removing Radon from Water Using Granular Activated Carbon," are available by writing Jerry Lowry, Department of Civil Engineering, 455 Aubert Hall, University of Maine, Orono ME 04469. Each pamphlet costs $2. (For more information on clean water and water filters, see chapter 51, Outdoor Pollution.)

If you suspect you've been exposed to high levels of radon, the American Lung Association suggests you see your doctor right away.

PRODUCTS USED AT HOME

Who would think that some of the products that make our lives easier and more convenient—products ranging from mothballs to paint—might actually pose a health threat?

These days, unfortunately, quite a few people are thinking that way, including scientists at the Environmental Protection Agency, the Consumer Product Safety Commission (CPSC) and the American Lung Association.

And one fear is that exposure to potent toxic chemicals *may* increase cancer risk. Unfortunately, nobody knows for sure. "For most consumer products, available laboratory and human evidence is insufficient to determine whether they pose a cancer risk," says a report on cancer risks by the Office of Technology Assessment.

Worse than the unknowns is the fact that some products are *known* to contain carcinogens. It might not be so bad if we used some of these products outdoors, where the ventilation would carry away the fumes. But in an indoor environment, our exposure to them may be concentrated.

It must be emphasized that no one knows for sure whether using these products in the home poses a *significant* hazard. "The difficulty in assessing cancers associated with exposure to consumer products is that the dose is usually low and the exposed population tends to be very large," comments the Office of Technology Assessment report on cancer risks. "At this time it is impossible to assess the contribution of consumer products to the overall cancer rate . . . [but] there is too much ignorance for complacency to be justified."

What's a consumer to do? Where to begin cleaning out the castle?

Some important clues to the most potent sources of carcinogens in the home were provided by a major study of indoor pollution by the Environmental Protection Agency.

In 1979, a group of EPA researchers decided to study exposure of householders to indoor, outdoor and air and water pollutants. (This now-famous study is referred to as the Total Exposure Assessment Methodology Study—the TEAM Study, for short.)

Researchers deliberately chose to study households in widely varying cities. Some, like Los Angeles, California, and Elizabeth and Bayonne in northern New Jersey, had heavy concentrations of industry. As a control, they chose what they thought was one of the cleanest cities in the world, Devil's Lake, North Dakota, which has no industries and which is swept clean by arctic winds.

The researchers provided 600 householders in the different cities with personal air monitors to carry with them all day, sampling the air they breathed for hazardous chemicals (including carcinogens). Breath analyses were periodically conducted on all of the subjects to check blood levels of the chemicals to which they were exposed.

As results started to come in, the researchers were surprised: *No matter how clean or dirty the city, indoor pollution levels were far worse than outdoor levels.*

The study's director, Lance Wallace, Ph.D., an environmental scientist with the EPA's office of research and development and formerly a visiting scientist with Harvard University's Energy and Environmental Policy Center, explains, "In New Jersey, even though outdoor pollution was as high as one could expect, the indoor levels were still 2 to 5 times higher—and sometimes 100 or even 1,000 times higher than outdoors."

The other big surprise was that the chemicals they expected to find only in big city homes were showing up in North Dakota homes, even though there were no polluting industries in Devil's Lake.

What could it mean?

By the end of the five-year study, the conclusion was certain: "We're pretty sure that the main sources of these chemicals are personal activities, building materials and personal products," says Dr. Wallace.

Six of the chemicals that they found in home air and in breath analyses are carcinogenic. One of those, benzene, is a known human carcinogen, and the others are animal carcinogens and therefore a possible threat to humans.

Fortunately, the researchers were able to identify probable sources for most of the carcinogens—from which much can be learned. They're listed below, along with some ideas for reducing levels in your home.

GENERAL HOUSEHOLD PRODUCTS

They lurk in kitchen cabinets, attic closets, basement shelves and garage workshops. What's in them? Dr. Wallace's team found benzene in paints, "not at high levels but high enough to be measurable." (Cigarette smoking was the worst source of benzene.) Carbon tetrachloride, another animal carcinogen, was tracked to industrial strength cleansers and insecticides, although other sources may be possible.

The TEAM study wasn't the first to find carcinogens in household products. One example of a carcinogen that was removed from consumer products is trichloroethylene (TCE), a solvent that was widely used in aerosol products.

Similarly, there's an ongoing controversy over methylene chloride, another potent solvent that has been used not only in paints and paint strippers but also in aerosol hair sprays, cosmetics, and even decaffeinated coffee. The Consumer Product Safety Commission (CPSC) says that the chemical poses "one of the highest risks ever calculated for a consumer product." The Food and Drug Administration (FDA) has proposed banning methylene chloride from aerosol hair sprays, and the CPSC wants to designate it as a hazardous substance, but that could take time.

Suggestion: Dr. Wallace says that these kinds of products should be stored carefully or thrown out. And here are some other tips.

- Make sure that the products you keep are sealed tightly and kept in a ventilated garage or outdoor shed.
- Avoid aerosols. If you must use them, be sure the nozzle is pointed in the right direction.
- Always follow label directions.
- Whenever possible, replace strong chemical products with less toxic formulas (see below).
- Take special care to avoid or minimize use of pesticides (see below).

Moth crystals, room deodorizers and toilet-bowl cleaners are made primarily of para-dichlorobenzene, a chemical that was recently discovered to be an animal carcinogen. "They don't actually clean the air—they affect the central nervous system and deaden your nose," Dr. Wallace explains. "They evaporate slowly and are designed to stay at an elevated concentration in indoor air."

The researchers found that half the homes studied in New Jersey had elevated levels of para-dichlorobenzene. Further testing showed that even if the substance was kept in a shut closet, levels were elevated throughout the houses.

Even more disturbing, the researchers found that within a short time after the chemical was placed in a home, their subjects' blood levels of the chemical (as measured by breath analysis) rose dramatically. "That means it was collecting in blood and fat," says Dr. Wallace. "We could estimate a half-life in the body of at least 20 hours"—with unknown health consequences.

Suggestion: Avoid using these products. Ventilation is the best air freshener. Look for nontoxic substitutes (see below).

PERSONAL ACTIVITIES AND PRODUCTS

Cigarette smoking turned out to be the primary source of benzene, a known human carcinogen, that was found in many homes. Smoking also generates styrene, a mutagen and possible carcinogen. Family members beware: In homes where a smoker lived, there was 50 percent more benzene in the air. It's not news that passive smoking increases the risk of cancer (see chapter 63, Tobacco). "In the last two years, two studies, one American and one Swedish, have shown that children of smoking parents die of leukemia at a higher rate than children of non-smoking parents. In the Swedish study, if the mother smoked ten or more cigarettes a day, children's death rate from leukemia doubled," says Dr. Wallace.

One category of indoor pollutant that's received a great deal of attention recently is the trihalomethanes, including chloroform, which are considered to be carcinogenic. Trihalomethanes can be created at municipal water treatment plants if chlorine reacts with organic debris in the water.

The concern is not just for the water we drink. We also may breathe trihalomethanes in our home's air. How do they get into the air? The TEAM study findings led to the hypothesis that running hot water—in a shower, dishwasher, and so forth—can cause them to vaporize.

The researchers found that chloroform levels in the air inside homes were *four or five times* that of outdoor levels. "We felt it must be coming from water. We decided it's probably the use of hot water in homes—especially dishwashing and clothes washing," says Dr. Wallace. The researchers also identified a factor that makes the situation worse: using a chlorine bleach in the washing machine or a chlorine scouring powder. "We found that the scouring powder and probably the bleach create more chloroform as they react with dirt and water," says Dr. Wallace.

Suggestion: Make sure your laundry area is well ventilated, and minimize or eliminate the use of chlorine bleaches. Also, remember that showers can be a significant source of trihalomethanes in the air—especially if several people in the house shower and afterward leave the door open without venting the steamy air. So keep your exhaust system in your bathroom going when you shower, and afterward, don't leave the bathroom door open—shut it and open some windows.

CLEANING OUT THE HAZARDS

No doubt you can conclude from all this that good ventilation is very important. But Dr. Wallace says source removal is the *best* solution. "Ventilation will reduce chemicals by maybe 20 percent, but source removal reduces them 100 percent," he says.

What about air cleaners? Some air-cleaning devices can help reduce indoor levels of certain carcinogenic pollutants, says Dr. Wallace. While the devices don't reduce organic vapors, they can reduce levels of carcinogenic particulate matter, like benzo(a)pyrene (which comes from cigarette smoke). Since radioactive material (from radon) can settle on air particles, air-cleaning devices may help alleviate that problem, too.

Not all types of air-cleaning units are effective, but some "new generation" models appear to do the job, according to tests conducted by the product testing staff of *Rodale's Practical Homeowner* magazine. These include machines that use a prefilter (to strain out particles), then an activated carbon filter, an electrostatic precipitator and/or a negative ion generator. The activated carbon filter "adsorbs" certain gaseous pollutants, the electrostatic precipitator electrically charges particles and sort of magnetizes them to plates inside. The negative ion generator also charges particles on floors and walls—removing them from circulating air. (Some of these units have fans and filters that eliminate the pollutants before they reach the floor.) Or, as mentioned earlier, you can open a window.

But what do you do if you just can't do without mothballs, room deodorizers and strong cleansers?

The good news is that there's a whole new environmental movement trying to help people come up with safe alternatives. One chapter of the League of Women Voters is actively involved. They've designed a whole program around "household hazardous wastes"—what's safe, what isn't, what to buy and what to avoid. For more information, contact the League of Women Voters of Massachusetts, 8 Winter St., Boston, MA 02108.

Just to get you started, here are a few less toxic substitutes for some of the products which the TEAM study found problematic.

Closet and room fresheners. You can use a box of baking soda in enclosed areas such as refrigerators and closets. Freshen room air by sprinkling a sweet spice, such as ginger or nutmeg, on the floor before you vacuum.

Toilet cleaners. To remove light stains from the toilet, mix borax and lemon juice into a paste. After flushing, rub the paste on, and let it set two hours before scrubbing.

Mothballs. Make a sachet of dried lavender, equal parts rosemary and mint, dried tobacco, whole peppercorns and cedar chips, soaked in real cedar oil. Take care to store and maintain woolens correctly.

You can find plenty of other ideas in a book put out by the League of Women Voters of Massachusetts and the Golden Empire Health Planning Center in Sacramento, California. The book is *Making the Switch: Alternatives to Using Toxic Chemicals in the Home,* and can be ordered from the Golden Empire Health Planning Center, 2100 21st Street, Sacramento, CA 95818. The price is $5, including postage and handling.

A WORD TO THE CREATIVE

Artists are supposed to suffer a little, but they're not supposed to get *sick.* Whether you dabble in oil paints, throw pots, build furniture or snap photographs, you may be exposing yourself to potentially toxic chemicals, some of which have been linked to cancer, says Nancy Seeger, author of the *Alternatives for the Artists* series. Good ventilation in your work area is very important. Also, make sure you clean up all dust, spills and residues and wash your hands thoroughly. Don't ever smoke or eat while working. Wear a protective covering and mask when so recommended, and at home, keep children under 12 away from the materials being used.

THE PESTICIDE PROBLEM

Among household products, there has been a special concern about pesticides, including insect killers and weed killers, in the house and garden.

A homeowner should be extra careful with these products, says Alexandre Tarsey, Ph.D., head of the technical support section in the insecticide-rodenticide branch of the EPA.

"Most pesticides are intended to kill pests—that's what the word means," says Dr. Tarsey. "Anything that interferes with the biological system of an insect can conceivably cause problems with the biological system of a human being."

Some pesticides pose a cancer risk, and hundreds more require further testing (see chapter 53, Pesticides in Food). Even products containing suspected carcinogens are not necessarily banned from household use. (For example, 2,4-D, a widely used garden weed killer, has been linked to tumors in rats and is a possible cause of non-Hodgkin's lymphomas in human beings.)

"For the homeowner, by far the most important thing is to read the label," says Dr. Tarsey. "The EPA has very specific rules about the use of each particular pesticide."

Some pesticides may be dangerous if absorbed through the skin; others may be a threat if inhaled. "You'll find that each label is a little different," says Dr. Tarsey.

Another caveat: "If the product is registered for rose bushes, don't use it on tomatoes or strawberries." (You don't eat roses.)

You should also look for natural alternatives to home and garden insecticides: predatory pests, gummy pastes that trap and products with a "mating" scent that trap bugs in a bag.

OFFICE WORKERS BEWARE!

Everything we've said about air pollution in the home applies to the office, too—and maybe more so. Along with many of the same polluting chemicals that are in homes, offices also may have other sources of particularly toxic chemicals: copy machine toners, felt-tip pens and markers, correction fluids, carbonless carbon paper and paints.

The American Lung Association is very concerned about the possible health effects of air pollution in offices as well as homes. You can contact your local American Lung Association for more information.

CANCER PREVENTION PLAN: INDOOR POLLUTION

- If you suspect asbestos, formaldehyde or radon is present, have your home tested.
- If asbestos is present, have it professionally encapsulated or removed.
- If formaldehyde is present, remove or treat the source or purify the air.
- If radon is present, ventilate your home.
- Use and store hazardous household products with care.

C   H   A   P   T   E   R 43

Iron

Can pumping iron defend you against cancer? Not the kind of iron in a set of barbells, of course, but the kind you find in foods like beef liver, the dark meat of poultry like turkey and chicken, a baked potato, and even blackstrap molasses. The answer just might be *yes.*

Why? Because a diet deficient in iron weakens the immune system, and we need a strong immune system, researchers believe, to help prevent cancer. Just how does this metal strengthen your immune system? Basically, it's iron's job to help the body form hemoglobin, the protein in the blood that carries oxygen. All cells need oxygen to thrive, including the white blood cells—the guys at the front lines of immune defense. Without enough iron to produce this vital supply of oxygen-carrying hemoglobin, your white blood cells may not be able to fight off invading infections.

And that's just the kind of situation in which cancer cells could set up camp, says Joseph Vitale, Sc.D., M.D., professor of pathology, Boston

216

University School of Medicine. "A chronic iron deficiency may lead to tissue changes and may produce premalignant cell changes," he says. "Such a weakened environment could be particularly inviting to carcinogens, which may lead to cancer."

Oddly enough, though, too much iron may be as harmful to the immune system as too little. That's because cancer cells—like all other cells—also require oxygen to grow. But the compounds that form when too much iron interacts with oxygen can be harmful to the cells.

BUILT-IN IRON REGULATORS

Fortunately, most of us have a built-in iron regulator that safeguards us from overloading our cells with iron. When infection strikes, our bodies produce a protein called transferrin that takes iron out of circulation, locks it in the bone marrow and liver and makes sure that only our immune system has a key to the supply.

For some people, though, this iron safeguard system fails to function. In one recent study sponsored by the National Cancer Institute, researchers followed more than 21,500 Chinese men for ten years. When they reviewed the records of 70 who later died of liver cancer, they found that the men's blood readings taken at the outset of the study looked almost identical. Each had a high level of an iron-binding protein (called serum ferritin) in the blood, along with low levels of the iron regulator, transferrin. And these findings seem to indicate that the men had higher stores of iron in their bodies.

The researchers could only speculate on the role iron plays in the growth of cancer. "An excess of iron may promote an excess of oxygen [free] radicals, which we know can destroy healthy cells," says Richard G. Stevens, Ph.D., cancer epidemiologist with Battelle Pacific Northwest Laboratories in Richland, Washington.

Still other people have never had the iron regulator to begin with. It is estimated that 1 in 300 people is born without the ability to shed excess iron and may be at a genetic risk for a condition known as hemochromatosis, a disease that results from iron overload.

KNOW YOUR IRON INDEX

How can you tell if you are in danger of iron overload? The best way to find out is to have your blood tested, suggests Barry Skikne, M.D., associate professor of hematology, Department of Medicine, University of Kansas Medical Center, Kansas City.

A high level of serum ferritin and a low level of transferrin may indicate an increased risk for cancer of the liver. If that's what your blood indicates, your doctor may suggest that you select supplements without added iron and perhaps cut back on iron-laden sources of food.

More likely than not, though, your blood test will probably indicate that you have normal levels of iron or that you are even a bit low. In fact, reminds, Dr. Vitale, many people, especially young children and women of childbearing age, are "so low in iron stores that they will need to boost their supply with supplementation."

Here's the best way to keep your iron stores at a healthy level and to steel your cells against invaders:

- Include some vitamin C in every meal to enhance iron absorption. Drink orange or tomato juice and serve vitamin C-rich vegetables such as broccoli, green peppers, Brussels sprouts and caulifower. Don't forget to season with lemon or lime juice or parsley.
- Spread your meat protein out over more meals. Eat smaller portions of chicken, fish and red meat combined with fresh vegetables and whole grains.
- Use iron cookware. Simply cooking spaghetti sauce for three hours in an iron kettle boosts its iron content almost 30 times.
- If you take iron tablets, do so between meals and with vitamin C for maximum absorption.
- Avoid combining iron-rich foods with other foods that may block its absorption. Foods such as eggs, tea, spinach, rhubarb, eggplant, beet greens and lentils can inhibit iron absorption.

CANCER PREVENTION PLAN: IRON

- A high level of serum ferritin and a low level of transferrin may indicate an increased risk for cancer of the liver. The best way to find out where you stand is to have your blood tested.
- Include some vitamin C in every meal to enhance iron absorption.
- Spread your meat protein out over more meals.
- Use iron cookware.
- If you take iron tablets, do so between meals and with vitamin C for maximum absorption.
- Avoid combining iron-rich foods with other foods that may block its absorption.

C H A P T E R 44

Jewelry

A hot topic in the 1960s was hot gold—not stolen jewelry but the radioactive kind. It seems that people began showing up with skin lesions, including squamous cell carcinoma (skin cancer) on their ring fingers, the very same fingers that had been wearing a gold ring for some 20 years. The rings were found to be radioactive and, strangely enough, most of them were turning up in western New York state.

That prompted the Bureau of Radiological Health of the Food and Drug Administration (FDA) to put together a committee to review the radioactive gold problem. They concluded that contamination did not appear to be a widespread problem, and the issue was all but dropped—until recently.

RECYCLED WEDDING RINGS

A few years ago, New York health officials became suspicious when a report of cancer of the ring finger resurfaced in the empire state. They decided to investigate.

Sure enough, after conducting a statewide screening program involving 160,00 pieces of jewelry, researchers at the New York State

RADIATING BRILLIANCE

Ever wonder why some jewels are so brilliant? They're zapped with radiation! That's what makes the turquoise a truer blue and the topaz a dazzling yellow. Will wearing these gems make *you* glow? Experts say no.

According to Gail D. Schmidt, M.P.H., health physicist for the FDA's Center for Devices and Radiological Health, some methods of irradiation used to upgrade gems may leave radioactive material that decays over time. However, he assures, "the amount of radiation emitted is sufficiently low that we do not generally consider irradiated gems a health hazard."

If you are fond of wearing cloisonné jewelry, you probably should leave it in the jewelry box once in a while.

A few years back, health officials discovered that about 10 percent of the cloisonné enameled jewelry imported from the Far East contained glazes made with radioactive uranium—a substance that's used to produce specific colors, including bright beige and golden yellow.

Here, again, the danger to the wearer is minute. Says Anthony Tse, Ph.D., nuclear engineer with the Nuclear Regulatory Commission: "There is really no cause for concern unless the radioactive enamel is in direct contact with the skin every day for long periods of time."

For example, he explains, if you wore a pendant or bangle bracelet with the radioactive enamel surface touching your skin for ten hours every week, in a year's time you would have received a radiation dose of 2,000 to 4,000 millirems to the small area of skin. "This corresponds to a skin cancer incidence risk of two to four in a million." If you have a clothing barrier between the enamel surface and your skin, the radiation dose—and risk of cancer—is even smaller than that.

Contaminated cloisonné is no longer allowed to be produced or imported, thanks to a 1984 ruling by the NRC. If you have some of this exotic colored jewelry, though, you can wear it in good health—just make sure the enamelled surface is not next to your bare skin.

Department of Health uncovered nearly 200 items "hot" enough to make the Geiger counter needle jump off the scale. Of the 135 individuals who were exposed to the contaminated jewelry, 41 had mild to severe skin problems and 9 had squamous cell carcinomas at the site of exposure. Furthermore, reported the researchers, "the incidence of skin cancer on the ring finger was 11 times that expected for men and 45 times that expected for women."

Why was western New York cursed with tainted gold? Researchers believe that in the 1930s, certain jewelers in that area got hold of gold "seeds," hollow gold tubes that were filled with a radon-decayed product and which, at that time, were used to treat cancerous tumors. When the radon decayed, the gold seeds were no longer of medical use and somehow ended up in the hands of gold manufacturers for recycling into jewelry. Unfortunately, neither the jeweler nor the customer could know that hidden in the recycled gold was a radon-decayed product that remained radioactive long enough to cause cancer for 30, 40 or even more years.

Does that mean it's goodbye to that great gold ring you purchased at the antique fair in New York state? Probably not, according to Karim Rimawi, Ph.D., director of the Bureau of Environmental Radiation Protection and one of the investigators of the New York survey, who states, "We haven't seen any further cases since publicizing the report in 1984." That doesn't mean that contaminated jewelry is not around somewhere. "The question is: Are we not looking hard enough or does no problem exist?"

Although unlikely, it's possible that hot gold exists in other states, admits Gail D. Schmidt, M.P.H., health physicist with the FDA's Center for Devices and Radiological Health. "Western New York is the part of the country where the most extensive radiation screening of gold jewelry has been conducted," but, Schmidt continues, "the possibility may exist undetected in other locations, since 30 to 40 radon-producing facilities are believed to have operated in various cities throughout the U.S."

Still, he doesn't recommend getting rid of your old gold made in the 1930s and 1940s. He does suggest, however, that you stop wearing it if you notice a persistent irritation. "See your dermatologist right away. Redness on the ring finger may turn out to be more serious than a simple sensitivity to jewelry."

CANCER PREVENTION PLAN: JEWELRY

- Stop wearing your gold jewelry if you notice persistent irritation.
- See your dermatologist right away if you have redness on the ring finger.

Mammograms

Mammograms, breast x-rays that screen for cancer, had a questionable reputation for a number of years. And rightly so, since the radiation required by mammography reportedly caused more tumors than it could detect. But new reports are in, and they're shedding a new, more positive light on this technique.

The amount of radiation used in today's standard mammography (called xeromammography) is about one-tenth what it was 20 years ago. It's less than two rads of exposure. (A rad is the way exposure to radiation is measured. It is the "unit of absorbed ionizing radiation." In other words, the higher the number of rads, the more radiation your body has absorbed.) "The radiation risk today is so small there literally is no risk," says Leon Speroff, M.D., chairman of the Department of Reproductive Biology at Case Western Reserve University School of Medicine, Cleveland, Ohio.

An even newer form of mammography is available at larger city hospitals. Known as the film-screen technique, it gives off a lower dose of radiation—one-tenth of a rad. And the senograph, a mammography

222

machine developed in France, delivers the lowest dose ever—a total of about one-fiftieth of a rad for two views.

MAMMOGRAPHY CAN SAVE LIVES

Despite the potential danger of radiation, you may face more risk by not having mammograms done regularly as you grow older. Recent large-scale, long-term studies are showing mammography to be a highly effective way to prevent deaths from breast cancer through early detection. In the Netherlands, annual mammographic screening reduced the risk of breast-cancer death among women age 35 or older by 50 percent in one city.

The first reports from a long-term study in Sweden may show even more positive results. In this ongoing study, 162,981 women were randomly put into one of two groups—they either received no mammography screening or they received a mammogram every two to three years. After only seven years, there was a 31 percent reduction in deaths from breast cancer and a 25 percent reduction in advanced disease.

It doesn't take much figuring to see why mammography is so effective. It finds cancers long before they can be felt by hand, either by a woman or her doctor. Most women, and doctors, can first detect a lump when it has grown to about ¾ inch in diameter. At this time, the cancer has been growing for eight to ten years. It has a 30 to 40 percent chance of having spread beyond the breast to the lymph nodes under the arm, and possibly to other parts of the body. Mammography, on the other hand, can find lumps that are just half this size, or even smaller. The chances of the cancer having spread at this early stage are cut in half.

A mammogram can't tell you for sure if a lump is malignant or benign—only a microscopic study of cells from the mass can do that. And mammograms, unfortunately, cannot detect all cancers. Palpation (examination by touch) remains necessary to detect the 10 to 15 percent that are not visible with mammography.

SCHEDULING RECOMMENDATIONS

The American Cancer Society recommends a baseline mammographic screening for all women between ages 35 and 40 (this will be compared with future mammograms), a screening every one or two years for women ages 40 to 49 and annual screenings for all women age 50 and over. The rate of screening steps up at 50 because cancer is more likely to show up at that age and because the breasts of women over 50 are less glandular and dense than those of younger women, allowing mammography to be more accurate.

Also, the National Cancer Institute recommends that routine mammography for women under 35 years of age should be limited to those women who have a personal or family history of breast cancer.

Mammograms are seriously underutilized in the United States. Most are done to confirm the presence of a lump found by palpation, not to find hidden lumps. It's estimated that less than half of women over age 50 have had a baseline mammogram and that only 5 percent of women in this age group have an annual mammogram.

The time is right to ask your doctor if you should have mammography, Dr. Speroff suggests. "The true benefits of mammography have just become clear. Not every doctor is going to learn about this overnight." But they might learn about it much faster if their patients tip them off.

WHAT TO EXPECT FROM A MAMMOGRAM

Usually, you visit a radiology laboratory, diagnostic clinic, doctor's office or hospital outpatient clinic for a mammogram. The x-ray itself takes only about five minutes, but you'll probably need a half hour to complete the whole procedure.

You need no special preparations, but it's a good idea to wear a two-piece outfit instead of a dress, so you can disrobe to the waist gracefully. Also, don't wear talcum powder or skin cream on the breasts because these products can produce a suspicious-looking area on the x-ray.

The pictures are taken one breast at a time. Each breast is slightly compressed between a small shelf projecting from the machine and a cone lowered from above. The radiologist takes two pictures of each breast—one from the side and the other from the top (giving a top-to-bottom view).

The result will be images of the interior of your breasts recorded on film. Odds are, the x-rays will not turn up any signs of breast cancer. But if they do, they can save your life by allowing your doctor to treat you before the tumors have a chance to spread.

CANCER PREVENTION PLAN: MAMMOGRAMS

- If you are between 35 and 40, you should have a baseline mammogram, against which later tests will be compared.
- If you are between 40 to 49, you should should have a mammographic screening every one or two years.
- If you are over 50, you should should have annual screenings.
- If you are under 35, you should have mammograms only if there is a family history of breast cancer.

C H A P T E R 46

Marijuana

Cannabis is the scientific term. The people who use it are more likely to call it pot, dope, hash or reefer. But it all smokes down to the same thing: marijuana, the third most popular recreational drug in the United States after tobacco and alcohol.

Once regarded with nearly as much dread as heroin and believed to be the cause of "reefer madness," marijuana is a social climber that has all but shed its outlaw status over the past 20 years. In 1985, a National Institute on Drug Abuse survey found that almost 33 percent of the American population has tried marijuana at least once. Ten percent of the population uses marijuana currently (used marijuana in the month prior to the survey).

In 1982, the National Academy of Sciences' Institute of Medicine issued a report stating that marijuana use warrants "serious national concern," but that there is no conclusive evidence that it causes permanent long-term effects. Eleven states have decriminalized possession of small quantities of marijuana for personal use. And more than 30 states have recognized the therapeutic uses of cannabis by legalizing it for control of certain medical problems, such as the violent nausea associated with chemotherapy.

Because the scientific literature is inconclusive, a bitter debate has raged for years between those who assert that marijuana is relatively harmless and should be legalized and those who insist that it is dangerous and that laws against it should be strengthened. One of the key points of debate is the question of whether marijuana causes cancer.

There's no dispute about the immediate changes in the body that marijuana triggers. Small doses of marijuana can bring on the famous marijuana "high," relaxation combined with a heightened sense of touch, sight, smell, taste and sound. Other short-term effects may include a temporarily accelerated heartbeat and a rise in blood pressure. Higher doses can trigger more dramatic changes, including a dulling of attention, aggressive behavior or panic reactions. It should definitely not be used before driving or operating machinery.

Scientists believe that marijuana is not physically addictive to any significant degree. However, it is "under suspicion" for contributing to a range of health problems, from decreased sperm count to possible adverse effects on heart function. The by-products of marijuana remain in body fat for several weeks, with unknown consequences.

AN UNPROVEN LINK TO CANCER

But are the millions of Americans who smoke marijuana upping their risk of cancer? The answer is yes, possibly, but the evidence does not yet prove the connection definitively.

Ironically, the most serious suspicions about marijuana and cancer are proven indictments against tobacco, a very legal substance. Many scientists concur in the "educated guess" that marijuana promotes lung cancer, much as tobacco smoking does.

Marijuana has been called a "living chemical factory," it contains some 400 substances, which convert to over 2,000 chemical compounds when smoked or burned. Most lung disease is caused by inhaling foreign substances into the lungs, the American Lung Association points out. The smoke produced by marijuana cigarettes contains many of the same compounds as tobacco smoke, and may be even more irritating to the lungs.

The major difference between tobacco smoke and marijuana smoke is the "psychoactive" ingredient. Tobacco's activator is nicotine, which affects the central nervous system and cardiovascular system and lungs. In marijuana, the ingredients that stimulate these systems are a unique and little-understood class of chemicals called cannabinoids.

The most important cannabinoid is THC (full name: delta-9-tetrahydrocannibinol).

Like nicotine, THC is not proven to be "mutagenic"—that is, it does not appear to alter cells, and therefore would probably not cause lung cancer. But there are other substances in marijuana smoke that are mutagenic and are proven carcinogens. Marijuana smoke, in fact, contains more known carcinogens than tobacco.

That fact is enough to persuade leading scientists that regular marijuana smoking may contribute to lung cancer. In 1982, the National Academy of Science's Institute of Medicine issued a comprehensive 15-month evaluation of the health-related effects of marijuana, entitled *Marijuana and Health.* Arnold S. Relman, M.D., editor of the *New England Journal of Medicine,* who chaired the investigating committee, sums up the findings of their report on the subject of lung cancer: "Since marijuana smoke has many of the components of tobacco smoke," explains Dr. Relman, "the committee thinks that prolonged heavy smoking of marijuana would probably lead to cancer of the lungs and serious impairment of pulmonary function. The committee carefully points out, however, that there is so far no direct confirmation of this inference."

Here is the kind of evidence on which some people conclude that marijuana can cause lung cancer.

- Marijuana smoke contains substances such as carbon monoxide, ammonia and several other compounds, many of which are known as respiratory irritants. Worse yet, the smoke also contains N-nitrosamines, benzo(a)pyrene, and benzanthracene, three known carcinogens. Scientists who examined the makeup of marijuana smoke found that it was quite similar to tobacco smoke, but because marijuana smoke is less combustible, it contains about 50 percent more carcinogenic hydrocarbons. Another study found that marijuana smoke had 70 percent more carcinogenic benzo(a)pyrene than tobacco smoke.
- When "tars" from marijuana smoke are painted on the skin of mice, they produce abnormal tissue in the skin glands. In some of the studies, however, marijuana tars were less mutagenic than tobacco tars.
- Cells from human lungs grown in a laboratory and exposed to marijuana smoke stimulated irregular growth in the respiratory system. This abnormal growth resembled precancerous lesions that could contribute to the development of lung cancer.
- Young, chronic hashish smokers have abnormalities in the cell tissues lining the larger air passages in the lungs. These abnormalities may be precancerous. (Hashish is a stronger form

of marijuana.) This kind of damage is usually seen only in older, heavy tobacco smokers—those who have been smoking for 10 to 20 years.

● Animals exposed to marijuana smoke for one year suffered irreversible lung irritations, inflammations and damage following a 30-day recovery period.

Observations about the ways people in the United States and Europe use marijuana support the conclusion that it may cause cancer. Marijuana cigarettes are unfiltered, and smokers usually inhale more deeply than with tobacco. They often hold their breath after inhaling. Each "joint" is typically smoked down to the very end. These rituals are intended to maximize the "high"—but they also maximize the exposure of sensitive lung tissue to toxic substances.

Another reason to suspect that regular marijuana users are more susceptible to lung cancer is that many tobacco smokers have tried marijuana. Scientists fear that tobacco and marijuana may be a particularly dangerous and potentially synergistic combination—doing even more harm to the lungs than is done by the simple combination of the two substances alone.

THE HERBICIDE THREAT

Another possible factor that may contribute to the danger of marijuana smoke is a man-made factor: herbicides sprayed on marijuana. Some years back, there was furor over the U.S. government's policy of allowing paraquat to be sprayed on marijuana crops. Although it is not considered carcinogencic, paraquat is a toxic, potent herbicide that can cause grave, irreversible damage to various body organs, including the lungs.

According to Kevin Zeese, former national director of the National Organization for the Reform of Marijuana Laws, the Colombian government, in cooperation with the United States, is spraying not just paraquat but a variety of questionable chemicals on marijuana, including glyphosate, which the Environmental Protection Agency considers to be a possible carcinogen.

HOW DANGEROUS?

All that evidence sounds persuasive—but it is not considered definitive. There are studies of human populations in Costa Rica, Jamaica and Greece that indicate that there is no major statistically significant difference between cannabis smokers and nonsmokers with respect to health status. (However, these studies have been criticized on various methodological grounds. Smoking styles—including inhalation—may be safer in these countries, too.) The missing "links" from the evidence are the human and epidemiological (population) studies, which would, for example, show whether marijuana smokers in the United States are indeed more likely to develop lung cancer. These are the kinds of studies that cinched the case against tobacco smoking after 25 years of suspicions. "But it must be remembered that, in the case of tobacco smoking, debilitating lung diseases appear only after 10 to 20 years," notes the American Lung Association. Most marijuana smokers in the United States have not yet smoked that long. Therefore, it may be years before there is a noted increase of lung disease caused by marijuana smoke.

In the absence of that proof, some scientists say, the evidence should be kept in perspective. "The empirical proof [that smoking marijuana causes lung cancer] is not present," says John P. Morgan, M.D., medical professor and director of the pharmacology program at City University of New York Medical School. "When people say 'carcinogenic,' you have to remember what they mean is rubbing the tar on the skin of a rodent or putting it in a variety of preparations that might cause some cellular change. People don't *know* that smoking marijuana doesn't cause cancer. That's a political statement. People are very frightened."

Dr. Morgan adds, "Marijuana is a substance that has been used in this culture for a long period, and I don't know of a single cancer that can be attributed to smoking marijuana. That doesn't mean it didn't happen; just that, at this moment, there's no proof."

But the American Lung Association takes a strong stance against marijuana, based on the same evidence, explains Norman H. Edelman, M.D., consultant for scientific affairs for the American Lung Association, and professor of medicine and chief of the Division of Pulmonary and Critical Care Medicine at the University of Medicine and Dentistry of New Jersey-Robert Wood Johnson Medical School, New Brunswick, New Jersey.

"If you're doing a rigorous scientific study, you want absolute proof," says Dr. Edelman. "But if you're making health recommendations, it's ridiculous to wait for absolute proof.

"Cigarette smoking is the best example," he says. "We knew for a long time that cigarettes are irritating to the lungs and had cancer-causing elements in the smoke. But to prove it from an epidemiological point of view required many years. I think you can make the same argument about smoking marijuana. We know the smoke contains many irritating compounds, in higher concentrations than in cigarettes, including compounds associated with carcinogenesis. The question is, do you want to wait 20 years if you're dealing with a substance with no redeeming social value?" Dr. Edelman adds, "It's foolish of someone who smokes to wait until all statistics are in, because by that time they may have cancer."

HOW MUCH IS SAFE?

Would *occasional* users of marijuana also be at risk for lung cancer? That's another question that can't yet be answered in absolutes. Many scientists argue that there's no such thing as a threshold level of safety for carcinogens—that even tiny amounts can trigger changes. Dr. Edelman applies this argument to marijuana. "It's illogical to talk about threshold effects. There's no question that the risk will increase with the amount of exposure to any carcinogen. But there's no reason to believe that there is a threshold below which there is no risk. The less you smoke, the less risk. The more you smoke, the more risk. It's unlikely that there is some absolutely safe level."

SUSPECTED IMMUNE SUPPRESSION

There is one other possible, but far more tentative, connection that has been made between marijuana and cancer. That is the possibility that the active ingredient, THC, impairs immune function and therefore lowers the body's defenses against cancer and other diseases. There are studies which suggest that regular marijuana users have lower immunity, and some animal and cell studies indicate a correlation between marijuana smoking and reduced immune response. Monique Braude, Ph.D., research pharmacologist with the National Institute on Drug Abuse, who is evaluating the evidence on marijuana, says, "Among animals, it's well established that marijuana depresses immune function, but not as well established in humans. Alone, marijuana does not depress immune function badly enough. Still, it could be a risk factor in cancer patients who already have a depressed immune system." Also, Dr. Braude says, there is some concern that it could act as a "co-agent," contributing to lowered immunity "if it is taken at the same time as other drugs which depress immunity, like the drugs involved in chemotherapy."

CANCER PREVENTION PLAN: MARIJUANA

- Do not smoke marijuana.
- Do not smoke tobacco.

C H A P T E R 47
Moles

Moles that you're born with—congenital moles—carry a greater risk of developing into cancer than moles you get later in life. Size is often an indicator of future problems. Cancers called malignant melanomas develop in 5 to 10 percent of all congenital moles that measure an unbelievable ten or more inches across at delivery. Doctors recommend surgically removing them when the child is sufficiently developed, but before 12 years of age.

Most moles, however, are not congenital. Rather, they begin to develop during the first year, and by the time most people reach adulthood, they've amassed a number of them. Few of these will develop into cancer; most will begin to disappear as you age and eventually be completely gone.

Certain families seem to be more prone to getting moles than others. And of those, some seem to be at a much greater risk than normal in the development of malignant melanomas. (These same families are also at high risk for a number of other malignancies, including Hodgkin's disease, breast cancer and lymphoma.)

Check your family history for cases of melanoma associated with moles. If you find such a history, let your examining doctor know. Some other risk factors include fair skin and a record of sunburn in youth.

Doctors have designated such high-risk families as having Familial Atypical Multiple Mole Melanoma (FAMMM) syndrome. First-degree relatives of an affected person—brothers or sisters, parents and children—have a 50 percent greater risk of acquiring mole-related melanoma. Typically, persons in this group have large (greater than ½ inch), unusual moles, frequently located on the trunk. The moles can be either flat or raised, with uneven coloring and jagged borders. People in this group should work out a cancer surveillance program with their doctor.

The Skin Cancer Foundation and the American Academy of Dermatology recommend that most people have a total skin exam at least once a year. Those who have a record of skin cancer (or high risk) should be examined more often. These exams take only a few minutes in the doctor's office. Generally, the physician will examine your skin from head to toe, noting the size and location of your body's moles. Any that look suspicious will be noted so they can be carefully rechecked in future exams.

Having your doctor perform this service will serve two purposes. First, the doctor will find moles you can't see for yourself. Second, odd-looking moles can be identified and monitored. If abnormalities are diagnosed early, melanoma is almost 100 percent curable.

BIRTHDAY SUIT EXAM

You can do a similar examination at home on a more frequent basis. All you need is a good mirror, a well-lighted, private space like your bathroom and a simplified sketch of the human body. Basically, you will do the same thing that your physician does in the total skin exam, noting the arrangement and location of your moles. Don't forget to check between your toes, behind your ears, between the buttocks and in the genital area. You may want to enlist the aid of a friend or relative to help you check places that are too difficult for you to see clearly, like your scalp or some areas on your back.

See your doctor if you discover one or more of the following:

- A change in size, especially if it is sudden or seems to have grown quickly.
- Pain, soreness or itching.
- Moles that appear in clusters.
- Surrounding skin that becomes reddened or sore-looking; small red spots may appear that are not connected to the mole but are close to it.

- An existing mole loses its uniform, somewhat rounded shape, has ragged edges or develops "projections."
- Hardening or softening; the consistency of the mole itself changes.
- Flat moles that have become partially or completely raised.
- Color changes (usually the most obvious signs). The normal tan to brown color may take on a mottled appearance with various tones of brown to black, sometimes white, red or even a deep blue. The mole itself may seem to "bleed" color into surrounding skin.
- Scaling, crusting, bleeding; any changes in the surface of the mole that make it obviously different from normal.

The Skin Cancer Foundation has simplified the above advice into an easy-to-remember code. They call it the ABCD's of self-examination.

A for assymetry. Irregularly shaped moles should get attention.

B for border. Check the border for even, regular edges.

C for changes. Watch for changes in color.

D for diameter. Check the diameter for changes in size.

ABCD—it's as simple as that. Most moles aren't dangerous. It's learning to recognize the early danger signs that can make the difference between wellness and illness.

CANCER PREVENTION PLAN: MOLES

- Have a total skin exam at least once a year.
- Do a similar examination at home on a more frequent basis.
- See your doctor if you discover a change in the size of a mole; if you feel pain, soreness or itching; if surrounding skin becomes reddened or sore-looking; if an existing mole loses its uniform shape; if the consistency of the mole itself changes; if flat moles become partially or completely raised; if the mole changes color; if the color "bleeds" into surrounding skin; if there is scaling, crusting or bleeding; or if there are any unusual changes in the surface.

Nitrites and Nitrates

Repeat this: Nitrate begat nitrite begat nitrosamine begat mutagen.

No, you haven't just been inducted into a new religious cult. But you have recited the family history of a group of chemicals that animal studies have shown are among the most powerful causes of cancer. "People concerned with cancer should limit their nitrate intake," says Phillip Issenberg, Ph.D., of the Eppley Institute for Research in Cancer at the University of Nebraska Medical Center in Omaha.

While his advice is good, most people would not really know how to follow it. So picture a hand-embroidered tablecloth set with this: a crystal glass of cool, clear water, a platter of Italian-style mixed grille, *griglia mista,* which is made up of grilled sausage, thick sliced bacon, ham and smoked rabbit, along with a side dish combining sautéed zucchini, tomato and garlic fresh from the garden. Sound tempting? It loses some of its appeal when you learn that these foods contain the mutagens that may cause cancer. That's right. Vegetables, cured meats—even water—can contain nitrate, nitrite and nitrosamines. Nitrate and nitrite are very similar chemically—just one oxygen atom different. While nitrate alone is safe, unfortunately it has a tendency to break down into nitrite while food is sitting in the cabinet or refrigerator and while it is being cooked. Nitrate in food also can continue to break down into nitrite after it has been eaten. And nitrite can react with chemicals in your food and in your body to form carcinogenic nitrosamines.

According to the National Research Council (NRC), studies in Colombia, Chile, Japan, Iran, China, England and Hawaii have found that where there are high levels of nitrate or nitrite in the diet or drinking water, there is a higher incidence of stomach and esophageal cancer. These studies didn't measure each person's precise intake of nitrate and nitrite, so they can't be taken as definitive. Rather, they looked at the experience of certain high-risk groups—and found an ominous correlation.

According to the NRC, "The absence of evidence that nitrite is a direct carcinogen does not diminish the possibility that it can interact with specific components of diets consumed by humans and animals or with endogenous metabolites to produce N-nitroso compounds that induce cancer." Translation: Even without proof positive, we know enough about nitrite to say that it can interact with certain substances in food—or even with substances originating from our own bodies—to produce compounds that induce cancer.

These last suspects, the N-nitroso compounds, such as nitrosamines, occur when nitrate and nitrite break down, either in food or inside the body during digestion. Numerous studies have demonstrated that their link to cancer in lab animals is beyond doubt.

Roughly 300 of these nitrosamines have been tested by scientists for their cancer-causing effects. They've passed their tests with flying colors, though you might wish they'd flunked. The results showed that 80 percent of all the nitrosamines are capable of causing cancer in various tissues of one or more types of lab animals.

THE NITRITE SCARE

All this information really became a worry to people in the United States in the early 1970s, when government scientists found nitrosamines in some kinds of foods, including cooked sausage, cured pork, dried beef, cooked bacon and fish. Bacon got the worst rap because thin slices of the meat fried at high temperatures contained the highest levels. But, in fact, many popular foods of the American diet were threatened, because nitrate and nitrite were used extensively to give cured meats their rich color and—not to be overlooked—to prevent botulism, a lethal foodborne disease.

Nitrate was so popular with food manufacturers because, when it is used to cure meat, it decomposes to nitric oxide, which converts red and brown iron-containing pigments in the muscles and blood of the meat to bright red or pink compounds. This chemical action gives the meat a fresher appearance than the brown or gray look it would have without the additives. And the addition of chemicals also assured the manufacturer that the food could be transported and sold without the fear that a lapse in refrigeration could lead to fatal food poisoning.

Thus the U.S. government was put in the tricky position of weighing the toxic effects of nitrite against what was seen as a considerable benefit: preventing botulism. Given all the information, the Food and Drug Administration (FDA) considered a ban on nitrite in food.

And then a new study was completed, one which threatened to blow the lid off the nitrite controversy. A joint study by the Department of Health and Human Services and the Department of Agriculture found that it wasn't just nitrosamines that caused cancer. Nitrites by themselves also were indicted as carcinogens.

The FDA didn't want to act too hastily on the results of just one study, because a ban on nitrite could cost billions of dollars to the economy. So it had another group of scientists review the original study, which was done by a scientist at the Massachusetts Institute of Technology in Cambridge, Massachusetts. This group found that the original research might have been wrong about a lot of tissue samples that were analyzed and that diagnosis of some of the cancers had been questionable.

As a result, the FDA decided not to ban nitrite. But the FDA commissioner at the time still said that nitrite wasn't to be considered perfectly safe. Other researchers agreed with him. And while there is no concrete proof, many links between cancer in humans and nitrite have been found. And all the debate has definitely promoted a reduction in nitrite as a food additive.

Nitrite is now listed on food labels wherever it is used. And those who process food are now using less and less nitrite. For instance, the legal limit in bacon is now 100 parts per million, down from 200 parts per million a few years ago. Manufacturers add vitamin C to cured meats, because it inhibits the formation of nitrosamines in the lean part of bacon. And the federal government has approved another product that could make bringing home the bacon a little healthier.

Both the Department of Agriculture and the Food and Drug Administration have approved the use of alpha tocopherol, a form of vitamin E, as an optional ingredient in bacon. Vitamin E inhibits the formation of nitrosamines while the bacon is cooking. This process should reduce nitrosamine content in the fatty part of the meat by 70 to 80 percent, according to some estimates.

However, all this worry about nitrite and nitrate might someday be a thing of the past, because new methods of curing meats are being tested. One promising technique is the Wisconsin process, so called because it was developed at the Food Research Institute at Madison, Wisconsin. With this process, sugar and a harmless bacteria are injected into the bacon. When this meat is then left out at room temperature—the right conditions for botulism to form—the bacteria increase in number and give off lactic acid, which stops any botulism from growing. While the bacon isn't as "pretty" as nitrite-cured bacon, it does taste just as good. And it's safe.

According to Dr. Issenberg, the nitrate and nitrite controversy is a case where a problem was seen and a solution was found. "The levels of nitrite in processed meats have been reduced significantly in the last several years. It's at a point now where I would say that the major cancer risk from something like bacon is the high fat level, not the chemicals used to preserve it."

One health food crusader recommends that people avoid nitrite-treated meats. "I believe that nitrite-treated meats are problems in two regards: They increase slightly the risk of cancer, and they are generally loaded with saturated fat and salt. For these two reasons, I suggest that you eat salami, bologna, hot dogs and especially bacon rarely or not at all," says Michael F. Jacobson, Ph.D., of the Center for Science in the Public Interest.

Dr. Issenberg stresses that because no one knows what a "safe" level of nitrite or nitrate consumption would be, it's hard to make dietary recommendations. But he believes that as long as cured meats aren't a staple of a person's diet, there shouldn't be any problems with the additives. "A varied but balanced diet is the key," he says.

A balanced diet might include a salad rich in vitamin C with your meal or a glass of orange juice if you have bacon for breakfast. In fact, the vitamin C in the orange juice would help stop the small amount of nitrite left over after the bacon is cooked from turning into cancer-causing nitrosamines in your stomach. Eating something rich in vitamin C would be especially useful when you eat processed meats that don't have to be cooked—like salami in your sandwich. "It's important to remember that the vitamin C has to be eaten at the same time as the food with nitrite if you want to prevent nitrosamines from forming in your stomach. It won't do any good to take a vitamin C pill in the morning hoping for all-day protection," says Dr. Issenberg.

"NATURAL" NITRITE

A peculiar facet of the protective factor of a balanced diet is that fresh vegetables contain nitrite. But the danger isn't as great as it might sound. Most of these vegetables also contain vitamin C. "Most vegetables have enough of this, so there really isn't a problem of forming nitrosamines from eating vegetables. I think that a normal, varied diet with lots of vegetables poses no problem in terms of nitrosamines and cancer," says Dr. Issenberg.

SMOKED FOODS AND CANCER

Smoked foods (smoked oysters, cheese, sausages or fish) might be delicious, but they should be consumed as occasional treats or appetizers rather than as frequent main courses.

Why? Because the smoking process deposits mutagenic and cancer-causing substances on the surface of the food, according to the report, *Diet, Nutrition, and Cancer,* issued by the National Research Council. One study found a link between diets high in naturally smoked foods and cancer.

The cancer culprits are polycyclic aromatic hydrocarbons (PAH), and they occur any time an organic compound—including wood—is burned. But the carcinogen probably isn't much of a worry for most people in the United States, where natural smoked foods aren't usually considered a dietary staple, and those foods that are smoked are usually just smoked lightly for flavor. "If you go on a purely smoked foods diet, you should be concerned. But if you eat a little now and then, and have a varied diet, there is no problem," says Phillip Issenberg, Ph.D., professor at the Eppley Institute for Research.

Every bit as surprising as vegetables, drinking water also contains nitrate, which is converted to nitrite in the human body. In fact, sometimes water supplies are contaminated with *high* levels of nitrite. This contamination is mostly due to excessive use of fertilizers containing nitrate. When too much is put on a field, a good rain or excess irrigation will wash the chemical into the water supply. In fact, this runoff has been so bad that some town water supplies have been shut down because they were considered to have unsafe levels of nitrate.

According to Dr. Issenberg, people who rely on well water should have their water checked periodically. And if the level of nitrate is above 50 or 60 parts per million, steps should be taken to treat the water. Distillation is considered the best method.

People with city water shouldn't worry too much, however. The fact that some water supplies have been shut down because of nitrate contamination is a sign that the water is monitored closely. "State health departments have been cracking down more and more on public water supplies," says Dr. Issenberg.

FROM BABY BOTTLE TO BEER BOTTLE

Here's the lowdown on other recent nitrate controversies.

Baby bottle nipples. Canadian reports in the early 1980s showed that substances used to make baby bottle nipples contained trace amounts of nitrosamines. These carcinogens would migrate into the milk or juice in the bottle as the baby drank. Fortunately, the already low levels of these chemicals has been made even lower. And various nitrosamine inhibitors, in infant formulas, apple juice and orange juice (but not in milk) reduce the risk even further.

Beer. This drink did have high levels of nitrosamines at one time, but when scientists, the public and the manufacturers found out, new methods were developed for brewing beer. Now there are no nitrosamines in the suds.

Scotch. Six out of seven brands of Scotch whisky tested in 1979 contained very low levels of a carcinogenic nitrosamine. But while this substance can still be found in Scotch, it's present in such small amounts that it shouldn't be a problem. It would be difficult to drink enough Scotch to suffer ill effects from the nitrosamines. "You'd die from alcohol poisoning before you got cancer from nitrosamines," says Dr. Issenberg.

Tobacco. Tobacco smoke is a very complex mixture, with nitrosamines probably just being one culprit among many other carcinogens. Chewing tobacco and snuff, on the other hand, present nitrosamines as the big culprit. In fact, they have few problem chemicals besides nitrosamines. Yet they lead to all kinds of oral cancer—lip, tongue, mouth, esophageal and others. Therefore—and this statement cannot be made too frequently—stay away from all kinds of tobacco, because whether it is smoked and inhaled or chewed, tobacco is one of the more dangerous sources of nitrosamines.

If you don't eat cured meats excessively, if your water supply is good and you avoid tobacco, the amount of nitrite and nitrate you take in is probably safe. "While people should be concerned about their nitrite and nitrate intake, it's not really much of a problem for most people because, by now, nitrite levels are regulated to safe amounts," says Dr. Issenberg.

CANCER PREVENTION PLAN: NITRITES AND NITRATES

- Do not eat cured meat (ham, sausage and bacon, for example) as a staple in your diet.
- Do not smoke tobacco.
- If you use well water, be sure your drinking water has been tested for acceptable levels of nitrites.
- Eat smoked foods as occasional treats or appetizers, not as frequent main courses.
- When choosing smoked foods as a snack, select those that are labeled "smoke-flavored."

Obesity

A rat that has nothing to do all day but eat and sleep and sit around on the bottom of its cage gets about as big as the top third of a volleyball," says R. K. Boutwell, Ph.D., from McArdle Laboratory for Cancer Research at the University of Wisconsin.

And a round physique is the *least* of its problems—it also has an increased chance of getting cancer.

The same goes for mice. Two-thirds of the overfed mice in one study developed breast cancer in 1½ years. None of the mice that were fed normally developed that disease. Study after study has confirmed that obese rodents are more prone to cancer than their leaner counterparts.

But do these findings apply to obese *humans?* Could be. The matter is still in the early stages of investigation, but preliminary evidence seems to confirm this suspicion.

DOES OVERWEIGHT CAUSE CANCER?

The American Cancer Society conducted a large-scale investigation that brought a great deal of attention to the cancer-obesity link. The researchers kept tabs on 750,000 people for 12 years to see who would get cancer. And they found that people who were 40 percent or more over the average weight for their height were more likely to die from cancer. Overweight men had higher rates of death from colorectal and prostate cancer, and overweight women had higher rates of death from cancer of the endometrium, uterus, gallbladder, cervix, ovary and breast.

Cancer of the endometrium was the most prevalent cause of death for all the cancers studied. Women as little as 10 percent overweight had a 36 percent greater risk for this type of cancer. But for women 40 percent or more overweight, the risk skyrocketed to 5.5 times, which means their chances of dying were that much greater for this type of cancer. The researchers concluded, "The regularity with which obesity is found as a risk factor in a number of studies implies but does not prove that [overeating] may be a risk factor for a number of cancer sites."

Other studies tend to support these findings. A major study of 32 countries, for instance, showed that colorectal cancer and leukemia in men and breast cancer in women were common in areas where the average person ate more food. Researchers from the Johns Hopkins School of Public Health, Baltimore, Maryland, studied 6,763 men and found that those who were overweight had 2.5 times the risk of getting fatal prostate cancer.

While it looks likely that obesity is related to cancer, nobody knows exactly why. But scientists have suggested several theories.

"It could be that a larger person has more body tissue, and thus has more cells which could be at risk for cancer," says Demetrius Albanes, M.D., investigator of cancer prevention and control at the National Cancer Institute, Bethesda, Maryland. "Or consuming large amounts of food may expose people to more carcinogens that may be present in what they are eating. Another theory is that the faster basal metabolic rate associated with high caloric intake may increase cell division, which may increase your chances of developing a cancer." (Basal metabolic rate, or BMR, is the amount of calories that you have to burn to stay alive—to breathe, think and fuel your body's internal maintenance program.)

A more popular theory has to do with hormones. Many older overweight women have high levels of the female hormone called estrone. That's because after menopause, most of this hormone is manufactured in the fat cells. And the more fat cells there are, the more hormones can be manufactured. Some scientists believe that high levels of estrone cause cancer of the uterus and breast, perhaps by overstimulating these organs.

Or maybe obese people don't produce *enough* hormones to prevent cancer. "Obese laboratory animals have been found to secrete less cortisol, a hormone which turns body fat into glucose," says Dr. Boutwell. "That's because their body can use fuel from food—they don't need to mobilize body fat. Cortisol seems to have a protective effect against cancer."

Possibly, the type of food put into one's mouth does more harm than the fat it may form in one's body. A poor diet—with plenty of fat and sugar and small amounts of fiber—can promote cancer *and* cause obesity.

SHOULD YOU LOSE WEIGHT?

If you asked a group of scientists whether obesity causes cancer, you will hear no loud, hearty "yes!" Evidence *seems* to show a link, but science demands a proof-positive connection. It may be years before that link is proven to the satisfaction of the scientific community. In the meantime, if you are overweight you may well be at risk—not only of developing cancer but other diseases as well. While research studies further, the wise overweight person will begin to lose weight.

What is the ideal weight, health-wise? The Metropolitan Life Insurance Company compiled a chart to answer that question—it shows the weights associated with the smallest death rates. However, these tables may be misleading because they don't account for age. Scientists at the Gerontology Research Center in Baltimore, Maryland, analyzed the Met Life data on which the tables are based, and found that people with the lowest mortality rate tended to gain about a pound a year, more or less, between age 25 and age 65. They wove their new findings into a height/weight/age table (see the table, Desirable Weight by Age, on the opposite page).

Scientists still disagree as to which ideal weight table is ideal. Regardless, *no* printed table can tell you whether that weight is packed into heavy muscles or fluffy fat. But a table can help you and your doctor decide which weight you want to aim for.

THE FIVE BEST TIPS
FOR NATURAL WEIGHT LOSS

To lose weight, the rule is simple: Eat sensibly and exercise.

Simple to say, that is. But if that rule were simple to follow, weight loss books wouldn't be topping the best-seller lists.

CONTROL PORTIONS

Imagine consuming nothing but a chalky protein drink and some vitamin pills for breakfast and lunch every day until you're thin. It sounds grim, but it's exactly what some diet plans recommend.

Just how long would you expect to stay on such a diet? Not long, huh? It's just too boring and unappetizing. You're more likely to stick

DESIRABLE WEIGHT BY AGE

	METROPOLITAN LIFE INSURANCE COMPANY		GERONTOLOGY RESEARCH CENTER				
HEIGHT IN FEET AND INCHES*	WEIGHT IN POUNDS* AGES 25–29		WEIGHT IN POUNDS† MEN AND WOMEN BY AGE				
	MEN	WOMEN	25	35	45	55	65
4–10	. . .	100–131	84–111	92–119	99–127	107–135	115–142
4–11	. . .	101–134	87–115	95–123	103–131	111–139	119–147
5–0	. . .	103–137	90–119	98–127	106–135	114–143	123–152
5–1	123–145	105–140	93–123	101–131	110–140	118–148	127–157
5–2	125–148	108–144	96–127	105–136	113–144	122–153	131–163
5–3	127–151	111–148	99–131	108–140	117–149	126–158	135–168
5–4	129–155	114–152	102–135	112–145	121–154	130–163	140–173
5–5	131–159	117–156	106–140	115–149	125–159	134–168	144–179
5–6	133–163	120–160	109–144	119–154	129–164	138–174	148–184
5–7	135–167	123–164	112–148	122–159	133–169	143–179	153–190
5–8	137–171	126–167	116–153	126–163	137–174	147–184	158–196
5–9	139–175	129–170	119–157	130–168	141–179	151–190	162–201
5–10	141–179	132–173	122–162	134–173	145–184	156–195	167–207
5–11	144–183	135–176	126–167	137–178	149–190	160–201	172–213
6–0	147–187	. . .	129–171	141–183	153–195	165–207	177–219
6–1	150–192	. . .	133–176	145–188	157–200	169–213	182–225
6–2	153–197	. . .	137–181	149–194	162–206	174–219	187–232
6–3	157–202	. . .	141–186	153–199	166–212	179–225	192–238
6–4	. . .	. . .	144–191	157–205	171–218	184–231	197–244

SOURCES: Metropolitan "Height and Weight Tables," 1983, *Statistical Bulletin,* January–June 1983, Gerontology Research Center tables from Andres, Bierman, and Hazzard, *Principles of Geriatric Medicine* (New York: McGraw-Hill, 1985) pp. 311–318.

NOTE: Scientists have found that people with the lowest mortality rate tend to gain about a pound a year.

*Without shoes.
†Without clothing or shoes.

with a new eating plan through thick and thin if you gradually modify your usual meals. You don't have to give up your favorite dishes—just eat less.

Seem impossible? How could you pass up a second helping of lasagna, its cheesy splendor beckoning to you? You could call upon your will power, but any dieter can tell you how *powerless* will power is in the presence of lasagna.

The battle is easier if you overcome the temptation before you start to eat. Dish out the food in the kitchen. Any leftovers? Freeze them immediately so you have an easy meal for some other day. Or at least keep food away from the dinner table, so you don't grab for more automatically.

Then, eat slowly. Relish each morsel. Put your fork down between bites. Don't add food to your mouth before you have swallowed the previous bite. Talk. The idea behind these delay tactics is to give your stomach the 20 minutes it needs to tell your brain, "Enough food! I'm full." If you eat fast, so the theory goes, you will have eaten more food before the full message kicks in.

If you want a second helping, wait five minutes. A short "time-out" further prolongs your dinner and gives you time to decide if you're really hungry for that second helping after all.

Finally, enjoy an after-dinner drink in place of dessert. Mint tea is a low-calorie drink that can refresh your mouth and tell your taste buds that this meal has ended.

AVOID TEMPTATION

When do you eat the most?

Is it when you're sitting around alone on a Saturday afternoon with nothing to do? If that's the case, plan something to do at that time. Go for a walk. Invite a friend over. Learn to play a musical instrument.

Do you go ice cream crazy whenever your spouse eats a banana split in front of you? Ask him or her to eat it in the next room.

Do you overindulge in potato chips during your weekly bridge game? Why not take along some garden-fresh vegetables and a low-calorie dip?

If there is a time or a place or a situation in which you're tempted to binge, be prepared. Plan an activity that doesn't involve eating, or eat a food that is healthier and lower in calories. Which brings us to our next point.

CUT FAT

Weight problems aren't always a matter of how much you eat. *What* you eat counts, too. And fat is something you want to eat less of. In a study of rats, researchers at the University of Illinois in Chicago found that those who subsisted on a diet high in fat while they were young grew into overweight adults, even though they didn't overeat.

If you're a true-blooded American, you probably don't fare much better than the rats. Fat accounts for more than 40 percent of the calories in the American diet—about 135 pounds of fat per person per year. Nearly half of that comes from saturated (animal) fat, the most harmful kind. Nutritionists recommend cutting caloric fat intake to 30 percent or less, taking as much as possible from the unsaturated (or vegetable) variety.

Red meat, dairy products, creamy sauces and pastries are rich sources of saturated fat, so keep them to a minimum.

You can also reduce your fat intake through low-fat cooking. Cut away the visible fat from all meat and poultry before cooking. And peel the skin off that chicken—this simple step can cut fat content by up to one-half.

If you fry, avoid cooking with oil. Instead, try a nonstick pan or a nonstick vegetable spray. Or poach meat, poultry and fish in seasoned stock, flavored vinegars or water mixed with lemon juice or soy sauce. Better yet, cook meat on a broiling pan. Excess fat will drip into the lower pan, away from the food. Instead of frying chopped onions, steam them.

Also try low-fat substitutes for high-fat ingredients. Use stock, herb tea or juice instead of oil in marinades. Replace at least two-thirds of the oil in a basic vinaigrette salad dressing with pureed cucumber or plain low-fat yogurt. In recipes that call for ricotta cheese, use 1 percent low-fat cottage cheese instead—it can reduce calories by as much as 50 percent. Think up your own substitutes, and you can enjoy your favorite dishes while eating fewer calories.

EAT HIGH-FIBER FOODS

Eat more and weigh less? That's what one study from the University of Alabama, Tuscaloosa, implied. The researchers allowed people to "pig out" on high-fiber, "low-energy-density" foods, such as fresh fruit, vegetables, whole grains and beans. Another group had free access to low-fiber foods such as ham, roast beef, french fries and desserts. The first group spent more time eating, but took in half the calories (1,570 versus 3,000) of the second set of diners.

Fiber has been touted as a superhero in the weight-loss scene. High-fiber food takes longer to eat. Fiber has been shown to make you feel full longer by keeping food in the stomach longer and lowering levels of insulin, a hormone that stimulates the appetite. And that's not all. It has also been shown to escort certain dietary fats out of the intestine before they've had a chance to be absorbed. It's been estimated, in fact, that a diet rich in fiber could reduce the number of available calories one eats by about 5 percent, enough to dispose of about a hundred extra calories a day.

If you want to add more fiber to your diet, here are ten foods that are delicious, readily available, and high in fiber: 100 percent bran cereal, prunes, apples, lima beans, pears, nectarines, shredded wheat, peas, brown rice and unpeeled potatoes.

WALK

Cutting calories may not be enough. Start a diet and the weight begins to fall off at a brisk clip. After a few weeks, though, that brisk clip turns into an amble, then a shuffle. Eventually, it can become walking-in-place. When the basal metabolic rate wakes up one day and finds that you're dieting, it doesn't say, "Hooray!" It says, "Oh, oh. Something's wrong!" It thinks you're starving. And to protect you against this "impending starvation," it slows down. Every hour, it burns fewer calories—instead of a typical 70 an hour, for instance, it might drop to 60, or even lower. Multiply that by 24 hours a day, and you discover that a couple of hundred calories you *thought* you were dieting away actually are locked away in a kind of trust fund.

So the nonactive dieter finds himself the recipient of a double whammy: a restricted diet and a pinch-purse BMR that thinks it's saving his life.

The answer is simple: Walk your weight away. Mile for mile, you'll burn up about as many calories as if you were jogging. You'll also prevent your basal metabolic rate from doing you favors you don't need. An especially vigorous walk will actually *raise* your BMR for some time after you cease walking.

And with walking, you lose the right *kind* of weight. Weight lost with exercise is almost all fat, while dieting also tears away valuable body protein.

The importance of walking was demonstrated in a study of 11 chronic dieters who couldn't keep their weight off with low-calorie diets. Without changing their eating habits, they managed to drop an average of 22 pounds within one year simply by adding a walk to their

---

CANCER PREVENTION PLAN: OBESITY

- Those who are 40 percent or more over the average weight for their height are more likely to die from cancer.
- Overweight men have higher rates of death from colorectal and prostate cancer.
- Overweight women have higher rates of death from cancer of the endometrium, uterus, gallbladder, cervix, ovary and breast.
- Eat sensibly.
- Exercise.
- If you are overweight, lose weight.

daily routine. Weight loss didn't start until walks routinely exceeded 30 minutes a day.

So add a walk to your daily routine. If a half hour sounds too long, start with a ten-minute walk and work your way up from there. Also, build walking into your everyday life. Take the stairs instead of the elevator. Park at the far end of the parking lot. Walk to the newspaper stand Sunday morning. Or walk to work. Make up your own strategies.

Oral Contraceptives

They're effective, they're convenient, they're really quite popular—but even 25 years after their introduction, women still worry about the safety of oral contraceptives.

Indeed, in a recent Gallup survey, three-fourths of the women interviewed felt that birth control pills are risky. And what worries them most is that the Pill might cause cancer.

A common fear, perhaps, but it's as outdated as lovebeads, say experts. That's because the oral contraceptives, or OCs, of today are new and improved. These pills are less potent, with less risk of causing cardiovascular disease and—surprise—whether old or new, they may even *protect* you from certain forms of cancer. And today there are plenty of studies to prove it.

THE PARED-DOWN PILL

"Misconceptions about the Pill are astounding," says Elizabeth Connell, M.D., professor of gynecology and obstetrics, Emory University School of Medicine in Atlanta, Georgia. Yet, the birth control pill has been under more study than any drug in history. "You just can't compare the Pill of today to the Pill of 10 or even 5 years ago," she says. "And you certainly can't compare it to the Pill that first came out 25 years ago."

The original birth control pill, Enovid 10, had 150 micrograms of estrogen and ten milligrams of progestin (the synthetic version of the natural progesterone hormone). Today's Pill is pared down. It contains only 50 micrograms or less of estrogen and just one milligram of progestin. A third less estrogen means less chance of it causing strokes, blood clots, heart disease or other serious side effects. At the same time, a reduced amount of estrogen has decreased the "nuisance" side effects that range from breast tenderness to bloating.

These low-dose OCs may be lean but they are just as mean as previous pills when it comes to controlling fertility. The estrogen portion prevents ovulation by inhibiting the pituitary hormones that stimulate the ovaries to release an egg. Meanwhile, estrogen's partner, progestin, thickens your cervical mucus so sperm can't get through. If that's not enough protection, the Pill alters the uterine lining so even if ovulation occurs and an egg does become fertilized, it doesn't have a chance to get implanted in the uterus.

It all adds up to near-perfect protection against pregnancy, failing less than 1 percent of the time, if used correctly.

PROTECTION AGAINST CANCER

What's really placed the Pill in a positive light is the news that it can protect you from cancer of the ovaries and endometrium.

That's the word from the researchers who conducted the Cancer and Steroid Hormone Study, or CASH, a multicenter, population-based, case-controlled study sponsored by the Centers for Disease Control (CDC), Atlanta, Georgia, and the National Institute of Child Health and Human Development. CASH involved nearly 10,000 women aged 20 to 54, and is the largest and most respected study ever to investigate Pill usage and its risks of developing cancer of the endometrium, ovary and breast. Their results are providing welcome reassurance for countless women.

For starters, CASH researchers discovered that women who took the Pill for three months or more reduced their risk of getting ovarian cancer by 40 percent. The longer they used the Pill, the more they were protected. What was even more astonishing was that this protective effect showed up as much as ten years after the women first started using the Pill.

For endometrial cancer, the story is similar. Women who used the Pill for at least one year had half as much risk of developing endometrial cancer as women who had never used the Pill. Using the Pill for longer than that didn't seem to provide any extra protection. Again, the protective benefit appeared to linger—the risk of developing endometrial cancer remained lower in OC users for more than ten years even after they discontinued using them. Interestingly enough, the protective effect did not show up in women who had had a pregnancy.

What's going on here? No one is really sure, says past project director of the CASH study Peter Layde, M.D., coordinator of chronic disease activities with the CDC, but there are definite theories. "When the body is repeatedly stimulated by *natural* estrogen and progesterone hormones, it may make normal cells grow faster and abnormally until they become cancerous," he explains. "During pregnancy, the ovaries get to rest and do not have to produce estrogen and progesterone. The same thing seems to be happening with birth control pills."

Apparently, when the Pill introduces an artificial supply of estrogen and progesterone into the bloodstream, the ovaries don't have to do their job of meeting their "hormone quota." So they take a break. At the same time, the Pill may be protecting the endometrium by preventing rapid production of its lining. "Even a few months' rest may be enough to allow the ovaries and endometrium to regenerate and prevent carcinogenesis for a lifetime," says Dr. Layde.

That protective perk of the Pill is nothing to sniff at; experts believe it could save lives. CASH researchers estimate that more than 1,700 cases of ovarian cancer and approximately 2,000 cases of endometrial cancer are prevented each year by past and current Pill use among women in the United States.

Don't expect, however, to be popping the Pill strictly for cancer control—at least not yet, cautions Dr. Layde. "I wouldn't recommend taking the Pill for reasons other than for controlling fertility," he says. "The Pill may still exert a profound effect on the body over long-term use."

A BRIGHT PICTURE FOR BREAST CANCER

It's comforting to know that the Pill protects the ovaries and endometrium. But there remains in many people's minds a niggling fear about its association with breast cancer. Does taking the Pill increase a woman's odds of developing breast cancer?

"As a matter of fact, much Pill research has been directed at finding the answer to that very question," says Bruce Stadel, M.D., medical officer, Contraceptive Evaluation Branch, National Institutes of Health. "The incidence of breast cancer is so high that if the Pill had any effect on breast cancer, it would be of great importance." The good news is that it doesn't appear to. "So far, the substantial weight of evidence found through epidemiologic studies is that the Pill has no effect on breast tissue, positive or negative."

However, researchers have continued to check for a link to cancer. Each time they have found the same thing: Oral contraceptives appear to be safe in relation to breast cancer. In a large case-controlled study reported by the Drug Epidemiologic Unit at Boston University's School of Public Health, 1,191 breast cancer patients aged 20 to 59 were matched with 5,026 control subjects. The results? They found that women who had used the Pill for five years or more were not at an increased risk of developing breast cancer, even ten years or more after discontinuing their use.

The CASH study results are equally reassuring—and then some, reports Dr. Stadel. "Not only did we find no increased risk of breast cancer in relation to the use of the Pill before the age of 25, but the patients' age, family history of breast cancer, age at first pregnancy, the potency of the pills or how long they were used made no difference to relative risks."

What this means is that you probably can't pin the blame for breast cancer on the Pill. "The picture we are getting at the present time is that oral contraceptives present no problem to the breasts," says Dr. Stadel.

Studies, however, will continue. "A study of OCs and breast cancer in older women will need to be done sometime in the 1990s," reminds Dr. Stadel. Why? Because most breast cancer in the United States occurs after age 55, and few women currently older than that took the Pill when they were younger. So their relationship can't be studied yet. "In another five or ten years, we may be able to be even more sure that there is no relationship between the Pill and breast cancer," he says.

THE CASE FOR CONTINUING STUDIES

As one expert put it, we are in the middle of the story when it comes to oral contraceptives and cancer. So far, the story is getting better and better. Part of the reason is that we are learning more about the risk factors that play a role in cancer development. Without accounting for these various other factors in Pill research, the story is incomplete. For example, some studies, like the one conducted by a cancer researcher from the University of California School of Medicine at San Francisco, found an increase in superficial spreading melanoma (a virulent skin cancer) in women who had used the Pill for more than five years. However, more recent studies found no link between melanoma and Pill use. One plausible explanation for the difference, says Dr. Stadel, is that some studies did not take into account the fact that many women may have had long-term sun exposure, which is a known cancer risk.

Right now, experts are trying to dig through the latest chapter in the oral contraceptive/cancer story—the one that takes a look at cervical cancer.

Here, the plot appears to thicken, with fingers pointing at the Pill. Studies are showing that women who take oral contraceptives for many years show an increase in both cervical dysplasia (abnormal cells in the cervix) and invasive cancer of the cervix. According to experts, what may be occurring is that if a woman has abnormal cells, the Pill may prompt the cells to progress to a cancerous stage.

To get the whole cervical cancer story, though, you must read between the lines, explains Nancy Lee, M.D., medical epidemiologist, Division of Reproductive Health at the CDC. "The link could be accounted for because Pill users may be more likely to have multiple sexual partners than nonusers." The more partners, the greater the probability of that woman exposing herself to sexually transmitted viruses, a likely contributor to cervical cancer risk. What's more, she says, cervical cancer would be more likely to be detected among Pill users since they usually get a Pap smear each time they get a prescription.

Just how much of a risk of cervical cancer are we talking about, anyway? Not much, according to preliminary results from the ongoing study being conducted in 11 countries by the World Health Organization. Researchers did report a greater risk for cervical cancer among Pill users, with the risk possibly increasing the longer a woman took the Pill. "But it's not a very dramatic risk when you consider that there's a tenfold risk of lung cancer that shows up for smokers," reminds Dr. Lee.

All in all, she concludes, birth control pill users can rest easy regarding cancer risk. "I do not feel the current cervical cancer studies provide enough reason for women to abandon the birth control pill," says Dr. Lee. She does feel, however, that Pill users should get annual Pap smears, which can detect abnormal cells early and thus result in successful treatment.

Other doctors believe that getting more of the B vitamin folate in the diet could effectively counteract cervical cell changes which frequently appear with Pill use. Dr. Stadel is currently supporting research to determine just what part this nutrient may play in preventing cervical cancer.

WEIGHING THE RISKS

In the meantime, the bottom line on birth control pills is bright, assures Dr. Lee. "After reviewing all the evidence we have on the Pill, we have no firm or convincing knowledge that OCs cause any kind of cancer."

Aside from cancer risk, you also need to weigh the risk of pregnancy. "Many women forget that pregnancy and childbirth are more risky than the Pill," says Dr. Lee. In the Gallup survey previously cited, 65 percent of the people surveyed rated childbearing less risky or as risky as the pill. It isn't. It's about twice as risky. For each 100,000 women who use the Pill, there will be about five deaths related to the Pill compared to about ten deaths per 100,000 related to childbirth.

Despite all the reassuring news, it doesn't mean OCs are right for you. If you have sexual intercourse only sporadically, for example, it may not make sense to take OCs. Another type of birth control might be more sensible.

WHEN THE PILL IS PROHIBITED

Despite its reputation for safety, oral contraceptives are off-limits for those with a personal or family history of thromboembolic disorder (such as phlebitis), stroke, heart disease, benign liver tumor, cancer of the breast or reproductive system.

In addition, you should avoid using the Pill if you have high blood pressure, gallbladder disease, injury to the leg or impaired liver function, or if you are scheduled to have surgery in the next four weeks.

If you smoke, you should definitely consider another contraceptive. A smoker is 6 times more likely to have a stroke than a non-Pill user, but a Pill user who smokes is 22 times more likely to have a stroke than a woman who does neither.

To understand just how smoking skews safety statistics on the Pill, consider this. Of the 500 Pill-related deaths each year, if no one aged 35 and over used the Pill, and if no one who smoked used the Pill, the mortality figure would be reduced to 70 women.

That leaves the question of age. How long can you keep taking the Pill? Many doctors feel you can take the Pill past 40. In fact, says Robert Hatcher, M.D., professor of gynecology and obstetrics, Emory University School of Medicine, "the forties may be the decade in a woman's life when the Pill may prove most protective against ovarian and endometrial cancer." Eventually, it may be found that the period from age 35 to 50 is one in which the benefits of oral contraceptives are very high relative to the risk.

PERSONALIZED PILL PLAN

If you don't smoke and are free of serious health problems, your doctor will try to prescribe a Pill potency that fits your own body chemistry. "All women produce different amounts of estrogen and progesterone normally," says Stephen H. Paul, Ph.D., chairman of the Department of Pharmaceutical Economics and Health Care Delivery at Temple University in Philadelphia. If a pill doesn't fit, you'll know it from side effects.

If a pill has too much estrogen for your system, you may experience the more serious side effects like migraines, nausea or high blood pressure. Too little estrogen may cause you to spot or bleed at midcycle.

On the other hand, if your pill has too much progestin, you may be plagued with any number of annoying side effects like acne, vaginal infections, missed periods or breakthrough bleeding.

If you are a nursing mother, you are over 35 and a smoker or you cannot tolerate estrogen, your doctor may recommend the minipill. These pills contain only progestin and, while they don't invariably stop ovulation, they do thicken the cervical mucus and interfere with the uterine lining, which makes pregnancy improbable.

What could be winners in the OC category are the new multiphasic pills. Each tablet is packed with just enough estrogen so you won't ovulate. But what makes these pills different is that they contain booster amounts of progestin for you to take at differentpoints in the menstrual cycle in order to minimize breakthrough bleeding and annoying side effects.

The newest of these pills, the triphasics, dole out progestin in three phases during the cycle, which is said to mimic the way you naturally produce varying amounts of hormones each month. One of them changes the amount of estrogen as well.

The lowdown on the newest OCs is that they have about the same effectiveness as other low-dose pills. But are they safer? "Theoretically, lower doses would mean fewer side effects," says Joseph Goldzieher, M.D., professor and director of endocrine research, Department of Obstetrics and Gynecology at Baylor College of Medicine, Houston. "We

---

CANCER PREVENTION PLAN: ORAL CONTRACEPTIVES

- The Pill can protect you from cancer of the ovaries and endometrium.
- The Pill seems to have no effect on breast cancer risk.
- If you are concerned about the very slight increased risk of cervical cancer, you should get plenty of the B vitamin folate in your diet.

won't know for sure until studies are completed comparing the multiphasics to fixed low-dose OCs and higher-hormone pills." We'll also have to wait to see if the new pills protect against cancer as well as other OCs.

In the meantime, if you are looking for pregnancy protection now without paying a price later, the Pill may fill the bill—again. "The evidence is making the Pill an attractive option once more," says Dr. Stadel. Stay tuned, he says; the news about this form of birth control may get brighter. "I'm optimistic that if earlier pills with higher hormone doses showed no link to breast cancer, the story can only get better with the newer, lower-dose pills."

Outdoor Pollution

It wasn't so long ago that we believed our spacious skies, our amber waves of grain, our purple mountains and our shining seas could swallow up whatever we sprayed, dumped, littered or piped to them. America, with its vast resources, would surely remain The Beautiful.

Pollution came as one of the ugliest surprises of the second half of the twentieth century. Who would have predicted that dark clouds would descend over our major cities? That so many of our waterways would become undrinkable and unswimmable? That, even in rural areas, the earth itself would become suspect?

The spoiling of wilderness was a high enough price to pay for progress, but then came evidence of health threats: Los Angeles smog and respiratory disease; Love Canal toxics and leukemia; PBBs in Michigan cattle feed, linked to a variety of illnesses. And abroad, there was the chemical spill in the Rhine and the chemical plant tragedy in Bhopal, India. A litany of headlines, of human suffering—and of fears.

256

One of the greatest fears is cancer.

You've probably read that "environmental causes" account for 80 percent or more of cancer cases. But that statistic overstates the connection between *pollution* and cancer. When scientists say environment, they mean the *total* environment, which, along with pollution, means all nongenetic factors—like smoking, diet, exercise and income. Industrial pollution is only a fraction of that 80 percent. Just how small—or large—a fraction is the source of intense, ongoing scientific debate and research.

The pollution problem can seem overwhelming. But there are many things that can be done on an individual level and community level to stay informed, to protect your family and community—and our planet.

ARE YOU A GUINEA PIG?

Unknowingly, industrial workers have become our guinea pigs. Exposed to the highest levels and numbers of chemicals, they have developed health problems that put scientists on the trail of certain industrial chemicals as hazards.

Specific jobs became associated with specific cancers. Shipbuilders, who worked with asbestos, developed high rates of mesothelioma, an exceedingly rare cancer of the chest and abdominal membranes. Plastics workers developed extra cases of liver cancers, due to vinyl chloride. Metallurgical workers, exposed to arsenic, suffered skin, lung and liver cancer. Radiologists, exposed to x-rays, were at higher risk for certain cancers. And the list went on.

In addition to exposure on the job, people—even whole communities—have been exposed to toxic chemicals. Love Canal was only the most famous example. "There has been evidence from a number of hazardous waste site communities that show some relationship between the incidence of cancer, and other diseases, and chemicals," says Henry S. Cole, Ph.D., senior scientist with the Clean Water Action Project and research director for National Campaign against Toxic Hazards, both in Washington, D.C. Dr. Cole, an environmental scientist who was formerly with the Environmental Protection Agency (EPA), mentions a few. "There were studies linking people using highly contaminated lower Mississippi drinking water with the development of colon cancer, also studies that show lung cancer rates are highest in the 40 or so counties in the U.S. which have heavy concentrations of petrochemical plants. Anyone who says there's no evidence [linking pollution to cancer] is not looking at the facts," says Dr. Cole. "Animal workplace studies have identified dozens of chemicals that are suspected or known to cause cancer in humans. Those chemicals are showing up at waste sites."

But estimating the cancer risk to the general public based on occupational or isolated community exposures to high levels of chemicals is a task plagued with uncertainty. Usually, the public is exposed to far *lower* doses of carcinogens. Sources may be as familiar as the nozzle of the neighborhood gas pump, as obvious as the smokestack of a manufacturing plant, or as obscure as seepage from a hidden, remote toxic dump site.

Other uncertainties add to the difficulty of accurately estimating risk. For example:

- Only a small fraction of the more than 50,000 chemicals used in commerce have been tested to see if they promote cancer— and although most of the rest are probably not carcinogenic, it's impossible to say for sure. Also, hundreds of new chemicals are introduced into commerce each year, some of which may present a cancer risk.
- Cancers often don't show up until decades after exposure, so their causes aren't easily traced. We may be exposed to chemicals now that we won't discover are carcinogenic for years to come.
- Chemicals that don't pose much risk by themselves sometimes work synergistically, with other chemicals, to initiate or promote cancer or other diseases. Most government testing of chemicals tests them individually.
- Scientists must rely on animal tests as a source of data on many chemicals—but substances that cause cancer in animals don't necessarily have the same effects on humans.

With all those unknowns, it shouldn't come as any surprise that scientists' estimates of cancer risk from pollution vary widely.

"It is not surprising that the numbers vary widely. They vary even in the well-defined environment of the workplace," says David Ozonoff, M.D., chief of the environmental health section of the Boston University School of Public Health. In addition, two leading cancer epidemiologists, Richard Doll and Richard Peto, very conservatively estimate that about 2 percent—but maybe up to 5 percent—of all cancer deaths result from exposure to pollution.

The conservative estimate of 1 to 5 percent of cancer deaths would mean that, of 483,000 cancer deaths in the United States in 1987, anywhere from 5,000 to 24,000 deaths among the general public might be caused by pollution.

How should we view that statistic? Some scientists point out that the pollution threat pales next to cigarette smoking, which may account to 25 to 40 percent of all U.S. cancers. In fact, some experts attribute the rise in cancer rates in this century almost entirely to tobacco smoking. "Cancer rates [in the U.S.] have gone up, but when you remove the epidemic due to lung cancer, you find the cancer death rates really have not changed," says John Cairns, M.D., professor of microbiology in the Department of Cancer Biology at the Harvard School of Public Health in Boston.

The number of cancers caused by pollution, Dr. Cairns contends, is insignificant compared to deaths caused by smoking. "You have to worry about the big risk before you worry about the small risk. You don't say, 'My gosh, I may get killed by lightning tomorrow,' because very few people are killed by lightning, and some of the cancers [related to industrial exposure] are as rare as that."

But other scientists view the risks differently. "Even if you take the low numbers," says Dr. Ozonoff, "Even if you take 5 percent [of cancer deaths caused by industrial pollution] for argument's sake, and realize that makes . . . 50 people a day dying of [pollution-related] cancer, that's really pretty horrendous. If every day a mine accident or other industrial disaster killed 50 people, it would make headlines in every newspaper."

Dr. Cole concurs. "Who knows if [pollution] causes 10 or 30 percent of cancers?" says Dr. Cole. "Let's not forget for a minute that one in four Americans will have cancer in their lifetime. We know that some of these are preventable. Which means that industry has to do the preventing. It also means citizens will have to push industry and government to prevent release of these pollutants."

AIR POLLUTION

Automobiles. Chemical plants. Gas stations. Woodstoves. Incinerators. Sewage treatment plants. Manufacturing facilities.

What do they all have in common? They all spew pollution into the air, including known carcinogens ranging from arsenic to benzene, trichloroethylene to vinyl chloride. Each year, millions of pounds of potentially cancer-causing chemicals are emitted into our nation's air, according to the American Lung Association.

Some scientists say that lung diseases like asthma and emphysema may be the most important diseases related to general air pollution. So far, the epidemiological studies do not suggest a strong connection between general air pollution and lung cancer.

An extensive study conducted by the American Cancer Society concluded that "there is very little effect, if any, on lung cancer from general air pollution," according to Lawrence Garfinkel, vice president for epidemiology and statistics of the American Cancer Society.

Scientists hasten to add a number of qualifications to this conclusion. The risk, of course, depends on the type and proximity of pollutants. There are, for example, "hot spots," where cancer rates exceed the norm, especially around petrochemical complexes, smelters and coke ovens. In a major study assessing the problem, the EPA in 1985 estimated that 15 to 45 air pollutants may be responsible for between 1,300 and 1,700 cancer cases per year in the United States.

Another qualification is the possibility that air pollution in combination with other risk factors such as smoking may create a problem that's greater than the sum of its parts. "It's possible . . . though by no means certain, that some pollutant[s] of urban air may interact with cigarette smoke to increase the incidence of cancer over and above that which would be expected by the action of tobacco alone," say Doll and Peto.

Scientists are also increasingly concerned about indoor air pollution. The cancer risk from tainted air in the home may actually be even greater than the risk from air outside (see chapter 42, Indoor Pollution).

And then there's one great big exception to the general assurances about outdoor air pollution and cancer: the question of the ozone layer.

Ozone is a common pollutant that can cause respiratory problems in humans and, at much higher levels, is associated with an increased risk of tumors in animals. But that's not a major worry to most scientists. What's keeping them awake at night is that there may not be *enough* ozone up above us, in the stratosphere.

That's where a natural ozone layer shields us against ultraviolet rays of the sun. The ozone layer may be eroded by a class of chemicals known as chlorofluorocarbons. Used in refrigerants and aerosol sprays, chlorofluorocarbons waft up to the ozone layer and react with it chemically. The depletion of the ozone layer may permit more ultraviolet light to reach earth and may lead, in the long term, to increases in skin cancer rates. In the United States and around the world, government authorities are trying to work out agreements to stop chlorofluorocarbon production.

WATER POLLUTION

One top government expert on water quality calls surface and groundwater pollution the number one environmental problem of the 1980s.

Across the country, there is increasing awareness that the stuff pouring out of the tap isn't always *just* H_2O, and may be contaminated with dangerous substances ranging from bacteria to trace metals and synthetic organic chemicals. Some of these contaminants are carcinogens.

How do carcinogens get into our water? One source is industry, which may dump chemicals directly into water or bury them in the ground. Once buried, chemicals can seep into the water underground, which is the source of both well and spring water. Pesticides and other agricultural chemicals can also contaminate the water. Even disinfecting water with chlorine can cause carcinogens to form.

The result? You've probably read some of the headlines. Thousands of Louisianians, whose drinking water came from the mighty Mississippi, were shocked to discover a grim bisque of chemicals in their drinking water.

Similarly, in Woburn, Massachusetts, some residents found their water was contaminated with a chemical degreaser called trichloroethylene (TCE). The contaminant, an industrial waste product, has been blamed for higher-than-normal incidences of childhood leukemia in the area.

There are several studies that have shown an association between contaminants in drinking water and cancer mortality—but the degree of the risk is disputed. Authorities are concerned about a number of particular carcinogens:

Nitrites and nitrates. These are common in rural wells, because they're part of the runoff from manured or fertilized fields. They can also come from municipal and industrial wastewaters and septic tanks. They're associated with a sometimes fatal condition that diminishes the oxygen-carrying capacity of the blood in infants, and with stomach cancers, although there has been no clear link between cancers and nitrites and nitrates in drinking water (see chapter 48, Nitrites and Nitrates).

Trace metals. While some metals, such as magnesium, calcium and zinc, may actually be good for you, others can cause serious harm. You definitely don't want to find large amounts of arsenic or cadmium in your water, as these elements in drinking water have been associated with cancer. Asbestos, one of the worst carcinogens around, has also turned up in some water supplies, although drinking asbestos is not yet a proven cause of cancer.

Toxic chemicals. There's a whole alphabet soup of chemicals— including TCE (trichloroethylene), PCBs (polychlorinated biphenyls) and so on—that may be found in drinking water and that cause cancer in laboratory animals. What is known about their cancer risk to humans comes largely from accidental exposures, like New York's Love Canal.

Trihalomethanes. The commonly used water disinfectant chlorine poses a no-win choice: cholera or cancer? Chlorine kills bacteria in drinking water, but it can also react with organic debris in water to form compounds called trihalomethanes. One trihalomethane is chloroform, which has been shown to cause cancer in laboratory animals. There is some suspicion that trihalomethanes may increase the risk of cancer in humans.

Fortunately, there's a great deal you can do about water pollution that may affect your well, your municipal water supplies or your community water supplies.

GROUND POLLUTION AND HAZARDOUS WASTES

In the late 1970s, residents of a small neighborhood near Niagara Falls, New York, began to notice a great many health problems. There were a lot of miscarriages and birth defects in the neighborhood, and the state's highest rate of lung cancer.

The neighborhood, of course, was Love Canal. The residents' health problems were eventually linked to an abandoned chemical dump. Today, Love Canal is a ghost town. But there are other neighborhoods whose residents are frightened by their closeness to toxic waste sites. The EPA's preliminary list of waste sites is 26,000 long—and growing. At this writing, the EPA has placed over 950 of those sites on the National Priority List, meaning that they pose a threat or potential threat to public health.

What exactly is a hazardous waste site? It may be a landfill, an underground tank, an open chemical lake (called an impoundment) or just a few rusty barrels filled with wastes.

In some cases, waste disposal was a fly-by-night, negligent or even criminal operation. A manufacturing company in New Bedford, Massachusetts, for example, was recently indicted for secretly dumping 44,000 gallons of untreated waste water daily into New Bedford Harbor. "I think it's just sloppy management," the company's attorney was quoted as saying.

In other cases, industry took pains to dispose of wastes in ways they thought were proper but which were later found to be inadequate. Underground storage containers can leak; impoundments can catch fire, explode when new chemicals are added or give off noxious odors.

What exactly is in these sites? "They contain hundreds or thousands of chemicals which might be called hazardous," says Joel Hirschhorn, Ph.D., who directs the hazardous waste projects for the U.S. Office of Technology Assessment in Washington, D.C. Possible health risks run the gamut from rashes to nervous system disorders, from birth defects to cancers.

"That there is some threat [of cancer] is unequivocal," says Dr. Hirschhorn. "Most of the controversy centers around how bad it is and who is affected. There are very few epidemiological studies in this area."

Lois Gibbs, executive director of the Citizens' Clearinghouse for Hazardous Wastes, Inc. (CCHW) in Arlington, Virginia, concurs. "One of the biggest problems in this whole area is the scientists really don't know what low-level carcinogens will do to you—or to a baby—over a long period of time.

"My home turf is Love Canal, New York," Gibb adds. "In my home, four of the five chemicals that were found were carcinogens. The government said the levels were so low that they didn't pose any risk. I said, 'That's ridiculous!' My daughter has a rare blood disease and an 80 percent risk of getting cancer because of her exposure to benzene."

The hazardous chemicals can reach us in a variety of ways, including the water we drink and wash with. "There have been significant losses of drinking water supplies around the country from toxic waste sites," says Dr. Hirschhorn.

Washing with contaminated water may be an even greater threat than drinking it, notes Beverly Paigen, Ph.D., a research toxicologist at Oakland Children's Medical Hospital in Oakland, California, and a member of the board of directors of CCHW. "You can get twice as much exposure from a 15-minute shower than from drinking contaminated tap water," says Dr. Paigen. The chemicals can evaporate from the hot water and be inhaled. Other researchers agree. For ways to deal with this problem, see chapter 42, Indoor Pollution.

Toxic waste sites are a hazard not only to their immediate neighbors but to every citizen. Indirectly, because as taxpayers, we all pay for damages and cleanups. And directly, adds Gibbs, because "the fruits and vegetables on your dinner table could have been grown in an area with contaminated soils or water."

As you'll read, there is good news on the toxics front. Government and industry have stepped up their commitment to identify and clean up existing problems—and to prevent future Love Canals.

WHAT YOU CAN DO

"Don't drink the water and don't breathe the air," advises one humorist's lyric about pollution. Fortunately, that's not the only answer.

On an individual level, there are steps you can take to protect your family. Below, you'll read about some of them, like water filters for your home. (For information on air filters, see chapter 42, Indoor Pollution.)

Filters can be somewhat effective, but they are bandages and not cures. The larger pollution problem can't be filtered away. It will be cured only by individual, community and national commitment.

And you can play an important role. Look around you—at what's happening in your neighborhood and your community—stay informed and work with others to let your voice be heard. One day, perhaps, we won't need the filters to drink the water and breathe the air.

Here's how to start.

DON'T BECOME PART OF THE PROBLEM

Most hazardous wastes are created by manufacturers. But consumers, too, can add toxic substances to the environment, by careless use and disposal of everything from paints to insecticides. Some of these household products can contain carcinogens.

"When people dispose of these kinds of products, they often dump them in the 'back 40'—where they can leach hazardous chemicals," says Dana Duxbury of the Tufts University Center for Environmental Management in Medford, Massachusetts. "Or they put them out with the rubbish, and sanitation workers can be exposed to fumes or acids. Then the products may be incinerated, causing unhealthy emissions into the air, or put in landfill, from which they can leach into the groundwater."

There's a new movement coming up with better ways to deal with household toxics. Some states and communities even sponsor collection programs for household hazardous wastes, such as for waste oil and car batteries. The League of Women Voters has embarked on a national program to educate people about hazardous wastes. Contact your League of Women Voters for more information.

KNOW WHEN TO CHECK THE WATER

Testing your home water for contaminants is sometimes a good idea—but it's also expensive. How do you know when to test?

"If the taste or odor of your water changes, or if you live in close proximity to a potential source of pollution, such as a landfill, you might want to test," suggests Victor Kimm, deputy assistant administrator for pesticides and toxic substances for the EPA.

"If you notice you have skin rashes, but that when you go on vacation for a couple of days the rashes begin to clear up, that's a good indication you should check your water," says Lois Gibbs.

Dr. Cole adds, "Some solvents volatilize in the shower; you can breathe them, and may even be overcome by fumes. If you get dizzy in the shower, you should definitely get your water tested.

"If your neighbors had their water tested and found something in the water that's a carcinogen or a chemical that can cause problems at low concentrations, by all means get your water tested, too," says Dr. Cole. He adds, "If there's a hazardous waste site or Superfund site [a place the government has determined needs quick and dramatic attention] not too far away, you might want to get your water tested. And if it's a Superfund site, you can demand that the state and federal government do the testing." You may need to organize with your neighbors to get testing.

Municipal water suppliers are required to monitor their water. But in 1982 alone, there were 70,000 violations of drinking water standards by municipal systems. And there are many dangerous contaminants for which they are not required to test. So you can ask your water authority for the results of their routine tests, or you may want to do it yourself.

If you decide to have your well or municipal water privately tested, Kimm suggests you talk to local health officials about the kinds of contaminants you should be testing for. Or you can just ask for a test for "priority pollutants." "That's the list of chemicals that the government has found are risky to public health," explains Lois Gibbs. (Gibbs's organization, the Citizens' Clearinghouse for Hazardous Wastes, Inc., offers a list of priority pollutants and technical assistance for testing. See the box below for the mailing address.)

THINK ABOUT INSTALLING
A HOME TREATMENT SYSTEM

The testing company or a local health official can help you interpret the test results. Once you understand what you're drinking, you may want to think about buying a water treatment system.

SOME NATURAL RESOURCES

Here is a list of organizations that can supply information about pollution.

Water Pollution and Testing Filters

- Clean Water Action Project, 317 Pennsylvania Ave., S.E., Washington, DC 20003; (202) 547-1196.
- Water Quality Association, 4151 Naperville Rd., Lisle, IL 60532; (312) 369-1600.
- WaterTest Corporation, Box 6360, Manchester, NH 03108; 1-800-H2O-TEST (1-800-426-8378).

Air Pollution

- Your local American Lung Association.

Toxic Wastes and Testing

- Citizens' Clearinghouse for Hazardous Wastes, Inc., P.O. Box 926, Arlington, VA 22216; (703) 276-7070.
- Environmental Action Foundation, Wastes and Toxic Substance Project, 1525 New Hampshire Ave, N.W., Washington, DC 20036; (202) 745-4879.

Hazardous Wastes

- Your local League of Women Voters, or the national office at 1730 M. St., N.W., Washington, DC 20036; (202) 429-1965.

These systems are expensive, and they are not perfect, but they can improve the situation. One is an activated carbon system, which can remove chloroform, chlorine, some pesticides and organic chemicals from water. However, you'll need to buy a good system—a small unit on the end of a tap probably won't do the job, says Dr. Cole—and they require more frequent filter changes than the manufacturers may recommend. (If the organic material that collects on the carbon isn't cleaned, it may supply a food source for bacteria that may produce endotoxins, potentially carcinogenic substances.)

Some purifiers work through distillation, turning water to steam and condensing it back to water. Theoretically, this system removes all bacteria, but it doesn't necessarily remove chloroform and other organic chemicals, which can vaporize with the water and recondense.

Systems based on reverse osmosis can remove dissolved solids, viruses, hydrocarbons, asbestos, most pesticides and other chemicals— but they don't remove chloroform.

Some water problems require two or more units, says Douglas Oberhamer, former executive director of the Water Quality Association. "You may find you need a prefilter, an activated carbon unit and reverse-osmosis system or some other combination to take care of your water troubles," says Oberhamer. "A professional will be able to help you design the best system for you." For sources of more information on water filter systems, see the box on the preceding page.

Doesn't it seem simpler to switch to bottled water? That can work—but sometimes, Dr. Cole warns, "people may switch to a water supply that's just as contaminated. I think all suppliers of bottled water should do testing and labeling." Write to the supplier to ask for their water test results.

TRACK DOWN THE HAZARDS

If there's a major pollution problem in your area, a filter in your home won't fix it. "What people need to do then," says Lois Gibbs, "is find out where the source is and from there get the responsible party or the government to deal with that source of pollution." How? "People need to organize their neighbors," she says.

That's precisely what Gibbs did. She organized her neighbors, first in Love Canal, and then all across the country. The organization she established helps individuals and community groups deal with local pollution problems.

If you suspect a problem, play detective, says Gibbs. "I always advise people to find out where the closest dump site is; that includes your local garbage dump. In industrialized areas, they should look for ponds, pits and lagoons full of chemical wastes."

In some cases, the dangers are apparent. Sometimes you can see black smoke rising from a stack at the local factory, or an oily substance floating on the surface of a river or creek, or black "goop" bubbling from the ground near your home, says Gibbs. Many contaminated areas have a sweet odor in the air, or a chemical smell.

Next, research the site. Industries are required to report their emissions to the state and federal government. And a provision of the new Superfund Law, passed in 1986, requires industries to make public the chemicals they use and discharge. "People can ask the state or federal government for their reports," says Gibbs. Call a local elected official to obtain the name of the proper state agency to contact.

If there's no apparent owner of a waste site, you may have to do a little more legwork. Sources of information include the local planning board, county health department, local office of the EPA, and even the newspaper. They may have records of who owns the property and what was dumped when.

GET HELP WITH TESTING

The next step is testing the water, soil and/or air. Community groups often need help in knowing what to test for and how to judge the results. That's why it's so important for citizens to work together and demand testing. "Those getting municipal water can demand that the full range of chemicals be tested for, starting with the 129 priority pollutants under the Clean Water Act, plus any pesticides widely used in the area. I would demand that kind of information as a fundamental right," says Dr. Cole.

Pressure for testing can be put on the municipal water utility, says Dr. Cole. "If you get enough citizens together, you can say, 'We're not going to pay our utility bill; we're going to reduce it by the amount it costs to get the water tested.' We find those tactics can be very effective," says Dr. Cole.

People who live near a Superfund site should insist that the EPA test their homes, adds Dr. Cole. "One technique, which worked at a site in Ohio, was a petition. People living near a Superfund site went door-to-door with a petition demanding testing in their homes and sent copies to state legislators. As a result, the EPA did greatly increase the number of homes tested."

It's a good idea to also have a nongovernment expert to help you monitor and evaluate the tests. A science department of a university, with a toxiciologist on staff, can ensure that the testing is going to be useful.

Other sources of technical assistance include environmental groups—and the Citizens' Clearinghouse on Hazardous Waste, Inc.

CCHW also provides help with the next steps—public education and organizing local groups.

CANCER PREVENTION PLAN:
OUTDOOR POLLUTION

- Test your home drinking water for contaminants, or ask your municipal water authority for the results of their routine tests.
- If needed, install a good water filter.
- Determine whether there is a hazardous waste site or Superfund site in your community.
- If there is a danger of contamination, have the EPA test your home for toxic pollutants.

C H A P T E R 52
Pap Tests

It's Judith's thirty-first birthday. As on every birthday, she celebrates in a rather unusual way: She calls her gynecologist's office and asks the nurse to put her down for a pelvic and a Pap. "A clean bill of health is my best present," says Judith.

When her appointment arrives, Judith is relaxed—she knows just what to expect from the routine procedure. Her doctor should examine her breasts, then her vagina. Next comes the Pap test. With the blunt tip of a depression stick or a cotton swab, he takes two or three sample scrapings: one from the outer cuff of her cervix, one from the area just inside the cervical canal and possibly one from the vaginal wall. The cell samples are smeared onto a slide and sent to a lab for microscopic analysis.

That's that for another year, Judith thinks. She leaves the doctor's office feeling the same way she always does after having a pelvic and Pap—proud for undertaking something that was quick and painless and provides her the best protection against advanced disease.

Judith is right to feel good about the Pap test. By taking this measure, her doctor may be able to detect abnormal cell changes in the cervix at least eight years before a full-fledged cancer develops. What's more, a Pap smear can detect nearly 90 percent of potential cancers early enough to ensure her of a 100 percent cure.

There are no conclusive studies to prove that women like Judith, who get Pap tests for early detection of cervical cancer, are less likely to die from cervical cancer than women who don't have Pap tests. But what we do know is that ever since George Papanicolaou, M.D., first introduced the procedure named after him, the cervical cancer rate has dropped. Since the 1940s, the death rate from cancer of the uterus (cervical and endometrial) has plummeted by more than 70 percent.

FLAP OVER PERIODIC PAPS

"The Pap test is the most widely used and perhaps most effective cancer prevention tool we have," says Saul Gusberg, M.D., Professor Emeritus of gynecology at Mount Sinai School of Medicine in New York City, and past president of the American Cancer Society.

But a tool only works when it is used. And that means getting periodic Pap tests. A few years ago, the American Cancer Society (ACS), under Dr. Gusberg's direction, established the current Pap test screening guidelines, which recommended that all healthy women over 20 and those under 20 who are sexually active should have a Pap smear once every three years after two initial normal smears.

This new screening schedule represented a switch for the ACS, which had advocated annual Pap tests in the past. Why the increased interval? Because, explains Dr. Gusberg, statistical evidence indicates that cervical cancer tends to develop very slowly, taking anywhere from 10 to 30 years to develop into a life-threatening cancer. "Before it gets to that stage, precancerous lesions can be detected and it can be successfully treated," he says. Yet other physicians, as well as the American College of Obstetricians and Gynecologists, believe the Pap test should be an annual affair. They worry about the fact that 5 percent of cancers of the cervix will progress from a symptomless stage to an advanced, invasive cancer in 3 years *or less.* What's more, there's no way to tell the fast-growing lesions from the slow-growing ones.

More frequent periodic Pap tests could keep a better check on them, insists Alex Ferenczy, M.D., professor of pathology and obstetrics/gynecology at McGill University School of Medicine in Montreal, Quebec. In fact, he notes, some doctors have estimated that if screened on a three-year basis, 40 in 1,000 women with untreated, well-established lesions would develop invasive cancer, compared to 12 or fewer of those who undergo annual screening.

But the biggest push for annual Paps is coming because women are having more abnormal smears. It seems that while the incidence of invasive cervical cancer (the spreading kind) is down, there's been an increase in preinvasive cancer or neoplasia (precancerous changes). And cervical intraepithelial neoplasia (CIN), which is the presence of abnormal cells limited to the surface of the cervix, could lead to cancer if not detected.

What doctors are noticing is that practically all abnormal Pap smears are showing signs of a group of sexually transmitted viruses known as the human papilloma virus (HPV), commonly called the condyloma virus. Allowed to flourish, all of these viruses will cause abnormal tissue breakdown or growth. Some will form tiny, flat warts that can grow undetected on the cervix or in the vagina, in the male urinary opening or on the penis. Others form large, cauliflower-shaped warts.

At high risk for HPV and CIN are women who have early intercourse, those who have more than one partner, or those whose mate may not be monogamous—there's some evidence that men may be carriers of the HPV virus. "Believe it or not, possibly 85 to 95 percent of women could be in this high-risk group," says William T. Creasman, M.D., professor and chairman of the Department of Obstetrics and Gynecology, Medical University of South Carolina, Charleston. "We could reduce that risk with earlier and more frequent Pap screenings."

If that isn't enough reason for yearly Paps, consider this: An annual test could reduce the margin of human error in reading your smear. As it is, Pap smears have a false-negative rate—meaning they could say your cervix is normal when it's not—about 15 to 30 percent of the time. So the more frequent the test, the less likely you are to be walking around with undetected dysplasia.

Finally, Dr. Ferenczy is concerned that a three-year gap in Paps may "plant doubt . . . as to the seriousness of the tests and make it easier to ignore or simply forget them." In fact, he points out, women who are scheduled for annual exams don't actually get tested for two years. "If such patients are advised to have Pap tests at intervals of three to five years, testing may not be done for five or seven years, if at all."

LEARNING LAB LINGO

Despite the ACS recommendations, Judith is among the many women who prefer to stick to yearly Pap tests in order to "catch any cancer in time." At this year's exam, though, her confidence in the test was threatened. Her doctor called and told her that her cervical cells looked "atypical" and she was to come in to the office at once.

The call, naturally, sparked a series of scary questions for Judith. "What does he mean by atypical cervical cells? Do I have cancer?" Her

NEW TECHNIQUE MAY BOOST
YOUR DEFENSE AGAINST CERVICAL CANCER

Having an annual Pap smear is a smart way to protect yourself against cervical cancer. But Pap tests aren't perfect.

A new screening technique could help make cervical cancer a disease of the past. It's called cervicography, and it consists of taking a picture of the cervix by means of a special photographic instrument called a cerviscope. The slide, or cervigram, can later be magnified on a screen for experts in cervical cancer to read, much like the reading of an x-ray.

In a recent study of more than 3,000 women between the ages of 18 and 50, this new diagnostic tool was found to be 4.5 times more sensitive in detecting precancerous changes than the Pap test.

Another study showed false-negative rates (when cancer is present but not detected) for cervicography to be somewhat lower than for the Pap test.

"Because of the high false-negative rate, the Pap smear did not eliminate all cervical cancer as it was intended to," says Adolph Stafl, M.D., Ph.D., professor of gynecology and obstetrics at the Medical College of Wisconsin and inventor of the cerviscope. "By combining the two techniques, we might be able to eliminate all cervical cancer."

Dr. Stafl still recommends that a Pap smear be done every year. A cervigram would be necessary only a few times during a lifetime, in particular during early adolescence and with a first pregnancy, times when women are at highest risk for development of precancerous cells. "This is when a cervigram is helpful to see if the cells are changing and determine if the woman is at risk for cervical cancer," explains Dr. Stafl. The cervigram can then be kept as a permanent photographic record and used for comparison if the need arises at some point in the future.

Because the photographic equipment is relatively inexpensive, Dr. Stafl believes it will be affordable for most examining rooms. Already, cervicography is now being used in over 200 locations in the United States and in several foreign countries.

panic subsided only after she learned how Pap tests are analyzed and how to interpret the lab lingo.

She found out that when a smear slide is examined under the microscope, it's possible to detect an inflammation or infection of the cervix and endometrium as well as to see signs of abnormal changes in cells in the cervix. Cell changes may show up in daughters of women who took diethylstilbestrol (DES) during pregnancy, in women who smoke cigarettes and even in those who have a lower than normal intake of selenium, vitamins C and A and the B vitamin folate. But whatever the reason, the Pap smear then gets classified in one of two ways. It is either categorized into one of five classes and several sub-classes according to the severity of tissue change, or, increasingly, the abnormality found in the cells is more fully described.

Unfortunately, no two labs use the same classification. So at some labs, abnormal cells are referred to by classes such as Class I, II and III while at other labs, abnormal cells are referred to by descriptive words like atypical and suspicious.

If you are perplexed by your Pap test results, the following list may help you make sense of your smears.

- Class I; negative; normal smear with no abnormal cells.
- Class II; early dysplasia; slightly atypical. A catchall category for minor cell changes that can include inflammation and infection.
- Class III; suspicious; mild and moderate dysplasia; cancer precursor; cervical intraepithelial neoplasia (CIN). These cells are rated as either CIN 1 or 2, according to the proportion of abnormal to normal cells present on the slide sample as well as the degree of change in size and shape of abnormal cells. They may or may not be precancerous.
- Class IV; highly suspicious; severe dysplasia; CIN 3, carcinoma *in situ* (cancer of the surface of the cervix). Cannot definitely be called positive for cancer, may or may not be malignant.
- Class V; positive for cancer; suggests need for further diagnostic testing.

ARRESTING ABNORMALITIES

If you get a phone call like Judith did, telling you your Pap test is abnormal, don't panic. Quite a few women at some time in their lives will have smears that show mild, moderate and even severe dysplasia, but they don't develop cancer because their condition will be successfully treated.

"Think of a positive Pap as a warning sign for further follow-up," advises Dr. Gusberg. "Remember, any precancerous condition and even early cervical cancer is very treatable and curable."

In Judith's case, abnormal cells appeared on a Pap as a result of an infection, which her doctor treated with antibiotics. Other cases may require further diagnosis of dysplasia by looking for lesions and taking a tissue biopsy. If dysplasia is confirmed, the lesions will be removed.

Treatment may be repeated if your follow-up smear is not normal after several months. But even with a perfect Pap test after treatment, you'll need to repeat the tests yearly.

KEEPING YOUR SCREENING SCHEDULE

The Pap test can continue to be your best preventive weapon against cervical cancer, but only if you have it regularly throughout your lifetime. If you are over 40, it's probably been a lot longer than it should be since your last Pap test, because older women go to the gynecologist less frequently, says one specialist. But neglecting to get more frequent tests may be the reason so many older women fall victim to cervical cancer.

Here's a reminder to give yourself a Pap test present each and every year:

- Stick to yearly Pap tests, especially if you are at high risk for cervical cancer: you smoke, you or your mate has more than one sexual partner or you had early sexual activity.
- Ask your doctor to describe any positive Pap test and why your cervical cells may be abnormal.
- *Never submit to treatment on the basis of one Pap test.*
- A Pap smear does not always detect cancer of the endometrium and ovaries. Tell your doctor about any abnormal bleeding or pain.

CANCER PREVENTION PLAN: PAP TESTS

- Have an annual Pap smear.
- If the test is positive, have a second test.
- Don't smoke tobacco.

53

Pesticides in Food

When it comes to cancer protection, the old "apple a day" adage has taken on fresh relevance. Studies indicate that eating plenty of produce may protect against certain cancers (see chapter 38, Fruit, and chapter 64, Vegetables). But ironically, even as the public has become more aware of the importance of eating fresh-grown foods, unease about what's in some of those foods has also increased.

And that's because of pesticides, the tens of thousands of chemical compounds farmers use to kill insects and weeds, combat crop disease and enhance the color and size of crops.

Who could avoid worring about pesticides these days? Virtually every week, it seems, new seeds of doubt are planted in consumers' minds about contamination of our food and our environment.

Pesticides have figured in some of the top news stories of the past decade. It was the Alar uproar, in the mid-1980s, that first alerted many people to the fact that use of questionable chemicals is as American as apple pie. (Alar is a growth regulator, commonly used on apples, which is suspected of being carcinogenic.) Other pesticide headlines: the 1984 Bhopal tragedy, caused by a leakage of a toxic chemical from a pesticide plant in India; the sudden banning of several widely used, potentially carcinogenic pesticides, like ethylene dibromide (EDB); the discovery of pesticide residues in a wide array of food products and in groundwater.

There is an emerging national consensus that something must be done. In 1986, the Environmental Protection Agency (EPA) put pesticide pollution at the top of its list of the most urgent environmental problems in the United States. Even the agrichemicals industry is working with environmentalists to urge tightening of federal regulations. The president of one agrichemical company told the U.S. Senate, "Times change. It's time for the agrichemicals industry to change."

What effect do pesticides—on our foods and in our environment—have on our health? The answer is uncertain. Government regulators are the first to admit that most pesticides have not been adequately tested for health effects, including cancer, and basic testing may not be completed until well into the 1990s or beyond.

This issue may seem hopeless, lending appeal to the idea of not eating, drinking or breathing at all. But scientists emphasize that fear and fasting are definitely not the answers, especially when it comes to fruits and vegetables. These do have proven health benefits, and all indications are that people are better protected against cancer if they do eat produce than if they don't.

Also, questions about cancer risk concern not only farmers, farm workers and rural residents, who have higher exposures to pesticides, but all of us. It's hardly any wonder that, more than ever before, consumers are demanding some answers. Are carcinogenic chemicals being applied to our food, and why? How much of these chemicals are we exposed to? How might they affect our health? Since it may be years until the uncertainties are resolved, there's a more practical, immediate question: Can we protect ourselves from the unknowns of pesticides?

The experts say you can reduce your pesticide exposure. Later on, this chapter describes some sensible, easy ways to minimize your intake of pesticides from foods. Not just your washing and cooking decisions, but also your shopping decisions, can have a real impact.

THE PESTICIDE CRISIS: SILENT SPRING REVISITED

If all the recent pesticide headlines gave you flashes of déjà vu, it's not surprising. In 1962, biologist Rachael Carson warned of the dangers to wildlife, the envirnment and people in *Silent Spring* (Fawcett), the book that led to severe restrictions on the use of DDT. But a quarter of a century later, traces of DDT are still showing up in soil, water, wildlife, store produce—and headlines. In addition, there's a broad array of other substances in the news: aldicarb, daminozide, dioxin, malathion and 2,4-D, to name a few of the most controversial.

What are they? The term "pesticides" covers some 50,000 chemical compounds approved for use in the United States. These include chemicals that control insects (insecticides), rodents (rodenticides), mold (fungicides) and weeds (herbicides), as well as growth regulators and more. The EPA estimates that 1.11 billion pounds of pesticides were used in the United States in 1985.

Pesticides offer numerous benefits. They increase crop yields significantly. They can prevent spoilage and block pestborne diseases. But is it really necessary for farmers to use *so many* chemicals? Some people answer that question by tossing it back into the laps of consumers. When you're at the supermarket fruit bin, do you push away the scrawny fruit with holes and bruises and reach for the large, perfect round apple? Most shoppers do, so farmers feel they can't stay in business without pesticides.

The food industry insists that consumers have preferred to buy perfect food, leaving farmers with no choice but to use pesticides. "That's based on scant knowledge on the part of consumers," says Monica Moore, executive director of the Pesticide Education and Action Project in San Francisco.

Elizabeth Weisburger, Ph.D., D.Sc., assistant director for chemical carcinogenesis, Division of Cancer Etiology, at the National Cancer Institute, concurs. "Obviously, the most desirable situation would be not to use any pesticides. But if you look at the realities of the situation, people would have to accept fruit that's not so nice to eat, more likely to be spoiled, have defects—we'd go back to days when there were worms in apples. Many people today are not too in tune with that type of product."

However, that tune may be changing as the public becomes more aware of the problems with pesticides. A recent Food Marketing Institute survey found that chemical residues in food are a major concern to three-fourths of all shoppers.

THE PROBLEMS WITH PESTICIDES

"There is increasing evidence that some chemical pesticides pose long-term cancer and other risks to humans exposed to them through dermal contact, inhalation or the food chain," notes the National Academy of Sciences' National Research Council.

Richard Levins, Ph.D., professor of population science at the Harvard School of Public Health, Boston, explains. "Pesticides are invented to be toxic," he says. "They're designed to get into the organism [of the insect, for example], and they're not something the organism has encountered in the past. The systems of insects and humans have enough in common that they can often affect humans, too.

"We just don't know enough yet about how carcinogens work," continues Dr. Levins. "These chemicals have unusual chemical structures, different from anything seen before in nature. That's why I think it's a good rule to be suspicious of any pesticide."

The other big problem with some pesticides, says Marion Moses, M.D., one of the nation's foremost authorities on pesticides and health and medical director of the National Farm Workers Health Group, is that they can be persistent. "Pesticides used in agriculture pollute that air, contaminate the food supply and are contaminants of groundwater, an irreplaceable resource. Pesticides are found in human breast milk and in the blood and tissues of newborn babies," notes Dr. Moses.

No one disputes that pesticides can pose a cancer risk to the farm and factory workers who are exposed to large quantities in the manufacture, application or harvesting of crops grown with pesticides. Dr. Moses points to dozens of studies linking high pesticide exposure to cancers in agricultural workers. These include cancers of the blood cells (leukemia), lymphatic cancers, lung cancer and liver cancer. One of those studies found that farmers exposed to herbicides for more than 20 days each year had six times more risk of developing the blood cell cancers than nonfarmers. The herbicides were of a class that includes 2,4-D—an ingredient that's also commonly used to kill dandelions in lawns.

AN APPLE A DAY?

But most of us are not farmers, and what the average consumer wants to know is this: Can long-term exposure—like that apple a day— to tiny levels of pesticide residues contribute to health problems, including cancer? Nobody knows for sure. Even the experts—like Dr. Levins—say they have no hard data.

The Environmental Protection Agency permits about 50,000 chemical compounds to be used on crops in the United States. These include some 600 individual active ingredients. At this writing, about 10 percent of those 600 active pesticide ingredients are known or suspected carcinogens ("suspected" meaning that there is evidence of a carcinogenic effect, although contradictory evidence may also exist).

Hundreds of other active ingredients are unknowns—meaning adequate safety testing is not yet completed on most of them.

Why does the government allow known and suspected carcinogens, or unknown chemicals, to be applied to our food crops? Simply put, they feel the benefits are worth the risks. For each known carcinogenic pesticide, the Federal Insecticide, Fungicide and Rodenticide Act (FIFRA) mandates that the EPA perform an analysis to determine whether the social, economic and environmental benefits outweigh the potential risk to human health.

What impact does this policy actually have for you? Well, it can determine what shows up on the supermarket shelves and it's partly responsible for the 'apple flap' in the mid-1980s, with the controversy over one particular pesticide, daminozide, whose trade name is Alar.

Alar has been used for more than 20 years on a variety of agricultural products ranging from cherries to prunes, but mostly on apples. It regulates the growth of fruits so they don't fall from the tree until they're fully ripe. That means apples are firmer, redder, less bruised and scarred—cosmetic differences that consumers demand. Alar doesn't actually protect the fruit against any pests, like insects or weeds. The chemical penetrates the fiber of the plant, and *it can't be washed off.*

Since the mid-1970s, animal studies have linked daminozide to cancer. In addition, the breakdown product of daminozide (resulting from mixing with water or heating) is a chemical compound known to be a potent carcinogen.

The government became concerned when Alar residues turned up in a variety of processed apple products, including baby foods. In 1985, the EPA proposed a ban on the substance. Concern was especially high because infants and children eat more apple products than adults.

Before the chemical could be banned, however, the law required proof that it poses an unacceptable risk. The agency examined the animal studies and decided that evidence was not conclusive. Therefore, Alar was judged "innocent until proven guilty." Instead of a ban, the EPA placed some restrictions on Alar use and ordered the manufacturer to perform better safety studies. The agency also ordered the amount used on crops reduced by 50 percent.

"Alar is not the only bad apple," says Sandra Marquardt, information coordinator of the National Coalition against the Misuse of Pesticides. "It's only one of them." Variations of the Alar story have been played out with other pesticides in recent years. One chemical that the EPA decided to ban outright was ethylene dibromide (EDB), a fumigant. EDB had been used for decades on grain and fruit. After it began turning up in everything from citrus to muffin mix—and in groundwater—the government banned it in 1984. "I am still astounded at some of the uses of EDB, and how we could be so stupid," said one EPA administrator, as reported in the *New York Times.*

These controversies have put enormous pressure on the EPA to speed up the review process for old pesticides. Hopefully, the "unknowns" will become "knowns" before too long.

WHAT YOU CAN DO

Despite all this bad news, long-term studies indicate that a diet that includes plenty of fruits and vegetables may actually lower your risk of cancer.

"The fruits and vegetables cotain nutrients that have positive effects, particularly fiber, which reduces risk of colon cancer," says Dr.

Levins. "At the same time, they may have toxins which induce cancer. Opposing forces are at work. If people could eat pesticide-free fruits and vegetables, they would probably be even healthier."

While it's virtually impossible to eliminate *all* pesticides from your food, there is a whole range of relatively simple things you can do to reduce your exposure to them.

IN THE KITCHEN

Two simple ways to remove excess pesticides from fruits and vegetables are washing and peeling. This works for pesticides which do not enter the fruit by uptake through the soil and are not absorbed through the skin.

When you peel, the loss of fiber and nutrients is relatively small. Remove the outer leaves of lettuce, cabbage, Brussels sprouts and other leafy greens.

If you don't want to peel, you can wash instead. Washing with water removes water-soluble pesticides, so take extra care when washing fruits and vegetables. Rinse them long and thoroughly, and by all means use a vegetable brush.

Studies indicate that washing can be even more effective if you bathe the vegetables first in water with a little mild liquid detergent added. The detergent will act as an emulsifier, removing non-water-soluble pesticides, explains A. Karim Ahmed, Ph.D., research director and senior scientist of the Natural Resources Defense Council in New York City. Follow that bath with a vigorous clear-water rinse.

One more kitchen hint: If you're making foods that call for citrus peel, be sure to wash the fruit well first. Citrus products may be sprayed with even stronger pesticides than soft-skinned fruits, under the assumption that the peel is not eaten.

SUPERMARKET SENSE

How much pesticide residue is on supermarket fare? That's a question that the Natural Resources Defense Council looked into recently, when they collected information on ten common fruits and vegetables sold in San Francisco markets.

The good news: They found a majority of pesticide residues on the produce to be below federal tolerances. The bad news: 44 percent of the 71 fruit and vegetable samples contained residues of 19 different pesticides, and 7 of the 19 were known or suspected carcinogens. Three of the pesticides they detected—DDT, aldrin and endrin—were banned for agricultural use in the 1970s. They are still in use, however, for other applications, and today they still appear in our food. The organization concluded that federal and local monitoring of pesticide residues is spotty, and enforcement is weak. That's why it's a good idea to exercise a little reasonable vigilance when you shop.

Guideline number one is to be sure to select a diverse array of fruits and vegetables. "If you choose a moderate and varied diet, your chance of obtaining an overwhelming dose of any one material greatly decreases," says Dr. Weisburger.

Consider the tempting dilemma posed by luscious tropical fruits like papayas and mangoes, which are generally imported. These fruits, rich in vitamin A and beta-carotene, also have a bad reputation pesticide-wise. "Imported fruits generally have more residues of pesticides, especially the banned pesticides, like DDT," says Dr. Ahmed. "*Tropical* fruits and vegetables are my first candidates for being contaminated."

Does that mean you must cross them off your shopping list? Well, Dr. Ahmed says that he doesn't. "I eat an occasional mango. I wouldn't lose sleep over it; I'm not paranoid," says Dr. Ahmed. "But I would worry about people on a steady diet of papaya, like certain ethnic minorities for whom papaya is a staple. Just don't eat them as if they're going out of style."

The diversity rule is especially important if you have children. Dr. Ahmed says that one reason that the Alar issue was so disturbing was because of the quantity of apples children eat. "Young, growing children are more susceptible to chemicals."

The second guideline for supermarket shopping: Don't choose the shiny waxed fruits instead of the duller, less perfect-looking ones. "I think waxed products should never be bought by anyone," says Dr. Ahmed. "It's not clear that paraffin wax isn't carcinogenic itself. And many of the non-water-soluble products are retained on the wax." If you do buy waxed fruits or vegetables, peeling is definitely a good idea.

Perhaps the most important step you can take in your supermarket is into the manager's office, says Monica Moore. "Tell them you prefer to shop there, but that you're very concerned about pesticides in food. Take out your checkbook and show them how much you've spent in the store. They may respond," she says—just as national supermarket chains acted when consumers expressed concern over Alar on apples.

ORGANIC THINKING

"If you believe in eating lots of fruits and vegetables, and if you really wish to avoid pesticide residues, you've got to go to organic sources, those that can be verified as growing food without the use of pesticides," says Dr. Ahmed.

If you do decide to buy organically grown food, you may have to make an important change in the way you think about fresh produce.

"People should pay less attention to seeking perfection in fruits and vegetables, the feeling that they should look like works of art," says Diane Baxter, a staff scientist with the National Coalition against the Misuse of Pesticides. "Such cosmetic perfection is unnatural and achieved only with the use of potentially hazardous chemicals."

Sources of more healthful produce may not be as hard to find, or as expensive, as you might think. "The good news," says George DeVault, executive editor of *The New Farm* magazine, "is that there has been an increase in the number of smaller farms that are producing more naturally grown produce, especially within two to three hours of major metropolitan areas." Even in mid-Manhattan, urbanites can turn to "The Green Market." Farmers from Pennsylvania, New Jersey and New York set up stands throughout the Big Apple to sell New Yorkers fresher, and sometimes more naturally grown, produce.

DeVault attributes the proliferation of these kinds of farms to the increasing sophistication of Americans' tastes, demanding not just fewer chemicals, but also maximum nutrition, quality and freshness.

However, he warns that "organic," like "beautiful," is often in the eye of the beholder. Just because a product is advertised as naturally grown doesn't mean it's so—and just because chemicals are used doesn't mean it's dangerous. DeVault advises people who shop at farmers markets to talk with farmers. "Ask them about what they use in the way of sprays. Farmers may also use compounds based on natural bacterias or chemicals, like lime sulfur, to protect crops. Some purists say these aren't organic, but at least they're not potent, toxic synthetic chemicals," says DeVault.

To find a local source of organic produce, talk to someone at a health food store or contact the organic growers' association in your state. They have certification programs and can give you a list of reliable farmers. There are at least three states which offer "certification," with strict standards for organically grown produce: California, Maine and Oregon. If you live in those states, you can check at your local store to find products that have been certified.

GROW YOUR OWN

The ultimate irony of the pesticide problem is that, in the long run, pesticides may not be entirely effective in eliminating certain pest problems. Pests can develop a resistance to these chemicals and come back stronger than before.

Farmers, scientists and home gardeners are finding better ways. One alternative to pesticides is Integrated Pest Management Systems. This can mean using a beneficial insect that preys on the harmful ones. The system isn't as obscure as you may think; you may even know someone who has deliberately unleashed a few hundred ladybugs in their garden, to eat the aphids attacking their prize tomatoes.

"My own view is that we have to go for systems that require minimum intervention," says Dr. Levins. "One principle is to recognize that not everything that crawls on a plant is an enemy. The idea of an insect-free field doesn't make sense. We have to give up the illusion of complete control over a cultivated field."

As for home gardens, be careful with any garden sprays and lawn care products that you must use. Their ingredients are not necessarily safer than what is being applied to commercial crops. For example, 2,4-D, which may be linked to lymphatic cancer among farmers, is common in consumer lawn and garden products. Be sure to read labels and follow directions exactly. "If a product is registered for rose bushes, don't use it on tomatoes or strawberries," says Alexandre Tarsey, Ph.D., head of the technical support section of the EPA's Insecticide-Rodenticide Branch. "There's a good reason for that restriction," he says. Also obey the label instructions about protective clothing, such as gloves.

CITIZEN ACTION

No individual can resolve the pesticide problem single-handedly. But in communities, on the state level and nationally, we are moving, slowly but surely, toward solutions.

Local "networking" is a key part of the solution. Farmers, consumers and retailers are working together to make organic foods widely available. One model networking approach is that encouraged by Americans for Safe Food (ASF). Regional ASF groups have prepared directories of local supermarkets, shops and farmers who offer contaminant-free food. They have also put together a national directory of farms and outlets, from which people can mail-order organically grown produce and meats.

Supporting such outlets may have a greater impact than just preserving an individual's own health. "We're convinced that the issue of pesticides won't be taken care of administratively and legislatively," says Cesar Chavez, president of the United Farm Workers of America, whose union has undertaken a campaign to grow grapes organically and to stop the use of carcinogenic pesticides on grapes. "We're convinced that the best and fastest way to take care of it is through the market. If 'clean food' becomes widely available, the problem of pesticides will be over quickly."

CANCER PREVENTION PLAN:
PESTICIDES IN FOOD

- Bathe vegetables and fruits in water with a little liquid detergent added, then rinse thoroughly.
- Limit consumption of imported tropical fruits.
- Avoid shiny, waxed fruits.

Prescription Drugs

Medications are most often thought of as lifesavers, not life takers. And certainly as far as cancer goes, drugs have prolonged the lives of countless people who otherwise would have been overcome by their diseases. But drugs have their dark side too: Medicines cause perhaps 1 to 2 percent of all cancers. That's not many cases when you look at the big picture, but it's very significant if you're afflicted by drug-induced cancer.

Different types of drugs are suspected of leading to cancer, including hormones, psoriasis medicine and immunosuppressive drugs given to people who've had organ transplants.

CATCH-22: CANCER TREATMENTS AS A CAUSE

But surely the most peculiar aspect of drugs and cancer is the fact that some drugs used to fight cancer can actually cause it. Cynics can take this as proof positive that trying to prevent cancer is a waste of time because *everything* causes cancer—even the cancer cures. But that's how cynics are. The truth is that these anticancer drugs work miracles where nothing has worked before. And while they might increase a person's risk of cancer, they also increase a person's chance of living a longer, fuller life.

"You're taking these drugs because you have cancer already. But there is a slim possibility that by taking them you might develop more cancer. You really have no alternatives, do you?" says George Mandel, Ph.D., chairman of the pharmacology department of George Washington University Medical School in Washington, D.C.

ALKYLATING AGENTS

Some of the more common cancer-causing drugs are used to treat Hodgkin's disease. They belong to a class of drugs called alkylating agents, which are also used on a lot of other cancers, including breast and lung cancer. Alkylating agents work by messing up the ways that cancer cells multiply. They get inside the cells and fool with the DNA, RNA and other protein molecules that control survival and reproduction. Everyone has seen the models of molecules that look like they're made of pencils joined by Ping-Pong balls. Well, alkylating agents do what all high school chemistry students want to do: They rearrange the layout of the pencils and Ping-Pong balls to their liking.

Unfortunately, alkylating agents (and other cancer drugs) can't be controlled as precisely as doctors would like. The result is that they sometimes attack healthy cells. When the building blocks of these healthy cells are damaged, they can become cancerous. In Hodgkin's disease, this damage can lead to acute myelocytic leukemia (AML).

This risk is demonstrated by these figures: Of more than 3,000 people with Hodgkin's disease who were studied prior to 1962, not one had AML. But in the 12 years between 1961 and 1973, the rate of AML among Hodgkin's disease sufferers was 156 per 100,000. And the highest rates of AML arose just a few years after a therapy called MOPP, which included the alkylating agents nitrogen mustard and procarbazine, was first used to treat Hodgkin's disease. This suggests an association between the use of alkylating agents for Hodgkin's disease and the later onset of leukemia.

Other studies have supported this link. Patients with multiple myeloma cancer, ovarian cancer, lung cancer, stomach cancer and colorectal cancer have also been shown to be at greater risk of developing leukemia within four to five years of being treated with alkylating agents.

But while this side effect of alkylating agents is very serious, the drugs are often the only therapy that will work. And in effect they give a cancer patient the opportunity to live long enough to risk getting another cancer, says Dr. Mandel. "For example, a person with Hodgkin's disease would definitely die of the cancer without the drugs, and he may die later because of the drugs. But he'll have an opportunity to live a productive life for an extended period, and enjoy his family and friends," says Dr. Mandel. "Most people would choose to live."

RADIOACTIVE DRUGS

About half of the people diagnosed as having cancer in the United States undergo radiation therapy of one sort or another to treat their cancer. Radiation works by attacking the DNA of cancerous cells, destroying their ability to reproduce and live. External radiation, similar to x-rays, is the most common radiation treatment. But sometimes drugs with radioactive "markers" are given to cancer patients, either as treatment or to help with diagnostic tests. Unfortunately, the radioactive drugs can build up in the body over time and lead to various types of cancer.

ANTI-IMMUNE-POWER DRUGS

Another class of drugs that poses a cancer risk are immunosuppressive drugs that are used to keep people from rejecting transplanted organs. These people have 32 times more risk than the average person of developing a type of cancer called non-Hodgkin's lymphoma. Transplant patients are also at increased risk for skin cancers, Kaposi's sarcoma and lung cancer.

One common class of immunosuppressive drugs is adrenal corticosteroid hormones. (These aren't the sex hormones some athletes take, which are called androgens. These are also used by transsexuals and by doctors to treat some illnesses, but they have not been proved to pose a cancer risk.) Like all the immunosuppressive drugs, corticosteroids pose a problem if taken over a long period of time because they lower the body's defenses. But again, the benefits of the drugs for transplant patients is probably worth the risk. "Someone who needs a kidney transplant is facing a choice between two evils, and the drugs and the transplant are probably the lesser evil," Dr. Mandel says.

DIETHYSTILBESTROL

Female sex hormones, unlike their male counterparts, are risk factors in various types of cancer. Estrogens that are produced naturally by the ovaries may be implicated as a risk factor for some types of cancer. *Synthetic* estrogen, which for years has been used in birth control pills, has also been linked to cancer, though present-day birth control pills seem to have greatly reduced the risk (see chapter 50, Oral Contraceptives). Another important hormonal link to cancer is diethylstilbestrol (DES), a synthetic compound very similar to estrogen.

Synthesized in 1938, DES became popular in the late 1940s as a way to prevent miscarriage. This was during the baby boom, and the miscarriage rate among American women was one in four. Doctors freely prescribed DES as a way to prevent the problem, even though there was no real proof that it worked. Reports of harmful side effects had shadowed DES from the beginning, but it wasn't until the 1960s, after millions of women had taken the drug, that the real story began to unfold. That's when doctors began to notice a rare kind of vaginal and cervical cancer in young women. In 1971 a study reported that DES was behind the cancer. And it wasn't that the girls had taken it, but rather that their mothers had. The Food and Drug Administration later suggested that the drug should not be used by pregnant women, though the FDA never outlawed its use by pregnant women.

While DES daughters have been the focus of much of the cancer warnings surrounding the drug, DES sons might be at greater risk of getting cancer, too. DES is associated with an increased risk of men having undescended testicles, and there is a direct correlation between this condition and testicular cancer.

DES is still used to treat prostate cancer in men. "It's probably one of the best treatments around for men with prostate tumors. Any risk is probably worth it," says Dr. Mandel. "The main risk is for daughters of DES mothers. They should let their doctors know so that they'll give them regular tests for cancer," he says.

DES was used in animal feed for many years to make livestock gain weight. That practice has been stopped and does not pose a cancer threat.

PSORIASIS TREATMENTS

Psoriasis can be a devastating disease because of the scaly skin plaques it causes and also because it is not very responsive to treatment. So any therapy that holds hope of working is likely to be widely and readily received. A drug called 8-Methoxypsoralen is often used with long-wave ultraviolet radiation (PUVA) to treat psoriasis, sometimes with good results. While the evidence is still inconclusive, this treatment might also increase a person's risk of getting skin cancer.

"This is a scary drug and the treatment must be very carefully done," says Dr. Mandel. "There is not much clinical evidence that it causes cancer, but there is a lot of laboratory evidence that it interacts with the DNA to cause cell mutation. People should be very cautious about using this drug.

"But then again, psoriasis can be a nasty disease and it's hard to treat. People will have to make the choice," says Dr. Mandel. "Fortunately, it looks like some newer treatments coming along may turn out to pose less risk."

Dr. Mandel also suggests that people should avoid using any skin medicines or shampoos that contain coal tar for any extended length of time. This substance was first shown to be a carcinogen around the time of the Declaration of Independence, but its medicinal benefits have always been thought to outweigh its harmful effects. However, opinions about coal tar's usefulness and its risks are changing.

"First of all, it's not usually necessary. And it is known to produce skin tumors in mice, though again the evidence for humans isn't clear. Regular use for a long time could lead to cancer. So I suggest people avoid coal tar," says Dr. Mandel.

Even with these problems, when you take into consideration the number of drugs on the market, they don't pose an alarming cancer threat. If you're knowledgeable about the drugs, there's really not that much you have to worry about, says Dr. Mandel. "The Food and Drug Administration does a pretty thorough job of keeping carcinogenic drugs off the market," he says.

Protein

Back in 1890, the evening newspaper contained a health bulletin from the Department of Agriculture—experts there had determined that working men needed 110 grams of protein a day. Athletes at that time were fed diets containing 155 grams a day. Fruits and vegetables were thought to be poor sources of protein and thus were disregarded, being thought of little worth.

Yet some people—even in those days—were urging that this protein recommendation be cut in half. They said people were eating too much fat and protein, and should rely more on fruits and vegetables. The Reverend Sylvester Graham, a Presbyterian minister (who was later immortalized, having provided the name for the graham cracker), preached that people should eat a wide variety of simple foods. He advocated that bran be left in flour and baked into bread.

These theories, once considered wacky, now sound very much like today's nutrition guidelines from the Department of Agriculture. (The latest official protein recommendation is 56 grams a day for men, 44 for women.) Many nutritionists believe that we still eat too much protein and that most of us rely too heavily on animal protein, which is often very high in fat. High-fat diets have been linked with a number of cancers, including those of the colon and breast.

IS PROTEIN A RISK FACTOR?

A number of researchers are now studying whether fat is the only culprit or whether protein itself might be increasing our risk for certain cancers.

E. J. Hawrylewicz, Ph.D., director of research at Mercy Hospital in Chicago and professor of biochemistry at the University of Illinois College of Medicine, has found that laboratory animals who eat a high-protein diet get more breast tumors than do animals fed a normal amount of protein. In the experiments, both groups were exposed to the same carcinogen known to induce breast tumors, and both consumed the same amount of fat and calories. The only difference was protein, and that turned out to be a significant difference.

Dr. Hawrylewicz based these experiments on a very logical chain of connections. He already knew that hormones play important roles in breast cancer, both in animals and in women. He also knew that certain amino acids from protein go right into the brain and there turn into neurotransmitters that send out messages that control hormones.

He then conjectured that a high-protein diet might alter the level of those neurotransmitters at the brain switchboard, and that this change might increase or decrease the levels of hormones such as prolactin, estrogen and progesterone, and thus affect vulnerability to breast cancer. "This could be an explanation for why people in Western societies seem to have a very high incidence of breast cancer in comparison to, say, Oriental populations," explains Dr. Hawrylewicz.

When he and his colleagues looked at the hormone levels of the animals at different ages, they saw no differences. Yet one consistent finding was that those on the high-protein diet always reached sexual maturity at an early age. "This is analogous to Western cultures, in which age of menarche is earlier than elsewhere in the world," says Dr. Hawrylewicz. Early menarche (that's the onset of menstruation) is one of the risk factors for breast cancer. "In Japan, age of menarche is getting earlier and, at the same time, the breast cancer incidence is rising slowly in Japan."

It is during puberty that breast tissues of laboratory animals are most sensitive to a carcinogen, because that is when their cells are dividing very rapidly. When cells divide, the chromosomes "unfold" (normally they are all crumpled in a ball), and it is when they are unfolded that they are most exposed to a chemical that might cause an abnormality. And this is probably true not only in animals, but in women as well. Tragically, after the atomic bomb was dropped on Japan, women who had been adolescents at the time of the explosion had a much higher incidence of breast cancer than did the older women, says Dr. Hawrylewicz.

If all girls are sensitive at puberty, why should it matter at what age it begins? Because pregnancy ends the risk period and, presumably, the earlier a girl begins to menstruate, the more time will pass before she becomes pregnant. Late pregnancy is another risk factor for breast cancer.

Can we now say definitely that a high-protein diet alters neurotransmitters, thus changing the hormone picture in our bodies, thus causing early menses, thus increasing our risk for breast cancer? Dr. Hawrylewicz is cautious. "You need to be careful when you transpose to humans. All I can say is that our high-protein animals reached menarche sooner and that for women, early menarche is one of the risk factors for breast cancer."

MORE ABOUT PROTEIN

There may be something more in excess protein that increases cancer risks than simply the indirect effect of possibly causing early menstruation. Other scientists have found a link between high-protein diets in animals and various other cancers. At Cornell University, Ithaca, New York, researchers discovered that too much protein increases liver tumors, and at the Eppley Institute in Nebraska, studies have associated pancreatic cancer with high-protein diets. The picture is not completely clear, however. One researcher at the University of Illinois has found no relation between cancer and protein.

Many other studies have looked at animal fat and protein together. In Israel, a study of the diets of 818 breast cancer patients and two control groups revealed that the risk for women who ate the most animal fat and protein and the least fiber was twice as high as for women who ate the least animal food and the most fiber.

In Australia, researchers studying diet and colon cancer reported that "high consumption of protein and total energy [calories] is associated with greater than a doubling of risk in women." Risks for men in the high animal protein group were also twice that of low or normal protein consumers, but only after age 70.

All in all, it is too soon to make recommendations to people, says Dr. Hawrylewicz. "It's probably true," he adds, "that the average person in this country is eating excessive amounts of fat and protein. My personal diet has changed significantly. I eat far less fat and more fruits and vegetables. I don't know that the total amount of protein in my diet has changed, but we eat meat only in moderation."

CANCER PREVENTION PLAN: PROTEIN

- Eat high-protein foods in moderation.
- Reduce dietary fat.

C H A P T E R 56
Salt

Yes, some people believe salt contributes to cancer. But it's not the salt you sprinkle on your popcorn. The salt that some experts are concerned about comes in the form of salt-cured foods. And to tell you the truth, it's not clear whether it's the actual salt or the process of salt-curing that poses the risk. Many of the studies that implicate salt-cured foods in cancer also implicate smoked and nitrate-cured foods (see chapter 48, Nitrites and Nitrates). Whatever the reason, salt-cured foods are associated with an increased risk of stomach and esophageal cancer. The National Academy of Sciences and the American Cancer Society urge everyone to eat salt-cured, nitrate-cured and smoked foods only moderately.

People in other countries such as Japan and China eat more pickled and salt-cured food than people in the United States do. This may be the reason that much of the research into the link between salt-cured foods and cancer comes from Japan, where the traditional diet includes a lot of pickled vegetables and salted fish. Studies of Japanese people have found that these foods increase a person's risk of stomach cancer. Stomach cancer causes more deaths in Japan than all other cancers combined. It is five times more common in Japan than in the United States.

But salt-curing isn't a common preservative for foods that are a major part of the U.S. diet these days. So unless you're addicted to salt-cured fish, pickled foods or smoked foods, you probably aren't increasing your risk of cancer.

CANCER PREVENTION PLAN: SALT

- Eat salt-cured, nitrite-cured and smoked foods only moderately.

CHAPTER 57
Selenium

Is the salt in your cupboard fortified with selenium? How about the bread in your breadbox? Don't bother to check the labels because they're not. But maybe they soon will be. Some scientists who are investigating selenium's potential for cancer prevention believe that before the turn of the century, foods fortified with selenium could become a reality—if their theories prove correct.

The truth is, theories about whether the mineral selenium can protect against cancer have been brewing for years. And the evidence has been getting stronger and stronger. More than 55 published laboratory studies show that animals given selenium had a reduced incidence of cancer. Even more important, there is a wealth of research from around the world indicating a positive anticancer connection in humans as well. Scientists are now ready to perform the acid test of selenium's effectiveness: clinical trials.

"There is now sufficient evidence from laboratory experiments and epidemiological studies [statistical analyses of various populations] to get on with clinical trials to determine whether when one raises selenium levels in humans one reduces cancer risk," says Larry C. Clark, Ph.D., assistant professor of epidemiology at Cornell University's Department of Preventive Medicine in Ithaca, New York. Dr. Clark is one of the scientists involved in this latest project.

What he is talking about is the final stage of research that could establish once and for all what scientists have suspected for years: People who get adequate amounts of selenium in their diets are less likely to develop cancer.

HITTING PAYDIRT

What got researchers interested in selenium, anyway? Ask Gerhard N. Schrauzer, Ph.D., professor of chemistry at the University of California at San Diego, and he'll tell you it was just a lucky coincidence.

Back in the 1960s, Dr. Schrauzer was attempting to develop a blood test that might be useful for diagnosing cancer. He knew that blood samples from cancer patients reacted more slowly with methylene blue, a well-known chemical dye, than did samples from healthy people. Searching for an explanation, he discovered that the test actually was measuring levels of selenium: It uncovered an apparent lack of the element in people who had cancer as compared to those who didn't. He asked himself, "Could low levels of this nutrient put people at greater risk for cancer?"

At that time, coincidentally, scientists also found that soil contains varying selenium levels, and in areas where there is little selenium in the soil, crops are low in selenium, too. As a result, people in those parts of the world get less selenium in their diets and have low levels of selenium in their blood. Scientists developed a theory that these low selenium levels might lead to a higher risk of cancer. Then researchers began to test the hypothesis, and their studies have taken them around the world.

For example, one recent study focused on 24 regions in China, where selenium is very unequally distributed in the soil and therefore in the foods grown there. Researchers compared the blood selenium levels of 1,458 people from these regions with corresponding cancer mortality statistics. They found that cancer death rates were higher in regions where people had lower levels of selenium in their blood. This connection was found to be particularly true for cancer of the stomach, esophagus and liver.

REAL PEOPLE PROVIDE REAL PROOF

But statistics can only *suggest* a relationship between selenium and cancer risk. To prove it, you've got to study real people. One such study was done in Finland, a country known to be one of the world's low selenium areas. It compared women who had cancer with women who did not. Those with cervical and endometrial cancer were found to have *significantly* lower concentrations of selenium in their blood than those who were cancer-free. The researchers concluded that low blood concentrations of selenium "might be a contributing factor in the development of cervical and endometrial cancer."

But the scientists still had their doubts. Suppose blood selnium levels in cancer patients didn't represent a risk factor at all. Suppose, instead, that they were a *result* of the cancer. One way tofind out was to measure people's selenium levels when they were healthy, thenwait to see if those with the lowest levels developed cancer more often than those with the highest.

Perhaps the largest study designed to test this theory comes from Finish researchers. They took blood samples from 8,113 men and women between the ages of 31 and 59 who had no history of cancer. Then they kept track of these people for six years. By the time the study was completed, 128 of the participants had developed cancer. And, as expected, those people with the lowest selenium levels were found to be three times as likely to get cancer as those whose selenium levels were high.

And what's true for Finland is true for the United States as well. A similar experiment used blood samples collected over a period of time from people who were cancer-free. The study was performed by Walter C. Willett, M.D., an epidemiologist from the Harvard School of Public Health, Boston, and his colleagues. Over a five-year period, 111 of those who were tested developed cancer. When the scientists compared them to 210 people who were still free of the disease, they found that the risk of cancer for those who had the lowest levels of selenium was *twice* that of those with the highest levels. (The greatest risk involved prostate and gastrointestinal cancer.) And what's more, those individuals who had low vitamin A or E levels as well as low selenium levels showed even greater risk of cancer.

Scientists like Dr. Willett are continuing to pile up evidence of a selenium/anticancer link. In fact, he recently was "knee-deep" in toenail clippings—70,000 samples, to be exact—which he hopes will help to confirm the results of his previous smaller study. "Toenails are a very good source of information about people's selenium status," says Dr. Willett. (Considering all the "bloodletting" that has gone on in the interest of selenium research, his subjects are undoubtedly grateful!)

DIET MAKES THE DIFFERENCE

So why *do* healthy people have higher blood levels of selenium than cancer patients? What makes the difference? In an attempt to answer this question, Dr. Schrauzer, in collaboration with the Japanese

Cancer Institute, compared the selenium levels of both American and Japanese breast cancer patients with those of healthy women. But they also compared the *diets* of the women to see if selenium levels were, in fact, related to what these women ate.

Their results showed that healthy Japanese had the highest blood selenium levels, followed by healthy American women. Cancer patients—both Japanese and American—had lower levels, and women with recurring breast cancer had the lowest levels of all. What's more, the difference between the healthy Japanese women and their American counterparts was attributed to differences in their dietary intakes of selenium. "Japanese women get twice as much selenium from their diets as American women," says Dr. Schrauzer. "And breast cancer rates are much lower in Japan, indicating that there is a connection." In fact, Dr. Schrauzer believes that most Americans only get about one-half the amount of selenium they need for cancer protection.

How much selenium do we need to protect us from cancer? That's what scientists like Dr. Clark are trying to find out. "The hard issue is, too little selenium may put you at greater risk of developing cancer, but too much can actually be toxic. Somewhere between the two extremes is the optimal dose. That's what we're trying to determine now."

What Dr. Clark and his colleagues are doing is studying people who are at high risk for nonmelanoma skin cancer—people who have a history of the disease and a good likelihood of getting it back again. Already 700 people are participating in the experiment. Some of them are getting 200 micrograms of selenium. Others are not. Instead they are getting an identical tablet, but of *low*-selenium brewer's yeast. Five years down the road, the researchers hope to be able to report that the selenium-supplemented people were protected from recurrences without experiencing any toxic side effects from the selenium itself.

According to Dr. Clark, "If these clinical trials show hat selenium in nutritional-size doses can protect people from cancer without risk of toxicity, then we should be prepared with a plan to improve the selenium status of the American population. And one practical way of accomplishing that would be to fortify foods with selenium."

SELENIUM: THE LAW ENFORCER

So it looks like scientists have substantial proof that selenium works, but how does it do its job? The experts don't know for certain, but they've made some intelligent guesses. Its presence, like a cop on the beat, may simply serve to protect. That's the function most theories focus on. Selenium appears to have the ability to protect individual cells from attacks by chemicals and viruses that can cause cancer. Picture a normal, healthy cell, minding the body's business as nature intended. Along comes a chemical, looking for trouble. How can selenium protect that cell? It may be able to do the following things.

Disarm the bandit. Sometimes a chemical can't cause cancer until the body unintentionally turns it into a carcinogen. Selenium apparently alters this process, causing the chemical to be transformed into inactive compounds instead.

Defend against attack. Selenium may work something like a bulletproof vest, keeping a cell's DNA molecules safe from the chemical bullets that could damage them and induce a cancer.

Help restore order. It's not always possible to stop a chemical from inflicting harm. When the DNA has already been damaged, however, your body can repair it, if there is enough time. Selenium delays cell division long enough for this repair process to take place.

Now picture that healthy cell again. Imagine that a virus has slipped in through the cell's wall and taken up residence. Just like a parasite, this unwelcome visitor will demand a large share of the cell's nutrients and force that cell's enzymes to work for its own duplication. The virus can also alter the cell's DNA, causing it to become a cancer cell. What can selenium do? It can keep the virus from getting the upper hand by slowing cellular processes. It may also protect the cellular DNA against the virus-induced changes. But viruses are not the only cause of cancer. Chemicals may also bring about the malignant transformation.

Researchers have shown that even if selenium is able to disarm such chemicals, the healthy cell is still vulnerable. It can be mugged from within by a free radical.

Free radicals are powerful aggressors in molecular form. They rip off hydrogen atoms from other molecules and claim them for their own. The result of this foul play is the formation of new radicals, which can corrode cell membranes in the same way that rust eats away at iron. This corrosion leaves a cell vulnerable toall manner of attacks by cancer-causers.

Selenium takes the punch out of the new radicals, but in a roundabout way. It helps to produce a special enzyme that turns them into harmless water.

Suppose, however, that a cell becomes cancerous in spite of this nutrient's superb protection. Then it's up to the immune system to seek out and destroy that malignant cell. Although not fully understood, it is believed the selenium aids in this process as well.

In addition to all these functions, selenium also latches on to harmful heavy metals like mercury, cadmium and lead and escorts them out of the body.

PROTECTION NOW

The evidence seems pretty convincing. Dr. Schrauzer, in fact, says, "I believe that we can say with a high degree of assurance that selenium has a protective effect against cancer."

But the final verdict is yet to be announced. And the results of the clinical trials are not yet complete. How can you take advantage—today—of the protection against cancer that selenium promises to supply? Here are some guidelines from the experts, to get you started.

According to the National Research Council, a daily intake of 50 to 200 micrograms (that's *not* milligrams) of selenium is "safe and adequate" to meet your nutritional needs. But if you're interested in taking full advantage of selenium's potential for cancer prevention, Dr. Schrauzer concludes from his studies that 250 to 300 micrograms a day may be required for optimal protection.

Does this mean that we can't get enough selenium from our diets to protect us from cancer without stepping over the safety margin into the toxic range? The experts don't think so.

Oliver Alabaster, M.D., author of *What You Can Do to Prevent Cancer* (Simon & Schuster) says that 300 micrograms "is far below the level of 2,400 to 3,000 micrograms of selenium per day that has been shown to cause toxicity when consumed for prolonged periods."

And Patricia Hausman, a nutritionist and author of a book on supplement safety, *The Right Dose* (Rodale Press) agrees. In fact, she believes that the 200-microgram upper limit set by the National Research Council is rooted in what she calls "selenophobia." "For those who want to play it very safe, I would recommend a total intake of no more than 350 micrograms daily." (Of course, she includes in that figure *all* the selenium you may be getting—from foods as well as other sources.) And we all know that the favored way to get our nutrients is from the food we eat.

HOW TO EAT MORE SELENIUM

Munch a bunch of peanuts and you can be sure of getting a healthy dose of vitamin E. Nibble a carrot and it brings visions of vitamin A. But what foods should you eat to provide enough selenium?

How about a tuna sandwich? Made from ½ cup of tuna fish and two slices of whole wheat bread, it could provide 138 micrograms of this mineral. Just make sure you use water-packed tuna, because the oil-packed type gives you only half the selenium.

Not only tuna but all fish and shellfish are by far the richest sources of selenium. Organ meats (like liver and kidney), muscle meats, whole grain cereals and brazil nuts are other good sources. The mineral can also be found in many protein-rich foods. Just don't depend on fruits and vegetables for your daily supply—they usually contain only small amounts.

But *do* eat them. In fact, why not eat those peanuts and that carrot as well. In animal studies, both vitamin A and vitamin E have been shown to have synergistic or additive effects on selenium. What this means is that when researchers combined doses of vitamin E with selenium, the combination was more effective in preventing cancer than vitamin E alone.

WHAT ABOUT SUPPLEMENTS?

Can we get enough selenium from the foods we eat, or do we need the "insurance" that supplements can supply? There are no easy answers. The truth is, it's very difficult to estimate exactly how much selenium your diet contains.

People who live in certain regions of the United States (the northeastern, Pacific northwestern and southeastern coastal areas) are most likely to be shortchanged, because these areas have low soil levels of selenium. But according to Gerald F. Combs, Jr., Ph.D., associate professor of nutrition at Cornell University's Department of Poultry and Avian Sciences, Ithaca, New York, "The selenium intakes of most Americans fall within the 'safe and adequate' range." Experts believe we probably achieve safe levels because a lot of the food we eat isn't grown locally but trucked in from the nation's breadbasket, from Florida and California, from almost everywhere.

But, remember, "safe and adequate" amounts can be anywhere from 50 to 200 micrograms daily, which is less selenium than Dr. Schrauzer believes is adequate for cancer protection. He says it makes good sense for most healthy adults to take a prudent amount of selenium in supplemental form—100 to 200 micrograms—daily (a level found in a typical Japanese diet). He also suggests that if you shop for a supplement, you purchase the form of selenium usually found in foods—either selenium yeast or as selenomethionine. These utritional forms of selenium are more readily used by the body. As long as you do not exceed this dosage you need not worry about toxicity, says Dr. Schrauzer. A slice of wheat bread, for example, may contain from 50 to 100 micrograms of selenium. (Before taking any supplement, get the advice and approval of your doctor.)

"My family and I and many of my physician friends have been taking 100 to 200 micrograms of selenium regularly for the past ten years," says Dr. Schrauzer. "The toxicity of selenium is often exaggerated. The difference between protective and toxic doses is reasonably large, and the symptoms of toxicity are easily discernible." (These symptoms include garlic breath, brittle nails, hair loss and dermatitis.)

And, while other researchers, like Dr. Clark, do not advocate supplementation, he readily admits to periodically taking the same dose he gives to the people participating in his study. "I wouldnt ask others to do what I am not prepared to do myself. We haven't seen any toxicity in any of our patients who have been taking 200 micrograms on a regular basis for up to three years."

CANCER PREVENTION PLAN: SELENIUM

- Eat foods high in selenium, such as fish and shellfish.
- Eat foods grown in a variety of locations.
- Take a selenium supplement only with your doctor's okay.

C H A P T E R 58

Sex

Can you "catch" cancer from someone else? Not exactly. The type of contact involved in caring for someone with cancer isn't going to give you the disease. If it did, there'd be an epidemic among health care workers.

But there is strong evidence now that you can contract viruses that may make you more likely to develop certain kinds of cancer. Each of these viruses can be transmitted a number of ways—through blood tranfusions, from contaminated needles, from mother to child during pregnancy or breastfeeding. Findings also indicate that some of these viruses often are transmitted through sexual intercourse.

To date, this list of viral-linked cancers includes cervical cancer; rare cancers of the vagina, vulva and penis; adult T-cell leukemia; a kind of liver cancer associated with hepatitis B, and certain cancers of the nose, throat and lymph glands. And more, perhaps many more, are expected to be found.

Some other sexually transmitted viruses—those suspected of causing acquired immune deficiency syndrome (AIDS), for instance—don't have the ability to change cells, making them cancerous. Instead, they kill cells. Because AIDS kills infection-fighting white blood cells, the body's defense mechanism is weakened and therefore is unable to prevent cancer and infectious disease.

It's alarming to feel at the mercy of parasitic particles so small only a powerful electron microscope can detect them. But before you declare yourself celibate, you should know that, for the most part, these viruses seem to be relatively inefficient at causing cancer. Many more people are exposed to them than ever get cancer. For instance, it's estimated that 90 percent of the adult population of the United States has been exposed to the Epstein-Barr virus. In Africa, this virus has been associated with a type of nose and throat cancer. In the United States, this form of cancer is rare. In industrialized countries, the Epstein-Barr virus mainly causes mononucleosis, the "kissing disease," although many who are exposed to the virus develop no symptoms at all.

Researchers do, however, point out that their estimates of how many cancers are virus-related are truly *guesses,* and perhaps not as educated as we'd like.

"The advent of genetic engineering techniques has greatly facilitated methods for studying viruses," says Anthony Faras, Ph.D., director of the Institute of Human Genetics at the University of Minnesota Medical School, Minneapolis. "We're just now learning how to detect certain viruses or virus genes present at very low levels in human tissue. Even five years ago we would have missed many of them."

Another factor makes it difficult to establish a firm link between viruses and cancer. It is the extreme variation in latency periods—the length of time between exposure to the virus and onset of symptoms. Your runny nose and cough might let you know within ten days that you've picked up a cold virus. But some cancer-inducing viruses have latency periods of 30 years or longer. Or they may never produce symptoms at all.

One reason for prolonged latency is that a virus alone is usually not the sole cause of cancer. Other factors must also fall into place. If you have a genetic tendency toward cancer—that is, if close members of your family got cancer, especially at an early age—you're probably more susceptible to these viruses. Poor nutrition, smoking, alcohol abuse and illnesses could also prompt these viral infections to develop into cancer.

HOW A VIRUS DOES ITS DIRTY WORK

Viruses are among the smallest infectious agents known. They are little more than a membrane, or envelope, of protein-sugar molecules containing strands of genetic material. Dozens of viruses easily fit inside a typical white blood cell.

A virus can enter the body several ways. Cold viruses, for example, enter the cells lining the nose or lungs via nasal secretions on the hands or in the air. The virus that causes polio enters through the cells of the intestines through contaminated food or water. The yellow fever virus is transmitted to the blood cells by mosquitoes. And sexually transmitted viruses enter through the cells of the sex organs, colon, or, less frequently, the mouth and skin. The viruses are carried in semen and, in lesser amounts, in saliva and vaginal secretions.

Having broken skin—a nick, a cut, a tiny sore—increases your chances of becoming infected by a virus. But just as a burglar can break into a locked house, a virus can enter the body even without the easy access of broken skin. Researchers found that out when they were able to successfully infect perfectly whole and intact colon cells that had been grown in the laboratory with the AIDS virus.

Unlike criminals, viruses do not invade merely to ransack and loot. They break into cells to survive. Their genetic material is incomplete. They cannot replicate until they have entered a living cell, because they must use parts of that cell for their own reproduction.

Once in a cell, some groups of viruses can facilitate the insertion of their genetic material (genes), into the host chromosome, therefore actually becoming part of the cell's genetic material. This meshing and restructuring of material is the same sort of genetic engineering being done in laboratories today, "only much more sophisticated," Dr. Faras says. This process can alter the genetic "guidance system" of a cell, turning it into a wayward monster that multiplies rapidly, crowds out other cells and migrates to new locations in the body.

Sometimes the virus brings along with it a gene that can directly cause cancerous changes. The acute adult T-cell leukemia virus is one that does this. Once symptoms come on, the disease progresses very rapidly.

Other viruses have to play hit-or-miss. They're waiting to find a cell that has what's known as a "proto-oncogene," a gene already in the cell that can be activated to make the cell become cancerous. These cancers progress more slowly. Chronic adult T-cell leukemia is one of these cancers. So is a rare form of skin cancer, epidermodysplasia verruciformis. This is a familial disease caused by papilloma viruses.

"This disease is very interesting because it demonstrates that there is indeed a genetic susceptibility to these viruses," says Wayne Lancaster, Ph.D., associate professor of obstetrics, gynecology and pathology at Georgetown University, Washington, D.C. "It proves that certain families carry genetic weaknesses to specific cancer-causing viruses."

And some viruses have the potential to turn a cell into a virtual "virus factory." When the AIDS virus becomes active, for example, it

PROTECTING YOURSELF FROM AIDS

Even though it can't directly turn cells cancerous, the AIDS virus opens the body to a multitude of deadly diseases, including cancer. Estimates of the percentage of people exposed to the virus who will go on to develop symptoms keeps climbing. Some researchers now say 50 percent or more of AIDS virus carriers will eventually die as a result of the disease.

This means you must know how to make sure you don't get AIDS—or spread it to someone else—even if you are a healthy heterosexual.

"These days, doctors are not so reassuring, and they shouldn't be," says Warren Johnson, M.D., professor of medicine and public health and chief of the Division of International Medicine at Cornell University Medical College, New York City. "We have reached the point where, unless you are having sex with someone on whom you would stake your life, you should have him use a condom. We have reached a time where women as well as men should carry condoms, so that there is no lack of availability. We need to say, 'If we are going to have sex, we are going to be careful.' "

Added to high-risk groups of homosexual and bisexual men and intravenous drug users are prostitutes, those having sex with prostitutes and both men and women who have had large numbers of sex partners. The disease is passed on by both men and women; oral sex is considered a transmission route.

Geographic location is also important. "At this time, the AIDS epidemic is most widespread in New York City, San Francisco, Los Angeles and Miami," Dr. Johnson says. "If you live in one of these cities, and you're a woman who has had sex with a bisexual man or you had blood tranfusions before 1983, when AIDS virus testing became available, you might also be at some, although lesser, risk."

Should you be tested for the AIDS virus? Doctors don't seem to want to encourage unneeded testing of worried but low-risk people. But they do urge high-risk people to find out for sure and

reproduces itself so quickly that the new virus particles escaping from the cell tear so many holes in the cell membrane that the contents of the cell ooze out and the cell dies.

Some viruses cause symptoms and then fade away because they have been successfully fought off by the immune system. Some stick

to take responsible action to make sure the virus stops with them.

Testing and reporting procedures vary considerably from state to state, even from city to city. But many states have a federally funded testing program—with anonymity guaranteed—run by the Centers for Disease Control. (Call your state's 1-800 operator for its AIDS hotline number.)

"This is the only place to get tested if you are concerned about confidentiality," says Holly Smith, communications director for the San Francisco AIDS Hotline. "Using a family doctor or a blood bank testing center may mean that information becomes available to insurance companies and potential employers, who may discriminate against you as a result."

The tests are for the AIDS antibody. In some testing centers, if a first test is positive it will be followed by a more specific antibody test (Western Blot, for example) to confirm the results.

If both these tests are positive, they signal definite exposure to the virus. Is there anything an exposed person can do to stay healthy?

Some doctors say it might help to avoid things like severe physical or mental strain—extreme diets, lack of sleep, job-related worries, alcohol, caffeine, tobacco and recreational drug use, even excessive exposure to the sun.

"Trying to stay healthy will help as much as it helps with anything else," Dr. Johnson says. "Rational, well-balanced diet and activities are appropriate, but they're no magic bullet."

Several drugs are being used in experiments to see if they stop the progression from early treatable symptoms to fatal complications. These drugs, which interfere with the life cycle of the virus, are not widely available.

"Our ultimate goal is prevention," Dr. Johnson says. "What we'd really like is a vaccine to prevent people from being infected in the first place." With the AIDS virus, unfortunately, that goal is still too far off for comfort.

around forever and can cause symptoms off and on your entire life. In either case, tests can always tell if you've been exposed to a particular virus. Your blood will show evidence of antibodies, virus-fighting particles. Some people are carriers, and transmitters, of certain viruses, without ever showing symptoms.

CERVICAL CANCER
LINKED TO PAPILLOMA VIRUS

Why do virgins, nuns and lesbians almost never get cervical cancer? And why is the same disease virtually an occupational hazard among prostitutes? Why are women who use diaphragms somehow protected from cervical cancer, while the wives of men who visit prostitutes face an indignantly high risk?

For years, these findings have tantalized researchers. The figures seemed to show that women's exposure to sexually transmitted diseases somehow made them prone to cervical cancer. Until recently, just about any infection—from gonorrhea to genital herpes—was considered suspect. Now, with new laboratory methods that allow tissue samples from patients with cervical cancer to be analyzed for traces of viral infection, those diseases have been discarded as possible cancer instigators. Instead the focus has been on the apparent real culprits—certain members of a notorious family known as human papilloma virus.

These viruses cause a miserable array of warty infections—common hand warts, painful plantar warts which appear on the soles of the feet, the massive warts that butchers and meat handlers sometimes develop and fleshy growths in the throat that can grow so rapidly they can cause suffocation. None of these conditions is known to develop into cancer. However, the chronic, recurring wart disease, epidermodysplasia verruciformis, can progress to skin cancer in 25 percent of its sufferers.

Other strains of this virus *are* linked with genital cancer. They can cause small, flat warts on the cervix and, less frequently, on the vagina and vulva in women and, in men, on the penis and in the urinary opening. These warts can be hard to see. And sometimes there are no warts at all, even though the virus is present in cells of the cervix or penis.

Of the 40 known types of papilloma, 3—numbers 16, 18 and 31—have been strongly linked with cancer. These viruses have been found in nearly 90 percent of the cervical cancers sampled. They have also been found in secondary tumors, or metastases—cancers that have spread from the cervix to the lymph nodes. "Evidence is strong that these viruses are a significant risk factor in cervical and invasive cancer," Dr. Lancaster says.

The same viruses have been found in rare cancers of the vagina, vulva and penis. They are being searched for in warts and polyps in the urinary tract, colon and bladder. They have thus far not been linked to cancers in these locations.

These viruses are "biologically sexist." Women, especially, are their victims; men, merely their carriers. Why?

Researchers think that women have an area of tissue on their cervix that's particularly vulnerable to viral infection. Called the "transformation zone," it's located at the tip of the canal leading from the inside to the outside of the uterus. Cells in this area are constantly changing from mature glandular cells to mature squamous (skin) cells. Because they are always in a developmentally sensitive stage, they are vulnerable to viral infection. Most cervical cancers occur in this zone.

RISKS MULTIPLY WITH SEX PARTNERS

The most serious risk factors for developing cervical cancer are associated with exposure to the papilloma virus through sexual contact. Simply put, the more sex partners a woman has had, the greater her risk of developing cervical cancer. But there's no clear-cut rule to say just how a woman's risks grow as her number of sex partners increases. Only one study has addressed this question, and it showed that women who'd had more than six partners had a 6.1 times higher risk. Another pointed out that 90 percent of American women under age 30 would be considered at high risk because of their number of sex partners.

Cancer risk also seems to increase for women who became sexually active at an early age. One researcher judged the risk to double if a woman's first sexual experience occurred when she was 15 to 17 years old. Some researchers speculate that the cervix is particularly vulnerable to viral infections during these early years. Others consider age at first intercourse merely a reflection of a woman's number of sex partners. (And one study found that young women with a diagnosis of papilloma had a greater risk of cervical dysplasia, or abnormal cell growth. A small percentage of young women seem to be vulnerable to rapidly growing, invasive cancer that begins in the cervix.)

Usually, an abnormal Pap smear is a woman's first sign that she has been exposed to the papilloma virus. The smear will show signs of dysplasia. Even if it's only mild dysplasia, it's important that your gynecologist get a written explanation of the abnormality, including any signs of papilloma, from the pathologist who examined the cell sample. (Your gynecologist usually is not trained to make this diagnosis alone.)

Unless you're being treated at a university hospital where specific research is being carried out, it's hard these days to find out exactly which type (number) of the virus you've been exposed to. If you are concerned that it's one of the three types strongly associated with cervical cancer, your doctor can send a Pap smear preserved in a special solution to a laboratory specializing in viral classification. Specialists there will examine the cells and identify them by viral type.

Usually, when you have dysplasia, your doctor will examine your cervix with a lighted magnifying tube called a colposcope. With this, he can usually see the dysplasic lesions or warts. He'll remove them by dabbing on a caustic chemical that peels off the infected tissue. Although this treatment is standard, it's not the best. The method of choice is carbon dioxide laser treatment, which isn't widely available and is relatively expensive. The laser vaporizes the warts in a quick burst of energy.

If you're lucky enough to be a patient at a major research center, or if your doctor is simply very well informed, you may be asked to bring your husband in for a checkup, too. Such an examination could prove to be a lifesaver, especially if you've been treated for cervical dysplasia or even localized cervical cancer and the disease has come back. Husbands are seen routinely at the medical centers at Georgetown and the University of Minnesota.

"Here, if a woman comes in with dysplasia, her partner is examined by members of the urology department," Dr. Lancaster says. The shaft of the man's penis is examined with a magnifying glass for signs of papilloma warts. (At the University of Minnesota, the penis is sometimes first treated with a vinegar wrap to make the warts easier to see. The vinegar makes them look white.) If no warts are visible on the shaft of the penis, a sample of cells is taken from the man's urethra. A tiny cotton swab is inserted into the urethra and rotated. Cells stick to the cotton. In Minnesota, a semen sample may also be analyzed.

Studies have revealed that more than half of the husbands of women with dysplasia have been found to be infected with the papilloma virus.

If the warts are on the shaft of the penis, they can be removed just as they are from cervix—with a chemical peel or laser treatment. If the virus is found in the man's semen, it means the warts are located in the urethra, and there's no easy way to get at them. In this case, it's advised that the couple use condoms to prevent reinfection. In some cases of severe recurrent papilloma infections, interferon has been used successfully to control symptoms. Interferon, which slows viral replication, is currently being used against papilloma infections in a number of clinical trials. But it is not widely available for public use.

There's no doubt that everyone who has multiple sex partners should use condoms. The number of cases of papilloma warts diagnosed each year is climbing rapidly. It's estimated that there were a million new cases in just one year in the United States. Papilloma is just behind chlamydia, and well ahead of herpes, as the fastest-growing sexually transmitted disease.

OTHER RISK FACTORS

Tobacco is a known risk factor for many cancers. Women who smoke more than 15 cigarettes a day are twice as likely as nonsmokers to have cervical dysplasia or cervical cancer. And they are 3.5 times more likely to develop invasive cancers. Samples of cervical mucus taken from women smokers contain chemicals that cause cancerous cell changes.

And nutrition could play a role in cervical cancer, just as it may in other cancers or precancerous conditions. Poor nutrition may make cervical cells less able to withstand the mutagenic effects of some viruses or the carcinogens found in the cervical mucus of women who smoke. It can also weaken the body's immune system, making it less able to fight infection.

Lower-than-normal intake of selenium and vitamins C and A and the B vitamin folate have been found in women with cervical dysplasia or newly diagnosed cancer.

Researchers at the Albert Einstein College of Medicine in New York City found that women whose intake of vitamin C was less than 30 milligrams daily (only half the Recommended Dietary Allowance, and equal to about half a medium orange or two ounces of juice from concentrate) had a risk of developing cervical dysplasia ten times greater than that of women whose daily intake was higher.

They also found that women were three times more likely to have severe cervical dysplasia or cervical cancer if their vitamin A intake was below the group median of 3,450 International Units daily (equivalent to about ⅓ cup of shredded carrots or four dried apricots).

Folate also seems to play a role in dysplasia, especially in women using birth control pills, who may have lower body levels of this vitamin, according to researchers at the University of Alabama at Birmingham.

Their research involved 47 young women with cervical dysplasia. Half were given ten milligrams of folate (25 times the RDA) each day, while the other half received a placebo. After three months, the cervical dysplasia had regressed and the cervix returned to normal in 4 of the women in the folate group. There was no improvement in the placebo group. In fact, the dysplasia had worsened in 4 of the women. (Remember, however, that large doses of vitamins should not be taken without a doctor's supervision.)

MORE SEX-RELATED CANCERS

In some areas of the world, exposure to a virus has strong links with the later development of cancer. In other areas, there seems to be virtually no connection. That's the case with the Epstein-Barr, or mononucleosis, virus.

Epstein-Barr is best known in the United States and other industrial countries as the virus that causes mononucleosis, a fairly common but nonfatal infection. This virus, a member of the herpes family, is definitely found in saliva and is probably shed from the cells lining the nose and throat. It is transmitted usually by saliva carrying viruses or infected cells.

In less developed areas like Africa and China, Epstein-Barr has been connected with a cancer that attacks the nose and upper throat. In these countries, this cancer is the third largest killer of men and the fourth largest killer of women. The Epstein-Barr virus has also been linked to a common African cancer of the lymph system called Burkitt's lymphoma. Some researchers think very early exposure, coupled with the effects of the virus interacting with malaria infection, may promote these cancers.

In the United States, very few nose and throat cancers have been found to contain the Epstein-Barr virus. In this country, its most likely victims are people with very weakened immune systems, those with unknown defects in the immune system, such as those on therapy to prevent organ transplant or graft rejection or those who have AIDS.

"So many more people are exposed to this virus than get cancer that, in the U.S., it would not be considered a major risk factor for cancer. While it would be desirable to prevent the spread of the virus in the human population, its presence should be considered a negligible risk," says Bernard Roizman, Sc.D., professor of biochemistry and molecular genetics at the University of Chicago Medical School.

ADULT LEUKEMIA: CAUSE FOR CONCERN?

Two closely related viruses have been associated with the rare adult T-cell leukemia. They live and reproduce right inside the infection-fighting white blood cells. The viruses transform your white blood cells into malignant, fast-growing cells that interfere with the body's ability to make red blood cells. Bruises, brittle bones, fatigue and internal bleeding are the result.

In Japan, which has the world's highest incidence rate, adult T-cell leukemia accounts for 60 to 70 percent of all cancers of the blood system, possibly because the virus has been there long enough to have spread throughout the population. And those who have been exposed to the virus seem to be vulnerable to other infectious diseases even if they don't develop leukemia.

In the United States, it's been found that a higher-than-expected number of homosexual men, as well as drug addicts, have been exposed to this virus. Even though their numbers are small, scientists are concerned that this virus could spread through the population the same way AIDS does.

They're particularly concerned because this form of leukemia can take as long as 30 years to develop. They fear an epidemic of the disease could occur years after exposure, too late to take measures to control its spread. Studies are currently being conducted to see if blood transfusions should be screened for this virus.

SOME LYMPHOMAS LINKED TO VIRUS

A virus very similar to those that cause leukemia has been found to cause lymphoma, a cancer of the lymph glands.

In the United States, lymphoma is not a particularly common cancer. Hodgkin's disease, a form of lymphoma, and other lymphomas strike an estimated 48,000 Americans each year, according to the American Cancer Society. Hodgkin's causes about 1,500 deaths a year, and other lymphomas cause 23,400 deaths a year. But just how many may be associated with this virus remains unclear.

HEPATITIS B AND LIVER CANCER

The hepatitis B virus can cause a range of symptoms, including liver inflammation that can bring about several weeks of jaundice, nausea and fatigue. After such an infection the virus sometimes hides in the cells and turns the person into a carrier. Studies show that the risk of hepatitis B carriers developing primary liver cancer is much greater than that for the average population. (Another form of hepatitis, called hepatitis A, is caused by a different virus and is not associated with liver cancer.) Hepatitis B can also lead to long-term degeneration of the liver, which in some cases can lead to liver tumors. Only those who become chronic carriers of hepatitis B are at long-term risk for liver cancer.

The hepatitis B virus is found in semen and is transmitted through sexual contact. It's also passed through dirty needles and through blood transfusions.

There is a vaccine available for hepatitis B. It's generally given only to those at high risk, such as homosexual men.

RESEARCH GIVES FUTURE HOPE

The news is not all bad regarding the prevention of viral cancers. The good news is that finding a viral cause for some cancers means that vaccines against these cancers, and perhaps others, can be developed. In fact, the hepatitis B vaccine, which was developed before its link with liver cancer had been established, could be rightly considered the first "cancer vaccine."

British researchers have come up with an early version of a vaccine against Epstein-Barr, made of purified outer membranes of the virus. And there is an experimental vaccine which protects cows against the papilloma virus, which may help researchers to one day develop similar protection for people.

Tests to detect viruses in the blood provide considerable lead time for dealing with them before they can begin the deadly work of converting normal cell machinery into malignant factories. Drugs which interfere with the life cycle of a virus are now being tested against AIDS, and scientists expect to come up with better and better versions of these and other virus-fighting drugs.

CANCER PREVENTION PLAN: SEX

- If you have papilloma virus warts, have regular examinations for the presence of cancer, particularly cervical cancer.
- If your spouse has papilloma virus warts, you should be examined and possibly treated.
- If you have multiple sex partners, use a condom.
- Do not smoke.
- Eat a diet high in vitamins A and C and folate.
- If you are at high risk for hepatitis B, get a vaccination against it.

Sugar and Artificial Sweeteners

Sugar," calls the man to his wife.

"Over here, honey," she replies.

Is this couple using terms of endearment—or are they trying to hurt each other?

The answer depends on your perspective. Given the amount of controversy surrounding sugar (and all the other substances people use to satisfy their sweet tooths), one person's sweetness may be another's poison.

Whether due to the puzzling inclination people have to feel guilty about foods that taste rich, or because of real medical evidence, sugar and its substitutes have been blamed for a wide variety of illnesses—including cancer.

THE GOOD NEWS ABOUT CANCER AND SUGAR

Whether or not there is a relationship between cancer and sweeteners is a question that has been tossed back and forth so much that it sometimes seems even scientists don't know what's going on. Because tests are still being done on artificial sweeteners, the final word isn't in.

315

However, here are the most up-to-date facts available about whether or not your sweet tooth is a cancer risk.

First, the good news: Regular sugar, when eaten in average amounts, has generally *not* been associated with increased risk of cancer. The term regular sugar encompasses white, molasses, honey, brown, powdered and all other types. Experts say that there is insufficient evidence to support a *direct* link between sugar and cancer.

But if you are indulging your sweet tooth instead of eating other nutritious fiber-rich foods like fruits and vegetables, experts believe you may be *indirectly* increasing your cancer risk by missing out on the protection these foods could provide. And when your sugar cravings lead you to eat huge quantities of high-fat, high-calorie foods like pastry, you increase the potential risk even more. High-fat diets have been implicated in a wide variety of cancers, and obesity is also considered a cancer risk.

ARE ARTIFICIAL SWEETENERS SAFE?

What about sugar substitutes? Whether you're a diabetic or you simply want to lose weight, sugar substitutes may seem an attractive alternative to the real thing. Are they? The sugar substitute sorbitol is considered generally recognized as safe by the Food and Drug Administration (FDA). But the FDA is now awaiting the results of a scientific review of some recent studies which suggested possible health implications.

The safety of other common sugar substitutes including aspartame, saccharin and cyclamate, is equally unclear.

What is clear is their popularity. In 1978 the number of people using artificial sweeteners was 42 million. As of 1985, approximately 69 million Americans over age 18 consumed saccharin, aspartame or a combination of the two (cyclamate is currently off the market awaiting review for safety by the FDA). That's a jump of more than 60 percent in seven years—and those figures don't include teenagers and younger kids who seem to consume their share of diet soft drinks. So there's a real need for these food additives to be safe.

Artificial sweeteners are regulated by the FDA under a law called the Food, Drug and Cosmetic Act. This gives the FDA responsibility to ensure that the public health is protected when these sweeteners are sold. That's a big responsibility—and deciding which sugar substitutes are safe, and which aren't, has been a difficult task.

THE SACCHARIN STORY

Saccharin's history is very tangled: The government first declared it safe, then unsafe, and now the sweetener is in a sort of limbo waiting for the FDA and Congress to take further action on its status.

To add confusion to the issue, saccharin wasn't intended to be used as a sweetener in the first place. It was discovered by two scientists, Ira Remsen and Constantin Fahlberg, at Johns Hopkins University in 1879, purely by accident.

One version of the story goes that Fahlberg bit into a piece of bread and found that it was inexplicably sweet. Realizing that he might have contaminated it with chemicals from the laboratory, he went back and sampled the chemicals he'd been working with. He found that one of them did indeed have a sweet taste.

Saccharin was first used primarily to preserve food, and as an antiseptic. Then diabetics began to use it. Then canners got interested. And then the first troubles started.

The chief of the Bureau of Chemistry in the Department of Agriculture voiced his concerns about saccharin in 1907. Fortunately for saccharin lovers, President Theodore Roosevelt came to the sweetener's defense: "You tell me that saccharin is injurious to health?" said Roosevelt. "My doctor gives it to me every day. Anybody who says saccharin is injurious to health is an idiot."

While a lot of "idiots" were to later disagree with Roosevelt's statement, his view prevailed at the time and saccharin continued to gain in popularity and was given a special boost by the sugar shortages of World War I and World War II. At the time there were no strict food additive regulations comparable to the those now imposed by the FDA.

Then, in 1958, the Congress amended the Food, Drug and Cosmetic Act, which decides how food additives are regulated. The Delaney Clause, which stipulates that no new food additive can be used if animal or other appropriate tests show it causes cancer—no matter how little or much of the additive is consumed—was added to the act.

SACCHARIN FIRST LISTED AS SAFE

But it was decided that the new amendment did not apply to saccharin, cyclamate and many other additives. Instead they were included on a list of "generally recognized as safe" additives, because they were in use prior to the amendment's passage.

While some people over the years had called attention to saccharin as a possible carcinogen, it wasn't until 1970 that dangers were suggested, and taken seriously. Then in 1972, while awaiting the results of additional studies, the FDA decided to remove saccharin from its list of "generally recognized as safe" foods, though the sweetener remained on the market. By 1973 the results of two more studies, one by the Wisconsin Alumni Research Foundation and one by the FDA, had reported a possible link between saccharin and bladder tumors in rats. Rats and their offspring fed diets of saccharin developed a significant number of bladder tumors, said scientists. But questions still remained.

Then in 1974, the Canadian government started a large study to get to the bottom of the saccharin controversy. The Canadians implicated saccharin as a carcinogen in animals. Scientific experts reviewed the findings and the FDA reported in the *Federal Register* that they "indicate unequivocally that saccharin causes bladder cancer in test animals." On April 15, 1977, the FDA made public its proposal to ban the use of saccharin in foods and beverages. It did ease its order a little by saying that saccharin could be sold as an over-the-counter drug in the form of a tabletop sweetener—but only if it could be established that it had important medical uses, such as for diabetes or obesity.

As could be expected, the outcry from the makers of saccharin was swift and strong. But in addition to displeasing the manufacturer, the proposed ban made the American public very sour. Consumers wrote thousands of letters to the FDA and congressmen asking them to reconsider the ban.

CONGRESS OVERRULES FDA

At the time, saccharin was the only low-calorie sugar substitute available, and apparently the thought of not being able to have it in diet sodas, desserts and other prepared foods was too much for people to take. Congress reacted by imposing a moratorium on the ban (extended several times since), effectively overruling the experts at the FDA. This moratorium allowed saccharin to be sold as long as it had the warning which has now become as familiar, and probably as often ignored, as the warnings on cigarette packages: *Use of this product may be hazardous to your health. This product contains saccharin, which has been determined to cause cancer in laboratory animals.*

Congress also instructed the FDA to have further studies done on saccharin, to resolve the seeming controversy about how safe saccharin was. The first of these studies, done by the National Academy of Sciences, had unequivocal results: It determined that saccharin was a low-level carcinogen in animals, that it might by itself cause cancer in humans, and it might enhance the carcinogenic effects of other substances. That was in 1978.

LARGE STUDY POINTS TO CANCER RISK

Then came a large study done on saccharin, which was reported in 1980 by the National Cancer Institute (NCI), in cooperation with the FDA. It involved 9,000 people. While this study didn't find that there was an added risk of using artificial sweeteners for *all* the people studied, it did find that it was of possible risk to some groups of people. These included heavy users of artificial sweeteners, especially consumers of diet sodas and sugar substitutes, and heavy smokers who were heavy users of artificial sweeteners. Women who used artificial sweeteners twice or more a day also had a 60 percent greater risk of bladder cancer than women who never used them.

But other studies have been done which find little risk, and the controversy does not seem likely to end soon. One thing is certain, however: The FDA sticks by the 1977 recommendation that saccharin be banned.

"The agency believes that saccharin is a weak animal carcinogen," says Jim Greene, a spokesperson for FDA, "but we are unable to take any regulatory action because of the 1977 Saccharin Study and Labeling Act, commonly referred to as the moratorium."

Whether Congress will continue to grant moratoriums on the FDA ban is anyone's guess. What isn't guesswork, however, is that Congress isn't only concerned about the safety of saccharin when it makes its decisions—it's also influenced by public desires and other factors that don't pertain directly to saccharin's safety as a food additive.

But if the moratorium is lifted, the FDA would have to repropose the ban. This process would, of course, take some time. Nothing would happen overnight.

TO USE OR NOT TO USE

Does this mean you shouldn't use saccharin?

Early studies on animals and the very large study of saccharin's effect on people *imply* that saccharin is a potentially weak risk factor for bladder cancer in humans, according to the National Cancer Institute. And, at the American Cancer Society, Vice President for epidemiology and statistics Lawrence Garfinkel says, "Some people say there may be a significant risk associated with saccharin and cancer. Others say that if there is, it is minimal, and the risk is very small. No one has established any safe levels for artificial sweeteners, but certainly if you're going to use them, use them in moderation."

Garfinkel is involved with a large study comparing the weight gains over a period of a year in people who use artificial sweeteners and people who don't. "The results are showing us that the artificial sweetener users are more likely to gain weight. Maybe they have a false sense of security, or something. So, artificial sweeteners aren't really a benefit in terms of weight loss. The only medical benefit may be for diabetics."

CYCLAMATE BANNED

In a sort of perverse reversal of the saccharin saga, cyclamate is an artificial sweetener that the FDA has said does *not* by itself cause cancer—but it is currently banned, while saccharin isn't. But this isn't just a lesson in the confusing ways of bureaucracy. Cyclamate is still banned because some studies have raised questions about it possibly being the cause of other medical problems, and it may act as a *cocarcinogen,* that is, it may enhance the cancer-causing effects of other substances a person is exposed to. The trail of studies and accusations that led to this conclusion was, as you might guess, quite complex.

The discovery of cyclamate, however, was a simple matter of luck—about as scientifically inspired as the discovery of saccharin. Only in this case the sweet chemical was noticed not on a piece of bread, as was the case with saccharin, but on a cigarette a University of Illinois scientist had absentmindedly left on a pile of crystal powder he was working with. That was in 1937, but cyclamate wasn't introduced in beverages and foods until the early 1950s. It was originally sold in tablet form so diabetics could have a low-calorie sweetener. But then the idea of diet foods became popular and cyclamate sales took off like a rocket. Most often cyclamate was mixed with saccharin, because, for one reason, both together had a better flavor than either did alone. Consumption reached a high of 18 million pounds a year, with sales of about $1 billion.

All this popularity grew in spite of recommendations by the National Academy of Sciences—over the years—that people restrict their use of artificial sweeteners. In 1968, the academy told the FDA that while reasonable quantities of cyclamate probably didn't pose any hazard to humans, more studies were needed to assure its safety.

A LINK WITH BLADDER CANCER?

Then in 1969, more evidence became available that cyclamate, or a cyclamate/saccharin combination, might cause bladder cancer. This evidence set the FDA in motion, and it was quite a roller coaster ride.

- The FDA banned cyclamate as of February, 1970.
- Oops! Then the FDA flip-flopped and said that cyclamate could be put into foods if they were labeled drugs.
- Sorry, fooled again. In September of 1970 the FDA changed its mind again and banned cyclamate completely, giving stores two weeks to get it off their shelves. It's been off the shelves since.

Are you confused? Well, you haven't heard the half of it, because cyclamate may yet reappear on the market. The manufacturer of cyclamate has been trying for years to get the FDA to legalize cylcamate again. In 1973 Abbott Laboratories petitioned the FDA to let them market cyclamate only in special dietary foods—taking into consideration 400 reports that Abbott felt would clear cyclamate. The NCI and the FDA decided that the evidence didn't vindicate cyclamate.

Abbott continued to petition the FDA until 1980, when the FDA commissioner ruled again that the safety of cyclamate had not been demonstrated. But he also ruled that its carcinogenic qualities hadn't been proved either.

Abbott proved to be very tenacious in its fight to have cyclamate approved, and in 1982 they reapplied in a joint petition with the Calorie Control Council to the FDA, asking for a permit to use cyclamate in beverages, processed fruit, gelatin, jellies, jams, toppings, salad dressings, chewing gum and confections, and as a tabletop sweetener. The FDA had its Cancer Assessment Committee examine the new data.

CONFLICTING STUDIES

This committee came to the conclusion that "There exists no credible evidence for the carcinogenicity of ingested cylcamate . . . on the basis of all studies on these substances using mice as experimental subjects." The same thinking applied to rat studies which had at one time been thought to indict cyclamate as the cause of cancer of the bladder in rats.

In search of a second opinion, the FDA had the National Research Council look into the issue. Given the Orwellian history of cyclamate, it's not surprising that their study came up with a decision that still left cyclamate the victim of a technical knockout. The NRC agreed that cyclamate by itself is unlikely to cause cancer in humans. But they found two separate studies, one of rats and one of mice, that indicate cyclamate might enhance the cancer-causing effects of other substances and lead to bladder cancer. However, they recommended additional studies of this possible promotional effect of cyclamate.

The question of whether or not a person should consume cylamate is really a moot point: It's still an illegal food additive and can't be sold.

Although a new evaluation of prior studies is being done now that might possibly clear cyclamate of being a carcinogen or cocarcinogen, it's doubtful that it will reappear soon on store shelves. Cyclamate has been implicated in a host of other health problems, including genetic damage and testicular atrophy.

THE LATEST PRODUCT: ASPARTAME

Aspartame—usually recognized as NutraSweet—is the latest artificial sweetener to charge into the sugar substitute market. It was first approved in 1981 for use as a tabletop sweetener and in some packaged foods, like cereals. Then it was given the go-ahead for soft drinks. Now it's hard to turn around in a grocery store without bumping into something that contains aspartame.

Part of its appeal seems to be that many people perceive it as being "natural" because it is synthesized from two amino acids that occur naturally in food. But in reality, the human body probably metabolizes aspartame differently from naturally occurring amino acids. When humans digest amino acids contained in food—the protein in meat or beans, for example—it is digested slowly, and along with other amino acids, not just the two present in aspartame. But when a person eats aspartame, he is quickly exposed to just the two amino acids.

Aspartame could be a definite health risk for phenylketonurics, people with a rare disease that makes them unable to process the amino acid phenylalanine normally, but otherwise the FDA has deemed it safe for human consumption. But as might be expected, FDA approval was not a simple matter.

Aspartame was first approved for use in dry foods and as a tabletop sweetener in July, 1974. But the validity of the data that the manufacturer submitted for approval, as well as the safety of the product, was challenged. As a result, aspartame wasn't marketed at that time. The FDA submitted the challenged studies to an outside panel of pathologists for their opinion, and in 1978 the panel confirmed their validity. In 1980, a scientific board of inquiry found the evidence did not support charges that it increased a person's risk of brain damage, mental retardation or endocrine dysfunction. But this review committee cited a study in which rats fed aspartame developed brain tumors and recommended that one more long-term animal test be done to check the carcinogenicity of aspartame. "This study was carried out in Japan. The results were negative," says an FDA spokesman.

The FDA commissioner at the time, and the FDA's Center for Food Safety and Applied Nutrition, didn't believe that further studies were needed, and aspartame was approved for use in dry foods in July, 1981. In July, 1983 it was approved for use in carbonated beverages. It's now on sale everywhere.

Because there is so much controversy about whether or not aspartame is carcinogenic (in addition to the fact that it has been linked to other health problems), people who want to use it might be wise to follow the advice of Michael F. Jacobson, Ph.D., executive director of the Center for Science in the Public Interest. He says that if you haven't noticed any problems after ingesting aspartame, a few servings a day probably won't put you at significant risk for health problems. But Dr. Jacobson says that "no one should be consuming five or ten aspartame packets or aspartame-sweetened sodas a day. Pregnant women and infants should avoid aspartame."

CANCER PREVENTION PLAN:
SUGAR AND ARTIFICIAL SWEETENERS

- Do not indulge your sweet tooth at the expense of nutritious fiber-rich foods like fruits and vegetables.
- Use all artificial sweeteners in moderation.
- Limit consumption of aspartame or aspartame-sweetened soft drinks.

Sunglasses

By now you've probably heard a lot about using sunscreens to protect your skin, but what about your *eyes?*

That's right. Just as your skin is vulnerable to the sun's harmful ultraviolet (UV) rays, so are your eyes. The good thing is that you can protect them quite easily.

The eyelids are the part of the eye most affected by too much sun, says Rene S. Rodriguez-Sains, M.D., an ophthalmologist at the Manhattan Eye, Ear and Throat Hospital in New York City.

People at highest risk of developing this type of cancer live where the sun beats ferociously for many days of the year. And the nearer the equator, the greater your risk. People who have outdoor jobs, like farmers or deckhands, and are exposed to the sun for long periods of time on a daily basis, are also at risk.

As with many other kinds of cancer, time is an essential ingredient in prevention. Years and years of repeated sun exposure take their toll on the eyelid and can result in a form of cancer called basal cell carcinoma.

The sun also can wreak havoc on the eye itself, causing an extremely rare form of cancer in the conjunctiva, the tissue lining the eyelids and protecting the eyeball. The first hint of trouble may be a constant feeling of having a speck of dust in the eye.

Then a raised, gelatinous, veined growth might appear. Eye irritation continues. Most people decide to have the growth surgically removed after the cancer becomes visible.

Another, much more common, condition that may occur in the same area of the eye but is not malignant is known as ptergyium. It is a benign growth that looks and feels much like its more cancerous counterpart and is also caused by overexposure to the sun. The growth, however, lacks veining; treatment for both conditions is similar.

Eye cancer doesn't have to happen. Wearing sunglasses or eyeglasses that have been treated to block out UV light protects both the conjunctiva and the eyelid.

"Sunglasses originally were designed to block out glare," says Dr. Rodriguez-Sains. "And that's certainly a desirable thing. However, few people are aware that over 40 percent of sunglasses do not filter out the most damaging kind of light, the ultraviolet rays.

"In fact, regular clear prescription eyeglasses can be treated to filter out 90 percent to 100 percent of UV rays, and without a darkening effect," adds Dr. Rodriguez-Sains. "Simply request that your optician give you the appropriate UV-filtering lenses."

But you don't need to have a prescription in order to get sunglasses with this same feature. "Just look for a small tag on the sunglasses that says 'Z-80.3 Standard.' That means that those lenses meet the guidelines for UV filtration set by the National Standards Institute. If you don't see the tag, check the temple of the glasses themselves, where the same information may be printed," he suggests.

Lens color isn't really a factor in UV filtration lenses, but it can be if you are selecting ordinary (untreated) sunglasses. Contrary to expectation, darker lenses allow greater, deeper UV penetration because their denser color forces the pupil to open up. "We only suggest that people select sunglasses with gray or brown lenses," says Dr. Rodriguez-Sains, "because these colors cause the least amount of color distortion. In treated or untreated lenses, polarization helps to reduce glare and won't interfere with the effectiveness of the UV filtration, either."

Sunglasses of this type are a little more expensive than the kind you pick up at the local drugstore. But if you fall into the high-risk category—if you just can't resist the sun on warm summer days or if you work at a job that repeatedly exposes you to the sun—try to see the cost as an investment in your health.

CANCER PREVENTION PLAN: SUNGLASSES

- Buy sunglasses marked with a small tag that says Z-80.3 Standard. These lenses meet the guidelines for UV filtration set by the National Standards Institute.
- Have regular prescription eyeglasses treated to filter out UV rays by asking your ophthalmologist to apply the treatment when you buy your next pair of glasses.
- Choose sunglasses with lenses that are dark gray or brown; these colors cause the least amount of color distortion.
- If you live where the sun shines for many days of the year, particularly near the equator, be especially careful to get sunglasses that provide proper protection.

Sunscreens

Suppose someone stopped you on the street and offered to sell you an ointment that he claimed would practically guarantee you'd never get basal cell carcinoma—one of the most common forms of skin cancer? Or malignant melanoma—a rarer but deadlier form of the disease? How much would you be willing to pay for a tube of this miracle formula? $20? $50? $100?

Well, for about $5 you can get your hands on a product that, while it may not ensure a cancer-free life for your skin, comes pretty darn close. And you don't have to patronize a street-corner huckster to buy it, either. Walk into any drugstore, supermarket or five-and-dime and you'll bump into towering displays of the stuff: sunscreens of various strengths, containing any of 21 different substances that disarm or deflect the sun's penetrating rays.

There are two kinds of ultraviolet light (UVL) that are potentially harmful, UVA and UVB. We know that it's UVB, the shorter wavelengths of solar radiation, that scramble healthy skin cells. The effects of UVA are less understood. These rays penetrate more deeply into the skin, causing wrinkling and premature aging. They, too, may contribute to skin cancer. Kindly-looking Mr. Sun may not be quite as deadly a cancer trigger as bomb-grade plutonium, but overexposure to sunlight ranks uncomfortably high on the Skin Cancer Foundation's lists of known carcinogens, especially for people with fair, sun-sensitive skin. Left to fend for itself, unprotected skin is virtually defenseless against over-exposure to this ubiquitous (it's everywhere) threat.

CANCER PROTECTION IN A BOTTLE

Luckily, compounds such as zinc oxide (which forms a protective, opaque shield against sunlight) and chemicals such as para-aminobenzoic acid, cinnamate, benzophenone and others (which absorb ultraviolet rays) modify the penetration of the sun's rays. You might say that sunscreens are to skin cancer what insect repellent is to mosquito bites—your single, most effective form of self-defense, short of staying indoors.

But trying to choose a sunscreen from the dizzying array of products available leaves many people bewildered—with good reason. Words like "benzophenone" may leave you yearning for a Ph.D. in chemistry. How can you tell what's right for you, an SPF of 8, 12 or 15? What *is* an SPF, anyway? To cut the confusion, follow this simple formula: R-E-P-A-I-R.

R: READ LABELS

Most of what you need to know about a sunscreen is on the bottle or tube. You just have to decipher the terms. The most important feature is strength, or Sun Protection Factor (abbreviated SPF). Simply put, the SPF number is a ratio of the amount of time you can spend in the sun during the course of the day *wearing* the sunscreen and *not* wearing the sunscreen. Scientists who developed sunscreens assigned number 15 to products that allow people who turn red after 15 minutes in the sun to stay out four hours, or 15 times longer. A sunscreen with an SPF of 15 blocks out about 98 percent of the sun's damaging rays—about twice the protection you get from wearing an ordinary white cotton shirt. Because an SPF of 15 is practically a total sun block, anything higher—say a sunscreen product labeled with an SPF of 23 or 30—may be overkill, according to the Skin Cancer Foundation (a non-profit group of physicians and researchers with a special interest in sun protection) and Thomas B. Fitzpatrick, M.D., of the Department of Dermatology, Harvard Medical School, Boston, a leading authority on sunscreens.

"A sunscreen with an SPF of 23 does not give an additional SPF of 8. However, the stronger sunscreen could compensate for poor application," explains Carol Taylor, spokesperson for the foundation.

By comparison, a sunscreen with an SPF of 2 gives minimal protection. It is a common misconception that sunscreens with such a low SPF will provide appropriate protection. As far as cancer protection goes, the Skin Cancer Foundation grants its Seal of Acceptance only to sunscreens with an SPF of 15 or greater, indicating that such products, in the foundation's words, "aid in the prevention of sun-induced damage to the skin."

The next thing to consider is the active ingredients in your sunscreen of choice. Compounds with all sorts of tongue-twisting names abound. But, according to the Skin Cancer Foundation, this multitude of agents can be classified into four main categories.

- PABA (para-aminobenzoic acid) and its chemical relatives, called PABA esters, including glyceryl, padimate A (also known as amyldimethyl PABA) and padimate O (also known as octyl dimethyl PABA). PABA also happens to be a B vitamin.
- Cinnamates (octyl methoxycinnamate and cinoxate), which are related to cinnamon flavorings in mouthwashes, chewing gums, toothpastes and other consumer products.
- Benzophenones, which include oxybenzone, methoxybenzone and sulfisobenzone.
- Anthranilates, which are moderately effective at screening both ultraviolet A and B.

You will often notice that PABA compounds and cinnamates are combined with UVA screens. That's because PABA compounds and cinnamates absorb ultraviolet B type radiation but not ultraviolet A, which is less understood than UVB. Benzophenones absorb ultraviolet A but not B. So combining ingredients gives you a "broader spectrum" of coverage and may offer more protection.

The SPF that's best for you—and the chemicals used to achieve it— depend primarily on your skin type, as well as how much time you spend in the sun and whether you have certain allergies. In fact, knowing your skin type is probably the most important part of choosing an effective sunscreen.

Additional protection is also available in the form of physical sunscreens containing talcum, zinc oxide or titanium dioxide. These are usually opaque creams, gels or lotions that reflect and scatter all wavelengths of sunlight.

E: EVALUATE YOUR SKIN TYPE

Choosing a sunscreen is much like choosing a shampoo. Just as shampoos are formulated for different types of hair—dry, oily or normal—the right sunscreen will depend on your skin type (specifically, how much natural pigment, or melanin, it contains and how your skin behaves in the sun.) Dark-skinned people have a built-in SPF of about 8. Tanned skin has an SPF of 2 or 3. Palefaces have little or no built-in protection. Generally speaking, the fairer your skin, the lower its natural SPF, and the higher the SPF you should apply. The table, What's Your Skin Type?, on page 330 will help you to evaluate your skin and determine how much protection it needs.

If in doubt, it's best to overestimate your skin's sensitivity and go for a higher SPF—for a couple of reasons. For one, to avoid any risk of overexposure. For another, the SPF listed on a label is the strength obtained in a lab, under artificial ultraviolet light. Outdoors, under real-life conditions, the SPF is usually lower.

What's more, SPF labeling is done on the honor system. You have to take the manufacturers' word that what you see is what you get. Unfortunately, says Dr. Fitzpatrick, some products test out at SPFs much lower than they claim. So choosing a higher SPF allows for such short-comings. The table, SPFs of Some Sunscreens, Indoors and Out, on page 334 can help you decide which product may be best for you.

"Ideally, everyone should use a sunscreen product with an SPF of 15," writes Jeffrey L. Marx, M.D., a dermatologist at New York University Medical Center. "At the very least, people with Types I and II skin, who tan poorly, should use 15, and people with Types III and IV should use a product with an SPF of 6 or 8."

You may also need to wear a lotion with a higher SPF on areas of the skin that, because of custom or changes in swimsuit design, have never been exposed to the sun before and have little of the protection that prior exposure bestows, according to Dr. Fitzpatrick.

No matter what type of skin you think you have, you should always wear a sunscreen with an SPF of 15 or higher, especially if you:

- Spend a lot of time in the sun, including time spent doing errands or shopping as well as playing sports, gardening or other work or hobbies that often take you outdoors for long stretches or for short periods of intense exposure.
- Are outdoors when the sun is strongest (between 10:00 A.M. and 2:00 P.M. standard time, or 11:00 A.M. and 3:00 P.M. daylight saving time).
- Experienced blistering sunburns as a child (increasing your risk for skin cancer).
- Have a parent, brother, sister or other close relative who has or has had skin cancer (also a risk factor).

If you are allergic to cinnamon-flavored toothpaste, gum or mouthwash, you may also have to avoid sunscreens containing cinnamates. If you're allergic to benzocaine, procaine, certain antihypertensive drugs and diuretics, hydroxyzine, sulfa drugs or para-phenylenediamine (used in some hair dyes), you may also be allergic to PABA or PABA compounds, which cross-react with those agents. An allergic reaction to products containing PABA products may produce redness, itching, stinging or burning a day or so after the sunscreen is applied. If PABA

WHAT'S YOUR SKIN TYPE?

SKIN TYPE	SENSITIVITY TO ULTRAVIOLET LIGHT	SUNBURN AND TANNING BEHAVIOR
I	Very sensitive	Always burns easily and severely (painful burn); tans little or none and peels.
II	Very sensitive	Usually burns easily and severely (painful burn); tans minimally or lightly, also peels.
III	Sensitive	Burns moderately; tans about average.
IV	Moderately sensitive	Burns minimally; tans easily and above average with each exposure; exhibits IPD (immediate pigment darkening) reaction.
V	Minimally sensitive	Rarely burns; tans easily and substantially; always exhibits IPD reaction.
VI	Insensitive	Never burns; tans profusely; exhibits IPD reaction.

SOURCE: Developed by Madhu A. Pathak, Ph.D., Thomas B. Fitzpatrick, M.D., John A. Parrish, M.D., and David B. Mosher, M.D., of Harvard Medical School and Massachusetts General Hospital, Boston, Mass., and Franz J. Grieter, M.D., of Vienna, as cited in "Skin Cancer in the Sports World" by William Hanke, *Skin Cancer Foundation Journal* (1985).

*SPFs higher than 15 are not appreciably stronger and will not necessarily give you more protection than a product rated 15.

irritates your skin, look for PABA-free sunscreens such as Piz Buin (pronounced "pitz bween") -8 and -12, Piz Buin Creme-15 or Parsol. The information in the box on the opposite page will help you determine if PABA irritates your skin. Also, see the table, SPFs of Some Sunscreens, Indoors and Out, on page 334 lists several PABA and PABA-free sunscreens.

If you have other contact allergies, you may have to avoid sunscreens with preservatives, lanolin or certain fragrances, possible troublemakers for people with sensitive skin. If you don't want to smell like

EXAMPLES	RECOMMENDED PROTECTION FACTOR
People with fair skin, blue or brown eyes, freckles; unexposed skin is white.	15 or higher*
People with fair skin, red, blond or brown hair, blue, hazel or brown eyes; unexposed skin is white.	15 or higher*
Average Caucasian; unexposed skin is white.	10 or higher
People with white or light brown skin, dark brown hair, dark eyes; unexposed skin is white or light brown.	6 to 8 or higher
Brown-skinned people; unexposed skin is brown	6 to 8 or higher
Blacks, unexposed skin is black.	None indicated

PATCH TEST FOR PABA ALLERGY

If you suspect you are sensitive to PABA, you can ask your dermatologist to confirm this by performing a type of allergy testing known as patch testing. Or you can conduct your own patch testing by applying a sunscreen containing PABA to a small patch of skin, preferably on the underside of the forearm, and covering the area with a Band-Aid or other adhesive bandage. After 24 hours, remove the Band-Aid and expose the area to 15 minutes of sunlight. If the test is positive, you will experience redness and swelling the next day where the Band-Aid was applied—and that means, of course, that you shouldn't use PABA.

the beach, you'll probably shy away from sunscreens with "tropical co-conut" scents. And if you have oily skin, avoid oil-based sunscreens (which can clog pores and promote formation of oil plugs) and use alcohol-based products instead.

If you spend a lot of time in the water or perspire heavily, look for a waterproof or water-resistant sunscreen, such as Bullfrog Amphibious Formula Sunblock, Coppertone Super Shade Sunblock Lotion-15, Eliza-beth Arden Suncare Creme-15, Piz Buin-8 and -12, Piz Buin Creme-15, PreSun-15, Sundown-15 and Total Eclipse-15, to name a few. "Water-resistant" means the sunscreen is formulated to withstand 40 minutes of immersion in water. "Waterproof" means it should withstand 80 min-utes of immersion. Both resist sweating. You still must reapply these sunscreens every so often, though, because sunscreens don't always perform as well under actual conditions as they do in the lab. Consult the table at the end of this chapter for the water resistance of various brands.

P: PLAN AHEAD

Don't wait until you're out in the noonday sun enjoying the annual Fourth of July barbecue and pool party to reach for your sunscreen. *Real* sun protection begins long before you drag the gas grill up from the basement or shop for a new swimsuit.

"You should start using a sunscreen regularly in the spring, when you have no tan left to protect your skin," says Frederick Urbach, M.D., professor of dermatology at Temple University School of Medicine, Philadelphia.

You should also apply sunscreen at least 15 minutes to a half hour before venturing outdoors, to give your skin ample time to soak up the protective ingredients. By the time you walk to the beach, spread your blanket, check the water (or check out the crowd), get out your radio or book and pour yourself a cold drink, you've already been out in the sun half an hour. If you're going skiing, keep in mind that sunlight ricochets back and forth between the snow and your skin, reflecting more than half of the sun's rays.

So next time you pack up your troubles and head for the beach—or upwardly mobilate to the ski slopes—plan ahead. Packing a sunscreen should be part of your preparations for any outdoor excursion. That includes bicycling, bird-watching, competing in the boomerang play-offs, fishing, flea marketing, flower collecting, horseback riding, hot air ballooning, snorkeling, white-water rafting—even attending the com-pany picnic.

A: APPLY LIBERALLY—ALL OVER

Where sunscreens are concerned, an ounce of prevention is worth, well, a whole lot of cure. So don't be stingy. Whatever sunscreen you choose, apply it generously. Otherwise, you'll only get a part of the SPF you think you're getting. One study showed that people tend to apply sunscreens only half as thickly as needed to achieve the SPF printed on the labels of the products they use, leaving them only partially protected. And don't forget to apply sunscreens under sheer clothing, such as gauzy shirts and beach coverups, or clothing that's apt to get soaked. Wet clothing—from swimming or perspiration—allows penetration of the sun's rays. (Dry, tightly woven clothing, on the other hand, serves as an excellent sunscreen. A pair of blue jeans, for example, has an SPF of about 1,700. That makes a denim cap a practical and effective sunscreen for your scalp, which is also vulnerable.)

Use a stick-form sunscreen or SPF-rated lip balm for other vulnerable areas such as your lips, lipline, nose and ears—the most common sites for basal cell carcinoma. Zinc oxide may also be used for these small but oh-so-sensitive spots. To protect your eyes and eyelids, wear sunglasses—preferably wrap-around style, paired with a visor or broad-brimmed hat. Makeup containing protective SPF ingredients—along with a good sunscreen—may also help women protect their faces from sun damage. (Some dermatologists recommend that women make a habit of wearing a sunscreen under their foundation makeup on a day-to-day basis.)

I: IGNORE BRONZED BEAUTIES AND TAN-O-PHILES

With heightened awareness of the unhealthful effects of too much sun, tanning as we know it may be out of vogue in a few years. If fear of cancer doesn't stop some people, fear of wrinkles will. As a result, sunscreens are by far among the hottest-selling grooming products on the market. So you shouldn't feel like an oddball for protecting your skin. Once applied, nearly all sunscreens are invisible. Only you will know you're wearing one. And you'll be glad you did.

"Some people feel they've wasted their money if they go to Barbados and come home without a tan," says Perry Robins, M.D., associate professor of clinical dermatology and chief of the Mohs Surgery Unit at New York University Medical Center and president of the Skin Cancer Foundation. "But in fact, a tan is a time bomb."

Dr. Robins should know—he's performed surgery on more than 17,000 people with skin cancer, almost all caused by overexposure to the sun. "So use a sunscreen and forget the souvenir tan," says Dr. Robins.

Dr. Thomas B. Fitzpatrick at Harvard tells people, "If you can't tan, don't try—and always protect your skin with sunscreens, every day—beginning in childhood."

"The first line of defense against malignant melanoma is to reduce sun exposure through sun avoidance and judicious use of sunscreens," states a report published by the American Council on Science and

(continued on page 336)

SPFS OF SOME SUNSCREENS, INDOORS AND OUT

TRADE NAME	ACTIVE INGREDIENTS	TYPE
PABA sunscreens		
Pabanol		Clear lotion
PreSun 15	PABA in ethyl alcohol	Clear lotion
PreSun 15		Gel
PABA-ester sunscreens		
Block Out	Isoamyl-p-N, N-dimethyl aminobenzoate (padimate A)	Lotion/gel
Original Eclipse	Glyceryl PABA and octyl dimethyl PABA	Lotion
Sea & Ski	Octyl dimethyl PABA	Cream
Sundown	Padimate O and oxybenzone	Lotion
PABA-ester combination sunscreens		
Bain de Soleil-15	Padimate O, oxybenzone and dioxybenzone	White cream
Blockout-15	Octyl dimethyl PABA, octyl methoxycinnamate and octyl salicylate	Creamy lotion
Clinique-19	Octyl dimethyl PABA, octyl methoxycinnamate and benzophenone-3	Milky lotion
Coppertone Super Shade Sunblock Lotion-15	Octyl dimethyl PABA and oxybenzone	Milky lotion
Elizabeth Arden Suncare Creme-15	Padimate O and oxybenzone	White cream
Estée Lauder-15 Ultra Screening Creme	Octyl methoxycinnamate and benzophenone-3	White cream
PreSun-15 (water-resistant)	Padimate O and oxybenzone	Milky lotion
Rubinstein Gold Beauty-15	Ethyl-hexyl-p-methoxycinnamate and octyl dimethyl PABA	Yellow gel
Shiseido-15	Titanium dioxide, octyl dimethyl PABA and benzophenone-3	Lotion
Sundown-15 (sunblock)	Padimate O, octyl methoxycinnamate and oxybenzone	Milky lotion
Total Eclipse-15	Octyl salicylate, octyl dimethyl PABA and oxybenzone	Milky lotion

SUN PROTECTION FACTOR (SPF)		RESISTANCE*	
INDOOR SOLAR SIMULATOR	OUTDOOR SUNLIGHT	TO SWEATING	TO WATER IMMERSION
15	6–8	Fair	Poor
15	15	Excellent	Poor
15	10–12	Good	Fair
6–8	6	Good	Fair
8–10	4–6	Fair	Fair
7–8	4	Fair	Poor
8–10	4–6	Good	Fair
15–18	9	Good	Fair
15	5–8	Good	Fair
15–19	7–8	Good	Fair
15–18	9–10	Excellent	Good
15–20	14	Excellent	Excellent
15–10	9	Good	Fair
15–20	8–10	Excellent	Good
10–12	9	Fair	Poor
15–20	8–10	Good	Good
15–20	10–11	Excellent	Good
15–18	10–14	Excellent	Good

(continued)

SPFS OF SOME SUNSCREENS, INDOORS AND OUT— *Continued*

TRADE NAME	ACTIVE INGREDIENTS	TYPE
Non-PABA sunscreens		
Piz Buin-8	Octyl methoxycinnamate and benzophenone-3	Cream
Piz Buin-8	Octyl methoxycinnamate and benzophenone	Milky lotion
Piz Buin-12	Octyl methoxycinnamate and benzophenone-3	Cream
Piz Buin Creme-15	Octyl methoxycinnamate and benzophenone	Cream
Ultra Vera-20— Chesebrough-Pond's	Octyl methoxycinnamate and 2-hydroxy-4-methoxybenzophenone	Milky lotion
Physical sunscreens		
RVPaque	Zinc oxide, cinoxate, red petrolatum, talc, kaolin and iron oxide	Cream
Shadow	See above	Cream

SOURCE: Adapted from information supplied by Madhu A. Pathak, Ph.D., and Thomas B. Fitzpatrick, M.D., of the Department of Dermatology, Harvard Medical School, and Massachusetts General Hospital, Boston, Mass., and individual sunscreen manufacturers.

*Ratings: Excellent = SPF value retained is 90–100% after stress of 45 minutes swimming.
Good = SPF value retained is 75–90% after stress of 45 minutes swimming.
Fair = SPF value retained is 50–75% after stress of 45 minutes swimming.
Poor = SPF value retained is less than 50% after stress of 45 minutes swimming.

Health, a national consumer education group directed by physicians and other health care professionals. "There are strong reasons *not* to cultivate a tan."

R: REAPPLY OFTEN

One of the nicest things about wearing a strong sunscreen is that you don't have to remember to turn over every 15 minutes as though you were working on a tan. But you *do* have to remember to reapply a sunscreen liberally and frequently—every 60 to 90 minutes at the least, more frequently if you're frolicking in the pool or working up a good sweat. Even waterproof or water-resistant sunscreens rub, sweat and wash off. (Newer formulas last longer in water than their older counterparts. So if you have a sunscreen that's more than about three years old, replace it.)

| SUN PROTECTION FACTOR (SPF) | | RESISTANCE* | |
INDOOR SOLAR SIMULATOR	OUTDOOR SUNLIGHT	TO SWEATING	TO WATER IMMERSION
15–20	10–12	Excellent	Good
20–22	10–12	Excellent	Good
15–20	12–14	Excellent	Excellent
20–22	15	Excellent	Excellent
12–15	6	Fair	Fair
10–12	6–8	Good	Good
4–6	2–4	Good	Fair

Waterproof or not, sunscreens shouldn't lull you into a false sense of security. Arthur Rhodes, M.D., assistant professor of dermatology at Harvard Medical School and chief of dermatology at the Children's Hospital in Boston, cautions against using sunscreens to prolong your time in the sun. "All sunscreens permit at least some UV radiation through the skin. Prolonged exposure, even with sunscreen use, may result in damage to the skin," says Dr. Rhodes. "In other words, a sunscreen is not a paper bag. You're still exposed."

So use your head—don't get red.

CANCER PREVENTION PLAN: SUNSCREENS

- Wear a sunscreen with a Sun Protection Factor appropriate to your skin type (the fairer you are, the higher the SPF number should be).
- When you swim or perspire heavily, wear a sunscreen that is water-resistant or waterproof.
- Apply sunscreen 15 to 30 minutes before going outdoors.
- Reapply sunscreen every 60 to 90 minutes.

Testicular Self-Exam

The American Cancer Society says the first sign of testicular cancer is usually a slight enlargement of one of the testicles and a change in its consistency. Pain may be absent, but often there is a dull ache in the lower abdomen or groin, together with a sensation of dragging and heaviness.

But even if these symptoms aren't present, it is a good idea to perform a monthly three-minute exam to check for lumps on the testicles. These lumps can be an early sign of the cancer.

The best time to perform the self-exam is after a warm shower or bath, when the scrotal skin is most relaxed, says the American Cancer Society. Then you should follow these guidelines from Richard Berger, M.D., urologist at the University of Washington Medical School, and chief of urology at Harborview Medical Center in Seattle. Check each testicle, one at a time. Hold the testicle with both hands, so it doesn't slip around. Then massage the surface of the testicle lightly, using both hands, and covering the whole testicle. If you feel any hard lumps, see your doctor immediately. (It's important that you know the location of the epididymis, a sausage-shaped organ that runs up and down the back of the testicle that feels like a bump when you touch it. There's a slight groove between the testicle and the epididymis. This organ is not cause for worry, though if you're in doubt, see a doctor.)

When a lump is found, the affected testicle must be surgically removed—that's the only way to determine the kind of malignancy causing the trouble, and also to stop it. However, malignancies are almost always confined to one testicle. The remaining testicle is perfectly capable of maintaining sexual fertility. And in the very rare cases where both testicles have to be removed, any potency problems can be corrected with testosterone shots, says Dr. Berger.

Though the risk of testicular cancer is low, says Richard D. Williams, M.D., a specialist in urological cancers, the self-exam is worth it. ''There're only certain parts of the body we can actually feel for cancer. So I tell men, 'Why not do it?' '' Dr. Williams says.

If you do the self-exam and find cancer early enough, says Dr. Berger, it is virtually 100 percent treatable.

CANCER PROTECTION PLAN: TESTICULAR SELF-EXAM

- Perform a testicular self-examination each month.
- The best time to perform the exam is after a warm shower or bath, when the scrotal skin is most relaxed.
- Check both testicles, one at a time, by massaging the surface lightly, using both hands.
- If you feel any hard lumps, see your doctor immediately.

Tobacco

The tension mounts as John reclines on his La-Z-Boy. His wife, Jane, knows he's going to light a cigarette. And—oooh!—it makes her mad. The smoke gets in her eyes and her hair, and it stinks up the whole house. But if she asks him to stop smoking, *he'll* be mad. "It's none of your business," he'll snap.

His smoking *is* her business. Because, according to the Surgeon General's report, it increases her risk of getting lung cancer, too.

John is at great risk, his wife at somewhat lesser risk—but both risks are real.

HOW BAD ARE CIGARETTES, ANYWAY?

Bad.

"My pet peeve is that people hear so much about the adverse effects of different things, they lose a sense of perspective," says Wayne C. Vial, M.D., of the pulmonary section at Dallas Veterans Administration Medical Center and the University of Texas Health Science Center at Dallas. "They read about saccharin and nitrosamines and such and think that everything causes cancer. But the fact is, cigarettes are so much worse than anything else."

In fact, cigarette smoking is the leading cause of cancer in America today. Each year, cigarettes kill more Americans than do all of the following combined: heroin, cocaine, alcohol, fire, automobile accidents, homicide, suicide and AIDS, according to a researcher from the University of Michigan, Ann Arbor. All of these deaths—about 129,000—are caused by cancer that results from smoking.

Virtually every scientist agrees that smoking is *the* major cause of cancer in America. The tobacco companies try to cloud the issue by coughing up a few 100-year-old smokers to imply smoking is safe. Nevertheless, scientists can point to *thousands* of studies that point to the connection between smoking and cancer.

Exactly how much do cigarettes increase an individual's risk of getting cancer?

"The risk depends on how many years a person has been smoking, how many cigarettes he smokes each day, how much tar is in the cigarette and how deeply he inhales," points out Dietrich Hoffmann, Ph.D., the associate director at the American Health Foundation, Valhalla, New York.

Even minimal exposure will boost the risk a little. "A person who smokes just one cigarette per day will have a somewhat higher likelihood of having tobacco-related cancers, compared to a nonsmoker," says Paul F. Engstrom, M.D., vice president of cancer control at Fox Chase Cancer Center, Philadelphia.

And the more you smoke, the greater the risk. "Let's assume somebody smokes two packs a day for 30 years," says Dr. Hoffman. "This smoker is at least 50 times more likely to get lung cancer than a nonsmoker."

The risk soars even higher for smokers who are exposed to certain materials. Smokers who work with asbestos, for instance, are 99 times more likely to get lung cancer compared to nonsmokers. And some types of miners who smoke are almost guaranteed to get cancer.

Lung cancer is the cancer most often caused by smoking. But smoking also can increase the risk of getting cancer of the mouth, throat, wind pipe, esophagus, pancreas, kidney, and bladder. How does smoking cause cancer in so many organs? To answer that question, let's follow a smoke particle in its journey through the human body.

THE JOURNEY OF A CARCINOGEN

Have you ever seen that brownish gunk that collects in the filter of a cigarette? It's called tar, and most of it lingers in a smoker's body long after a cigarette has been snuffed.

IF YOU MUST SMOKE,
HERE'S HOW TO CONTAIN THE DAMAGE

After having failed despite all pleas, bribes and nags to terminate your smoking habit, your doctor may urge you to switch to low-tar cigarettes and to smoke fewer of them.

While this advice is good, it's not foolproof.

"Low-tar cigarettes contain as much tar and nicotine as other cigarettes," says Wayne C. Vial, M.D., of the University of Texas Health Science Center. "They just register less tar in the tar test. You see, the government determines tar content by sticking a lit cigarette onto a smoking machine. A filter in the machine weighs the tar. But you can inhale more tar than the machine—if you take a deep drag and hold your breath, you're giving tar time to settle down and stay in the lungs."

Which is just what many smokers do when they switch to low-yield cigarettes—they inhale more deeply to get the nicotine they crave, studies show.

Cutting back on cigarettes may have the same effect. One study showed that people who dropped from an average of 29 cigarettes a day to 15 wound up with *more* nicotine in their sys-

And it's potent stuff. Each puff of smoke contains about 2,000 to 4,000 compounds, many of which, such as arsenic, formaldehyde, insecticides, nitrosamines and polonium 210, are proven cancer causers. Armed with these carcinogens, smoke can damage any body part in its path.

THE DESTRUCTIVE DESCENT

The first body part this smoke encounters is, of course, the mouth. As the smoke sweeps by, tar creeps into the oral lining, where it may stay for some time. Smoking may lead to cancer of the mouth, tongue, lip, cheek and throat.

"People who smoke have a risk at least six to ten times higher of getting oral cancer, compared to people who don't smoke," says Lawrence Garfinkel, vice president for epidemiology and statistics, who researches cancer at the American Cancer Society in New York City. And oral cancer is a very painful, distressing disease. The affected part of the oral cavity is removed. If it's tongue cancer, part of the tongue is removed.

The smoke particles that stick to the mouth can affect other parts of the body, too. "Saliva washes a considerable amount of the smoke's products out of the mouth," says Dr. Vial. "And when a person swallows

tems because they were inhaling more deeply, holding their breath longer and smoking cigarettes further down than they had before their wobbly-willed attempts to quit. Still, if they'd cut back even further—say to 5 smokes a day—would they have come out ahead?

Researchers from the University of California at San Francisco, the San Francisco General Hospital Medical Center and the Addiction Research Foundation in Toronto, Ontario, recently put that question to the test. They asked 13 smokers to drop from an average of 37 cigarettes a day down to 5. Each of those 5 cigarettes, the researchers found, delivered *roughly three times as many tobacco toxins (tar, nicotine and carbon monoxide)* as each cigarette did if smokers were blowing off two packs a day. As a result, the smokers reduced their toxic intake by only 50 percent—even though they reduced their cigarettes by nearly eightfold!

So what's a diehard smoker to do? "Smoke a cigarette with less tar, smoke fewer of them, but don't inhale more deeply or smoke the cigarette down to the filter," advises Dr. Vial.

that saliva, these products can have a large effect on the esophagus, the tube leading to the stomach. Cancer of the esophagus is much more common in smokers, compared to nonsmokers."

As smoke descends into the body, it irritates the lining of the breathing tubes. The body fights back with an arsenal of mucus.

"The glands in the respiratory tract produce mucus to protect the throat and the lining cells," says Dr. Vial. "The idea is to create a coat to prevent contact with the irritating smoke. But it doesn't always end up being protective. Excess mucus may cause chronic coughing or respiratory infections in some people. And smoke makes cells turn over faster. When cells multiply rapidly, there's more chance for them to multiply in an abnormal fashion and become cancerous."

Such irritation and multiplication may take place in the voice box, for instance. Have you ever heard a smoker with a raspy voice? Well, it might sound sultry, but the vocal cords may be sullied.

"Smoking irritates the vocal cords," says Dr. Vial. "It causes swelling and inflammation, which thickens the vocal cords. And just as altered strings change the guitar's sound, altered vocal cords change a person's voice. And the irritation may also lead to cancer."

As we mentioned before, the exact risk depends on a number of factors. But heavy smoking raises risks of throat cancers as much as 30 percent. And anyone who drinks a lot of alcohol in addition to smoking worsens already dismal odds of certain types of cancer.

So far, we've traced smoke to the throat and seen the vandalism it can perpetrate on the way. But you haven't seen the worst of it yet. Because smoke can do its worst in the lungs.

THE CLEAN-UP CREW GOES ON STRIKE

The lungs may be delicate, airy structures, but they have a hard-working clean-up crew. Unfortunately, smoke can overwork these defenses so much they finally go on strike, so to speak.

Take the cilia, for instance. Cilia are little hairs that line the air structures leading to the lungs. They beat in unison to sweep particles out of the lung. At least they work that way in a *normal* lung.

"As a person starts to smoke regularly, the cilia begin to beat at a slower frequency," says Dr. Vial. "As the smoking continues, the cilia become more and more damaged. Eventually they'll stop beating. Then they start to disappear. Finally, the cells with cilia are completely replaced by cells that have no cilia."

And consider the clean-up crew's alveolar macrophages. These immune cells actively pursue particles in the lungs and devour them, like the little scrubbing bubbles in commercials of yore. (See chapter 41, Immune System, for more about these little cells.)

"When we wash out the lungs of a smoker, we find a lot of alveolar macrophages," says Dr. Vial. "But these cells don't work as well at killing bacteria. They are are filled with a greenish pigment from smoke particles. Smoke overburdens and poisons these cells."

Scientists continue to find more smoking casualties in the lung. Recently, some scientists have discovered that cigarette smoking may be associated with lung cancer by depressing natural killer cell activity in the blood.

"Natural killer cells can kill tumor cells," says Barbara Phillips, M.D., from the division of pulmonary medicine, University of Kentucky Medical Centers and Veterans Administration Hospital in Lexington. "How? They may weaken the membrane of a cancer cell. Or they may engulf and eat a tumor. Or they may attract other immune cells to the area. Or maybe it does none of the above—we don't know yet. But we know that everybody has these killer cells. And a study I worked on shows that smoking depresses their activity."

Once all these defenses are down, particles are more likely to loiter in the lung and cause cancer. Not every smoker gets lung cancer, of course. But every smoker does experience some lung damage.

"I know of a doctor who, on an autopsy, can see from the lung tissue how long a person has smoked and whether he was a heavy or a light smoker," says Dr. Hoffman. "The point is, the lung tissue is stained and damaged in every smoker. It might not lead to cancer, but the damage is there."

The weakened defenses in the lungs also give more smoke particles a chance to hitch a joyride through the blood.

A RAMPAGE THROUGH THE BLOODSTREAM

"Once the compounds from the particles in smoke enter your circulation, they have the possibility of promoting cancer in any organ blood passes through," says Dr. Vial. "But of all these organs, only the bladder, kidney and the pancreas are linked significantly with smoking."

Why do these components affect some organs and not others? With the bladder and the kidney, the answer is easily explained.

"The kidney filters smoke particles out of the blood, into the bladder," explains Dr. Vial. "So these toxins are in direct contact with these organs in a concentrated form. And they're capable of causing cancer as they await disposal. We know that, because scientists have measured the mutagenic activity in smokers' urine. In other words, we've tested the effects smokers' urine has on bacteria. And we found that it's capable of causing mutations, or changes in the genetic properties of these bacteria."

How big is the risk for bladder cancer? Well, researchers at the Harvard School of Public Health, Boston, studied 3,287 people and found that cigarette smokers, in general, had twice the incidence of bladder cancer as nonsmokers. An individual's risk varied according to how many cigarettes were smoked and how deeply they were inhaled. Those who smoked two or more packs of cigarettes per day and inhaled deeply had nearly seven times the risk of nonsmokers.

But what about the pancreas? Smoking has been shown to triple the risk for this type of cancer. How does smoke affect this organ?

Nobody knows for sure, but some say the pancreas simply may be sensitive to certain smoke components in the blood. Others suggest that some of the smoke constituents are swallowed back up from the stomach into the pancreatic duct.

Dr. Hoffman describes another intriguing hypothesis. "Scientists have discovered chemicals called 'organ-specific carcinogens,'" he says. "There is, for instance, a chemical that will always cause nasal cancer in rats, wherever you apply it. You can paint it on the skin, inject it, let them inhale it, and it will always end up causing *nasal* cancer. A working hypothesis is that there are some organ-specific carcinogens in smoke. And it's possible that some may affect specifically the esophagus or the pancreas."

New preliminary evidence suggests the carcinogens in the blood may attack a woman's cervix as well. A study by researchers at the National Cancer Institute and five cancer-treatment centers around the country found the risk of cervical cancer is increased by approximately 50 percent in women who smoke 20 or more cigarettes per day.

INVOLUNTARY SMOKING

After reading about what smoke can do, you're probably proud if you don't smoke. But have you ever come back from a party smelling like Eau de Cigarette?

Yes? Then you actually have smoked, in a way. Scientists call it involuntary, or passive, smoking. And if you hobnob with smokers all day, you may inhale the equivalent of one or two cigarettes each day without lighting a match.

And the undiluted smoke that swirls from the tip of a burning cigarette between puffs is more toxic than that which goes through it, because it's unfiltered. In fact, this smoke has more than 50 times as much dimethylnitrosamine, a carcinogen, as filtered smoke. One study showed that a nonsmoker sitting at a crowded, smoke-filled bar inhales in one hour about as much dimethylnitrosamine as that inhaled by someone who smokes about 25 filtered cigarettes.

But let's get down to brass tacks: How risky *is* involuntary smoking? "The Surgeon General recently reviewed a number of studies on involuntary smoking and has concluded that exposure to other people's smoke increases a person's risk of lung cancer about 30 percent," says Mr. Garfinkel. "For those who are heavily exposed—if their spouse smokes a pack or more of cigarettes a day—the risk is doubled."

Granted, it's a relatively small risk. But it's nothing to sneeze at if you are one of the approximately 4,700 nonsmoking Americans estimated to die each year from lung cancer as a result of involuntary smoke exposure.

And the more smokers you encounter every day, the bigger your risk. So says a group of researchers from the National Institute of Environmental Health Sciences in Research Triangle Park, North Carolina. They set out to study the effects of exposure to smoke in early childhood on cancer risk in adulthood. And unexpectedly, they discovered that the effects of passive smoking accumulate during a person's lifetime. Cancer risk rises moderately if a person is exposed to household smoke during childhood or adulthood only. But if a person is exposed his whole life, his risk more than doubles. These researchers also found that overall cancer risk rose steadily and significantly with each additional household member who smoked. If three or more household members smoked, the nonsmoker had almost *four times* the risk of all smoking-related cancers.

Though smokers pooh-pooh the Surgeon General's warnings, nonsmokers are paying attention. Fueled with the evidence on passive smoking, various clean-air groups and coalitions have pushed for state restrictions on public smoking. And many have succeeded. Several states have passed strict regulations restricting smoking in public places. If a local health authority catches a New Yorker lighting up in a company conference room, for instance, the hapless perpetrator or his employer may be fined.

PIPES, CIGARS AND
SUNDRY TOBACCO PRODUCTS

There was a time when doctors advised smokers to switch to pipes or cigars to reduce their cancer risks. Those days are over.

Sure enough, the lung cancer risk is smaller with these forms of tobacco. One study showed that cigar smoking raised lung cancer risks twofold to threefold—a significant risk, but still smaller than the ninefold risk associated with cigarette smoking.

But don't think that cigars and pipes are safer. "The smoke in pipes and cigars is so irritating, most people who smoke them just keep the smoke in their mouth," says Dr. Vial. "So their lung cancer risk is smaller, but their risk for cancer of the mouth and larynx and throat is higher. But cigarette smokers who switch to cigars tend to inhale more. In this case, cigars are so much worse for the lungs, because they're unfiltered."

And if a person smokes four or more cigars and/or pipe bowls a day, it doesn't matter whether he inhales or not—either way his risk is elevated, according to University of Minnesota researchers. Smoking four or more pipes or cigars a day, they found, was equivalent to smoking about ten cigarettes a day.

And smokeless tobacco? Whether it be snuff or chewing tobacco, it's certainly popular. Currently endorsed by more than a few professional athletes, it's presently used by an estimated 22 million Americans—teenagers and college kids especially.

As far as your lungs are concerned, smokeless tobacco is safer than smoking. But regarding the teeth, tongue, mouth, esophagus, pharynx and gums, "drain cleaner could not be much more abrasive," Cooper Clinic dentist Jim Gallman, D.D.S., has said. Snuff can also increase your risk of getting cancer of the mouth by as much as *50 times*.

The cancer often grows precisely where the tobacco was placed. Usually it's placed between the cheek and gum. But not always—one Minnesota farmer who placed snuff in his ear for 42 years reportedly developed an ear tumor.

Snuff may cause irreversible damage. While lung cancer usually strikes people in their fifties, oral cancer often hits kids. "We are seeing cancer of the mouth and lip in teenagers who use chewing tobacco," says Dr. Engstrom. "There are reports of 16- and 17-year-olds who need to have their jaws removed because of oral cancer. And that's just after chewing snuff for three or four years."

There's yet another kind of smoke to worry about—clove cigarettes. These are becoming increasingly popular, especially among teenagers and young adults. In 1984, more than 150 million of these cigarettes were imported into the United States from Indonesia. While cloves are safe to eat, they're hardly safe to smoke. They contain about 50 to 70 percent tobacco. And they're even more harmful than cigarettes.

"These clove cigarettes that are becoming a fad have at least twice as much tar as cigarettes," says Dr. Hoffman. "And when you deeply inhale them, they make the lungs bleed."

Obviously, no matter how you dress up tobacco, you can't take it anywhere. "A carcinogen is a carcinogen."

THE POT OF GOLD

But here's some good news for a change: It pays to quit smoking. A study of 18,000 people showed that people who had smoked for as long as 20 years—but who had been off cigarettes for 10 years or more—had no greater risk of lung cancer than people who had never smoked at all.

"When you smoke, your lung is constantly challenged," says Dr. Vial. "So when you stop, you immediately reduce your risk, just by taking away the challenge. Then, gradually, the cilia in the lungs start beating normally again and start clearing out the sludge in the lung."

Of course, quitting smoking isn't easy.

"We're just now beginning to realize how addictive a substance nicotine is," says chest physician David P. L. Sachs, M.D., director of the Smoking Cessation Research Institute at the Palo Alto Center for Pulmonary Disease Prevention. "Ounce for ounce, nicotine has a stronger effect on the body than any drug being sold illegally on the street today. Many veterans of the Vietnam War have been able to get off drugs more easily than off their cigarettes."

If you need information on how to quit smoking, contact the American Cancer Society, American Lung Association or the National Cancer Institute.

But to give you a sense of what's out there, here's a list of the coping strategies clinicians recommend to help smokers give up their habit for good:

Chew away your withdrawal symptoms. People who have a strong addiction to nicotine can have severe withdrawal symptoms when they try to quit. We're talking irritability, disorientation, nervousness, hunger and coughing.

"I got to the point where it was hard to see anybody who quit cold turkey," says Nina Schneider, Ph.D., a research psychologist at the Uni-

IF YOU MUST SMOKE,
ARM YOUR BODY WITH VITAMINS

Have you ever wondered how so many people manage to smoke a pack a day or more and not get cancer? One reason may be the protective effects of certain vitamins.

Vitamin A and beta-carotene, a precursor of vitamin A, have proven their cancer-fighting ability time after time. Several studies suggest that people who have higher vitamin A intake have lower lung cancer incidence, even if they are heavy smokers.

In one study, 10 of 11 heavy smokers experienced a "significant" drop in the degree of their bronchial cell damage after six months of taking daily supplements of one form of vitamin A, even though they did not cut down on smoking during that time.

How does vitamin A withstand smoke's insidious influence? This vitamin regulates the process of differentiation, during which cells acquire individual characteristics. Since uncontrolled cell differentiation is what cancer is all about, inadequate vitamin A may be related to cancer development, according to researchers at the National Cancer Institute. Beta-carotene might capture free radicals, substances that damage lung cells. What's more, it even seems to reverse cancerous changes that a carcinogen causes!

Unfortunately, smokers may have lower beta-carotene levels in their blood, according to preliminary research done at the University of Texas Health Center at Tyler. "It could be that smokers just don't eat right, but it is possible that smoking depletes the very vitamin needed to repair lung damage," says Jerry W. McLarty, Ph.D., the chief investigator in the study. "Of course, studies say beta-carotene can decrease cancer risk two or three times. But a smoker's risk is ten or more times greater. So beta-carotene may improve, but not erase, the risk of smoking."

Scientists continue to discover how smoke and vitamins interact. New research suggests that smoke depletes vitamin E and inactivates B_{12} and folate. And it's been found that a localized deficiency of these vitamins can facilitate the development of precancerous growths.

Read chapter 65, Vitamin A, and chapter 66, Vitamin B, as well as chapter 38, Fruit, and chapter 64, Vegetables, to make sure you're getting maximum protection. If you smoke, you'll need all the protection you can get.

versity of California at Los Angeles who conducted a clinical study of smoking cessation. "When a person quitting cold turkey seeks help, you can spend hours just battling the constant withdrawal symptoms and the obsession with smoking. It was so much easier to treat people who used nicotine gum, which alleviates withdrawal symptoms and some of the urges to smoke. It weans smokers off nicotine, so they're not coping with their urges to smoke on a minute-to-minute basis. And it doubled their success rates."

Other studies have confirmed that nicotine gum (called Nicorette and available only by prescription) can indeed reduce nicotine cravings, but doctors point out that there is more to smoking than the desire for nicotine. There are behavioral aspects of the smoking habit that must also be confronted. What's more, there are some unpleasant side effects to the gum—among them lightheadedness, nausea, throat irritation, hiccups and excessive salivation. In conjunction with appropriate behavioral counseling, however, the gum can be an effective smoking deterrent.

Go through the motions. "Do you know how many times a smoker lifts his hand to his mouth?" asks Carolyn Price, M.D., at the Smoker's Medical Clinic in San Francisco. "It's about 8 times per cigarette, 160 times per pack. A heavy smoker may repeat this one movement over 300 times every day. And if they've been smoking for years, that behavior can really become embedded.

"So, if the patient feels very uncomfortable without a cigarette in his hand, I recommend SmokeBreak. This is a smokeless plastic cigarette that has the taste and smell of tobacco or menthol. It helps the patient recall the feelings associated with smoking and deal with the hand-to-mouth rituals."

"Don't leave yourself empty-handed when the cravings occur," says Tracy Orleans, Ph.D., former co-director of the Quit Smoking Clinic at Duke University Medical Center in Durham, North Carolina. "To keep your hands busy, fiddle with paper clips or a Rubik's Cube. During a work break, read a magazine or chew on ice chips. If you're hungry, suck on cinnamon sticks, munch on carrot sticks or chew sugarless gum."

Learn to relax.   "People will smoke in order to change their physical state when a stress occurs," says Dr. Schneider. "So when you quit, you have to learn instant methods to relax. One technique we have tried is: Take a quick deep breath; gently roll your head back slowly as you slowly exhale. It will help you relax when you don't have the time to do formal relaxation procedures. Many people in my clinic said this works. When the phone rings (this is a common trigger to smoke) there is no time for formal relaxation exercises. A quick breath or a minute of jogging in place may curb the craving."

Or you might try stretching exercises. It doesn't matter what method you use, as long as you can soothe yourself when you think you need a cigarette.

Reward yourself. "Most smokers will see immediate benefits when they quit," says Dr. Orleans, "and this positive reinforcement helps get them through the toughest times. They'll be able to walk further without getting winded. Food will begin to taste better, too. They'll feel less anxious and more in control of their lives than when they smoked."

Even if better health is its own reward, don't shortchange yourself for a job well done. "Give yourself presents," says Dr. Orleans. "After all, you used smoking a cigarette as a kind of reward for a long time. Now with the money you're saving from not buying cigarettes you can substitute other rewards."

Create a smoke-free environment. "It's almost impossible to quit smoking if your spouse continues to smoke in front of you," says Dr. Engstrom. "It helps if you quit together, so you can get that social support."

Don't surround yourself with smokers away from home, either. "Avoid situations where you know the urge to smoke will be irresistible," says Dr. Engstrom. "It might be at a coffee break or in a bar— know your own weak spots."

Dr. Schneider agrees. "It really helps if you're in a nonsmoking environment," she says. "The new work-site laws are the best thing to happen to smokers. They make it much easier to avoid temptation."

Exercise. At the very least, exercise is something you can do to keep your mind off smoking. But it may make quitting easier in other ways too.

"Exercise makes you feel good about yourself," says Dr. Schneider. "And it's a good outlet for stress."

And as you start to enjoy the activity, you may have another motivation to quit. "As you exercise, you'll notice that smoking decreases your performance," says Dr. Vial. "When people take up running or tennis for instance, and want to be good at it, they'll quickly realize that they 'ain't gonna be good' unless they quit smoking."

Learn to hate the habit. Dr. Sachs recently completed an extensive review of smoking-cessation strategies—physician-supervised plans plus do-it-yourself models—and what he found to be the most effective by far was a doctor-implemented approach known as "aversive smoking."

"What it boils down to is learning to hate the habit," Dr. Sachs says. "In your doctor's treatment room you smoke rapidly so that smoking ceases to be pleasurable."

Resolve never to touch a cigarette again. "I have worked with hard-core cigarette smokers, and smoking is much more than a habit. It's a drug dependence," says Dr. Schneider. "When you've watched people who're smoking even when they have a serious lung disease, and they're hacking away, it's hard to see smoking as just a simple enjoyable habit. Many people smoke who are unable to quit even though they dislike the habit.

"And just like a recovered alcoholic can't take one drink, an ex-smoker can't smoke just one cigarette. Even after years of quitting, a cigarette can trigger the whole addiction process," she says. "For a person who has been a regular smoker, trying to smoke occasionally leads back to smoking regularly. While people can slip and recover, it's always risking a full blown relapse."

CANCER PREVENTION PLAN: TOBACCO

- Don't smoke tobacco.
- Don't chew tobacco.
- Don't use snuff.
- Avoid "sidestream" smoke.
- Contact the American Cancer Society for a program about how to quit smoking.

Vegetables

It's almost dinnertime when you realize you haven't any vegetables in the house. You dash to the market. It's winter. The corn is mealy. The green beans are about to grow beards. Broccoli, the kids won't eat it. Zucchini, your husband will hit the ceiling. Carrots, you had them last night. You throw a pale green head of lettuce wrapped in cellophane into the cart. Nothing else there to inspire you. You settle for broccoli. You can bribe the kids to eat it with a promise of apple pie for dessert. You head for the bakery.

Although exaggerated, this scenario doesn't sound entirely unfamiliar; a lot of people think of vegetables as the *un*fun part of a meal, that spoonful of peas sitting in a puddle at the side of your plate.

The time has come to raise our vegetable consciousness—to think of aromatic vegetable soups and stews, of chili, of minestrone and of borscht (made with beets and greens), to think of acorn squash and sweet potatoes tenderly opened, steaming and dolloped with yogurt and chives, to think of golden baked potato and carrot puddings, and of peppers and cabbage stuffed with spicy vegetable rice. Time, also, to think of hidden vegetables—zucchini or pumpkin bread, spinach ravioli and carrot cake. Time, in other words, to put vegetables in the center of the plate. Because what your mother told you really is true: Vegetables are good for you. In fact, they may save your life (see the table below, Side-Dish Vitamins, for more information).

Did you know that, thanks in part to refrigeration and fresh foods in our diet, we have practically wiped out stomach cancer in the United States? One hundred years ago, gastric cancers topped the list of the ten deadliest cancers; today they are one of the least common. Further-

SIDE-DISH VITAMINS

VEGETABLE	PORTION	VITAMIN A (IU)	VITAMIN C (mg)	FIBER (g)
Acorn squash, baked	1 cup	874	22	4
Artichoke, cooked	1 med.	172	9	1.1
Asparagus, cooked	4 spears	498	16	0.5
Bean sprouts, soybean, raw	1 cup	0	11	1.6
Broccoli, cooked	1 spear	2,537	113	2.2
Brussels sprouts, cooked	1 cup	1,122	97	2.1
Butternut squash, cubed, baked	1 cup	14,352	31	2.6
Cabbage, finely shredded	1 cup	700	22	0.6
Carrot, raw	1 med.	20,253	7	0.8
Carrots, diced, cooked	1 cup	38,304	4	2.3
Cauliflower, cooked	1 cup	18	68	1
Celery, raw	1 lg. stalk	51	2.5	0.3
Corn, yellow, cooked	1 ear	167	5	0.5
Cucumber, unpeeled, sliced	½ cup	23	2	0.3
Green beans, small pieces, cooked	1 cup	833	12	1.8
Okra	8 sm. pods	489	14	0.77
Onions, yellow, cooked	½ cup	0	6	0.44
Peas, frozen, cooked, drained	½ cup	534	8	1.7
Pepper, red or green, raw	1 sm.	392	95	0.89
Potato, boiled in skin	1 med.	0	26	1.3
Pumpkin, canned	1 cup	54,038	10	4
Summer squash, sliced, cooked	1 cup	517	10	1.1
Sweet potato, baked	1 med.	24,877	28	0.9
Tomatoes, canned wedges in juice	1 cup	1,508	39	1.2
Tomatoes, cooked	1 cup	3,245	50	1.8
Tomato, raw	1 med.	1,394	27	0.6
Turnips, diced, cooked	½ cup	0	9	0.55
Yams, cooked	1 cup	0	17	· · ·
Zucchini, cooked	½ cup	216	4	0.45

more, this same miracle food that has protected our stomachs has, in study after study, been shown to shield people from all types of cancers. Research in Japan among thousands of people showed that the more vegetables they ate, including seaweed, the lower their risks for all cancers.

Many other studies have confirmed these results, including one in Massachusetts, this time with hundreds of senior citizens (a group usually at a higher risk for cancer). In New Jersey, the wonder food protected hundreds of men from lung cancer—even though they smoked! And researchers have noticed that, across the map, people who live in the southern half of the United States have been able to protect themselves against certain types of cancer, and they suffer a lower cancer rate than the Yankees up north. And this southern group includes all the retirees in Florida.

Best of all, this vegetable preventive against cancer is readily available without prescription and is recommended by such august bodies as the National Research Council, the U.S. Department of Agriculture and the National Cancer Institute. Vegetables really work!

HOW CANCERS FORM
AND HOW TO BEAT THEM

Cancer formation is a two-step process, explains L. Herbert Maurer, M.D., associate professor of medicine at Dartmouth Medical School. In the first step, a carcinogen infiltrates a cell and corrupts the DNA—the genetic material in the cell—inciting it to mutate. This first action is called initiation. Some of these mutations subvert the normal cell into a potentially malignant cell.

The second step is called promotion—substances that are not in themselves carcinogenic can, like governments that fund terrorists, support or promote the activities and growth of these subverted cells. In most cases, notes Dr. Maurer, 10 to 30 years will have elapsed between the first encounter with the carcinogen and the first detection of the cancer. This time lapse gives us ample opportunity to block the corruption of our cells and bring them back into line.

"There are several strategies we can use to bolster the body's defenses to stop these two processes from occurring, and vegetables may play an important role in each one," advises Dr. Maurer. Scientists are still pondering the whys and wherefores of just how vegetables work, which ones work best and whether some may have special anticancer effects. Evidence on the different powers of vegetables ranges from "Yes, we know this is true—many studies prove it; eat this, it will help you dramatically" to "Maybe there is something here; in any event it can't hurt you."

BLOCK THAT CARCINOGEN

One fact few would dispute is that vegetables contain certain vitamins, primarily vitamins C, E and A and beta-carotene, and the trace element selenium, which are known as antioxidants. These nutrients seem to help prevent a carcinogen from ever reaching its target cell or block its action after it gets there, explains Dr. Maurer. As antioxidants, they can help prevent the process called initiation and, as a result, help preserve the cell's DNA.

Any cook knows that a sprinkling of lemon juice (high in vitamin C) will keep apple slices from turning brown once they've been cut and exposed to oxygen. In the same way, these antioxidant vitamins have been shown to stop the corrosive effects of oxidation on our cells. Miraculously, these vitamin pals actually block potential toxins (such as the nitrites and nitrates in our food and environment) from shamelessly turning into carcinogens right inside our bodies. The evidence for the wonderful effects of these vitamins is so strong that manufacturers of processed meats are now starting to add vitamin C to their bacon.

Research on cancer prevention and diet is just beginning, but so far one of the most promising cancer-fighting vitamins just may turn out to be a family of nutrients that you don't normally get in your morning vitamin tablet—one you get just from vegetables.

PROTECTIVE BETA-CAROTENE

We're talking about carotenoids, one of which is beta-carotene. Researchers are extremely excited about these nutrients. In fact, Joel Schwartz, D.M.D., D.M.Sc., assistant professor of oral pathology at the Harvard School of Dental Medicine and assistant professor at Dana-Farber Cancer Institute, is very enthusiastic about the discoveries he and his colleagues have made.

They have found that beta-carotene will keep cancers from forming in the cheek pouches of hamsters that have been given a carcinogen that would normally cause oral cancer in those pouches. "Beta-carotene can inhibit both initiation and promotion—the two-step process in cancer formation—when applied locally to the pouch.

"Then," continues Dr. Schwartz, "we found that beta-carotene not only inhibits tumors from forming, but once they do form, it makes the tumors regress." Dr. Schwartz has also found that this regression is associated with a buildup of immunities that prevented the cancers from returning. "In particular, immune cells called macrophages will produce an immune product called tumor necrosis factor. This factor has been associated with the killing of both human and animal tumor cells. An algae extract that contains beta-carotene plus 15 other carotenoids produced an even greater amount of this factor than beta-carotene by itself. In addition, we've seen regression in tumors and asked the question, Will these tumors re-form? We've waited two months and compared them with controls [luckless animals who did not receive the beta-carotene treatment]. The controls had such massive tumors we had to put the animals to sleep, but with the treated animals there was only a small regrowth.

"We have evidence that beta-carotene works on other types of cancer than just oral cancer," says Dr. Schwartz, citing further studies that are just now reaching completion at Harvard. "It works not only on carcinoma [cancer of the epithelial tissue, which covers the surface of our bodies and the surfaces of internal organs], not only on isolated lesions that are invading deeply into the local tissue, but also on cancers that are spreading into connecting tissues (sarcoma).

"There is evidence that beta-carotene affects chemically induced tumors, so we've tried many different types of experiments and beta-carotene seems to be successful. Besides the enhancement of immune activity and tumor regression, it is also important to note that normal, healthy cells around the tumor remained unchanged, showing no obvious toxic effects from beta-carotene."

Beta-carotene, as its name implies, is the orange stuff in carrots and in other yellow fruits and vegetables such as acorn squash and sweet potatoes. It is also abundant in dark green leafy vegetables such as spinach, and in broccoli. Vegetables may contain many additional types of carotenoids, and some of these also may prove to be potent cancer blockers. For the moment, beta-carotene is simply the most investigated of the bunch.

In your stomach, beta-carotene splits in two, and these two parts turn into vitamin A. "This is a very sloppy process," explains Leonard A. Cohen, Ph.D., a cell biologist and the head of the section of nutritional endocrinology at the American Health Foundation in Valhalla, New York. "Not every molecule of beta-carotene turns into vitamin A. Far from it. Perhaps only 40 percent is converted. Retinol vitamin A (the nutrient you get from liver, eggs, milk and vitamin A pills) races straight for your liver, where it is stored for future use and may cause problems if you take too much.

"Beta-carotene, on the other hand, cannot get into the liver—it's too big—so it is stored in the fat layers under your skin. Did you ever notice that if you feed turnips to infants, their faces will sometimes take on an orange-yellow cast? It doesn't harm anything. It just sits there until it's needed. I don't think there's been a case in the annals of medical history of anyone who has poisoned himself by eating too many carrots," says Dr. Cohen. And that is fortunate, since the research shows that many of the good effects of this vitamin come not so much from vitamin A itself but from its now-famous precursor—beta-carotene from vegetables.

INCREASE CONSUMPTION

Surveys taken by the U.S. Department of Agriculture show that many Americans eat far too few foods containing vitamin A (beta-carotene and retinol). In fact, a quarter of us consume less than 60 percent

---

SEA VEGETABLES: AN ORIENTAL CONNECTION

Vegetables from the ocean that reduce cancer risks? Sounds outlandish, but researchers are finding growing evidence that the brown-colored seaweed known as kelp may offer protection from at least two types of cancer: breast and colon.

Population studies offer some of the evidence. The rest comes from laboratory research. According to demographic studies, the Japanese—who have low rates of breast and colon cancer and long survival rates if they do get cancer—eat kelp, harvested from cold waters, at just about every meal. In fact, kelp makes up an astonishing 25 percent of the Japanese diet. It appears on the table as a plain vegetable or garnish, as well as in soups, sweet cakes, jellies, sauces, and salads. Steeped, it makes an exotic tea. But that's not all. Combined with flour, kelp is kneaded into noodles.

Does kelp (the Japanese call it *kombu*) really hold a key to antitumor activity? The possibility is good, according to Jane Teas, who has a Ph.D. in pathobiology from Johns Hopkins University. While at the Harvard School of Public Health, Boston, she studied 116 young female rats that had been exposed to a potent breast cancer carcinogen. The rats were fed either a normal diet or one supplemented with sun-dried kelp. The results: 76 percent of the rats on the normal diet developed tumors, while only 63 percent of the rats on the seaweed did. What's more amazing, it took almost twice as long for the tumors to develop in the rats that ate the seaweed.

More good news: Another group of researchers, this time in Japan, got similar results. They observed a reduction in the number of intestinal tumors in young male rats that had been exposed to a carcinogen but fed a diet of kelp and algin sulfate, an extract of kelp.

Dr. Teas and other researchers aren't yet certain what "secret ingredient" in kelp slows tumor growth. According to Dr. Teas, maybe it's kelp's vitamins. Maybe it's the minerals. Or perhaps kelp's fiber escorts toxic substances from the body before they can do harm. Still another possibility is that kelp may contain a substance that stimulates the body's immune response.

of the Recommended Dietary Allowance (RDA) of this nutrient. Furthermore, the National Cancer Institute advises that even if you are getting the bare minimum RDA level, that may not be enough for cancer prevention. While we await the final results, the National Research

"Seaweed is a whole food, so it's difficult to guess what's in the whole food that's responsible for a particular reaction," says Dr. Teas. "But it may be fucoidan, a component of kelp's fiber structure. Studies indicate fucoidan alone will inhibit tumors. If that's the case, we could get even more protection from sea grapes, or fucus, found along the New England coast," she says.

Ready to add sea vegetables to your anticancer diet? You won't be alone. Seaweed is enjoyed by the Chinese, Koreans and Hawaiians. And, in limited quantities, the peoples of Ireland, Scotland and Wales have savored the subtly sweet flavors for centuries. Then, of course, there are the Japanese, who eat more sea vegetables today than ever before.

Where can you get sea vegetables? Oriental specialty shops are your best bet, but many natural foods stores carry them, too. Most of the sea vegetables sold in the United States come from Japan and are packaged in dry form. Names on the packages are *nori* or *laver, kombu, hijiki, wakame* and *arame*. Though each has its own flavor, you can use sea vegetables interchangeably in most recipes.

Preparing dried sea vegetables is remarkably quick and easy. First, freshen them in enough lukewarm or room-temperature water to cover for 2 to 15 minutes, depending on the variety. For most uses, *wakame* and *nori* take only 2 to 5 minutes; *hijiki* and *kombu,* 15 to 20 minutes. If the midrib remains firm even after soaking, trim it off and put it aside for making soup. Save the soak water; it lends body and zest to vegetable and beef stocks.

After freshening them, you can enjoy sea vegetables raw or cook them just as you would any other vegetable: sauté, steam or stir-fry. Initially, you may want to use them sparingly, say as a garnish or in salads, soups, stews or casseroles.

Store dried sea vegetables in plastic bags or glass jars in a cool, dry place. Freshened and cooked vegetables will stay tasty for a day or two in glass or ceramic containers in the refrigerator.

Council of the National Academy of Sciences recommends that we eat vitamin A-rich foods daily to lower our cancer risk.

Dr. Schwartz's experimental animals are never treated with a massive dose. Dr. Schwartz and his colleagues are looking for a treatment that can be prescribed for everyone without poisoning them. "I can't make dietary recommendations for others," says Dr. Schwartz, "but I take a spirulina algae compound, which contains numerous natural carotenoids other than beta-carotene." Dr. Schwartz is fully convinced of the wonderful effects of vegetables. "When you talk about inhibiting carcinoma, and all your controls are dead or have tumors and you have more than 50 percent of your treated animals surviving with regressed tumors, something unique is going on." That's how researchers talk when they're excited—and it doesn't happen very often.

Dr. Schwartz, is, of course, not the only vegetable enthusiast. Numerous experiments and studies support his evidence. A massive Japanese study suggests that eating vegetables every day can substantially reduce your risk of getting cancer—even if you're a heavy smoker. The study began in 1965 when researchers at the National Cancer Research Institute in Tokyo questioned about 100,000 Japanese men over age 40. They divided them into 16 groups according to whether they did or did not smoke cigarettes, drink alcohol, eat meat or eat vegetables every day.

The men were followed for almost 20 years, by which time about 30,000 had died, 8,000 of them from cancers. Not too surprisingly, by far the highest cancer death rate occurred in men who smoked, drank and ate meat but did not eat vegetables daily. This "high-risk" group had the highest rates of cancer of the throat, mouth, stomach, lung, bladder and skin of any of the 16 groups—in several cases, more than twice as high as any other group.

But perhaps the most interesting finding came from the men who shared the high-risk group's lifestyle—smoking, drinking and eating meat—but who also minded their mamas' commandment to eat vegetables every day. Among these men, the cancer-death rate was about a third lower than that of the high-risk group.

If you are not yet munching a carrot stick as you read this, here's still another cancer-fighting strategy from your vegetable allies.

THE BENEFITS OF FIBER

"Everyone agrees that the amount of fiber we're eating is low in comparison with countries where colon cancer is low and also in comparison with historical man," says Dr. Cohen. "We take in roughly 10 to 12 grams a day, according to researchers from Emory University, and in Finland, for example, they take in 20 or more. And in Finland, they have one-quarter our colon cancer rate."

"When people think of fiber, they often think only of bran," adds Peter Greenwald, M.D., director of the division of cancer prevention and control at the National Cancer Institute. "They may not realize that vegetables are a very good source of fiber. We recommend that people take in 20 to 30 grams per day. Most vegetables have 1 to 3 grams of fiber per serving (beans usually have 4 or more). Lettuce has almost no fiber. Many people think, 'Oh, I had a salad, that takes care of my fiber'—a lentil salad would be a better source." (See the table, Legumes for Fiber, below.)

George E. Demetrakopoulos, M.D., M.P.H., director of the Medical Nutrition Center of Greater Washington, D.C., recommends high-fiber vegetables to his patients, but cautions them against taking fiber supplements. "Foods that contain bran may not provide the best fiber. For cancer prevention, what you need are foods high in a kind of fiber called pentosans, found in such vegetables as cauliflower, onions, broccoli, endives, mushrooms, spinach, potatoes, eggplant, carrots, pumpkins or beans. Edible leaves like grape leaves and parsley are also good sources."

Above all, suggests Dr. Demetrakopoulos, take fiber from the whole food—don't separate it. "To my patients, I recommend two fruits, two servings of vegetables and one serving of whole grain cereal each day."

Dr. Demetrakopoulos has awarded his own personal vegetable Oscars based on natural talent (relative wealth of vitamins A and C and fiber). He gives five stars to sweet potatoes, celery, green beans, broccoli, tomatoes and peppers. Three stars go to zucchini, kale, lettuce and spinach. Eggplant, artichokes and collards get two stars. And, at the bottom, the white potato comes in with only one star.

LEGUMES FOR FIBER

LEGUME	PORTION	FIBER* (g)
Black beans, cooked	1 cup	7.2
Garbanzo beans, cooked	1 cup	10.6
Kidney beans, cooked	1 cup	9.0
Lentils, cooked	1 cup	6.0
Pinto beans, cooked	1 cup	6.8
Soybeans, cooked	1 cup	2.9

*Water-insoluble fiber.

BEANS OFFER GOOD PROTECTION

Eat beans, of course because they are high in fiber but also because, as members of the seed family, they may offer special protection against cancer. "Studies of different populations such as the Seventh-Day Adventists and the Japanese (whose major source of protein, until quite recently, was soybeans) show that eating seeds like rice and beans lowers the risk for colon, prostatic and breast cancers," says Walter Troll, Ph.D., a professor in the Department of Environmental Medicine at New York University Medical Center. Dr. Troll is interested in the possibility that protease inhibitors in beans may block cancers from forming. (Protease is an enzyme that may be produced in oversupply by tumors or things that are about to be tumors.)

All seeds contain these protease inhibitors, explains Dr. Troll, probably to discourage insects who cannot digest them and therefore tend to let the seeds grow in peace. People don't really digest these useful little cancer fighters either; protease inhibitors manage to survive the whole digestive process in our stomach, then appear in the colon fully active and are combined and excreted with the feces. Perhaps removing this enzyme from action is helpful in preventing cancerous cells. It seems to be there in the colon that beans and seeds do a lot of their good work, for colon cancer is one of the cancers protease inhibitors may prevent, in addition to breast and prostate cancer. "We need more study before we will fully understand just how they work," says Dr. Troll.

How about some tofu or lentil soup, while we're waiting?

CABBAGE HAS PROMISE

Cruciferous vegetables (which include Brussels sprouts, broccoli and cabbage) have been intriguing cancer researchers for hundreds of years. Michael Albert-Puleo, M.D., a partner in the Family Health Center of Medford, New Jersey, made an in-depth study of all the work on cabbage dating back to Cato the Censor of ancient Rome, who applied cabbage poultices to cancerous sores twice a day. It may seem incredible, but after all this time, scientists are still puzzled by the possible effect of cabbage—if there is one.

"Nothing is simple in this field," comments Dr. Albert-Puleo "We're really in the dark ages with diet and cancer prevention. Studies have shown that cruciferous vegetables activate a special enzyme system in the liver that is involved with breaking down and changing chemicals, including carcinogens, in the body and getting them ready for elimination."

"The evidence for cruciferous vegetables really started out with animal studies," adds Dr. Cohen. "Extracts of cruciferous vegetables were fed to animals and were found to inhibit tumors." Researchers then tried to do studies on human populations, with mixed results. "Sometimes you see things, sometimes you don't," is how Dr. Cohen sums it up.

At the State University of New York at Buffalo, where much of the original research on the cancer-cabbage connection originated, Tim Byers, M.D., associate professor of preventive medicine, explains that "there is reason to believe that there's something about them that is anticarcinogenic. The trouble is that there are hundreds of compounds in all fruits and vegetables, and we just don't know yet exactly which ones are protective and which are not. Even though cruciferous vegetables are an element in the dietary prescription of the National Cancer Institute, we don't really know whether they offer special protection or are simply good because they are high in fiber and beta-carotene."

Dr. Albert-Puleo is still intrigued. "There was one very interesting aspect that I'm trying to get people interested in exploring further," he says. "A couple of studies, one apparently done by the army in the 1950s, showed that when cabbage was fed to animals and they were then given a dose of radiation, the dose that would normally have killed them did not kill them. Perhaps cabbage might have beneficial effects for patients undergoing radiation therapy." Thoughts of Three Mile Island and Chernobyl come to mind, and suddenly, regular helpings of coleslaw (easy on the mayonnaise) sound mighty appealing.

"The whole thing with cruciferous vegetables is still highly experimental," explains Dr. Cohen. When the American Cancer Society says to eat cabbage, they're saying there is no harm in it; there's some evidence that it may be helpful, but it's by no means proven.

"It isn't like fat, for instance. Practically everyone now agrees that a high fat intake increases your risk for breast cancer, and if you lower the amount of fat in your diet, you're helping yourself. Twenty-five or 30 studies on animals prove that. But that kind of evidence just doesn't exist for cruciferous vegetables," according to Dr. Cohen. "If you want to look at the top of what we know without a doubt, it's the connection between breast cancer and fat. Down toward the bottom of what has been proven are things like cruciferous vegetables.

"It takes a lot of evidence and time to convince scientists. Look at the fat issue—it's just barely been accepted," he says. "I've been working on it for 13 years, and the original studies appeared over 50 years ago. In 1970, the idea of fat and cancer being linked was hardly mentioned. We were considered somewhat questionable—a fringe group. Now, though, finally, the rest of the medical research community has come around and begun to take it more seriously."

Dr. Cohen recommends we all eat cruciferous vegetables for two reasons: First, because there's no harm in them and they may work

GET THE MOST FROM LEAFY GREENS

If you drive through the French countryside in the spring, you will often see whole families out from town for the day to pick the wild greens that grow along the sides of the roads—free for anyone who knows their value. But you don't have to go to France to find the makings of a nutritious bowl of greens.

Next time *you* make a salad, send that iceberg lettuce back to the Arctic where it belongs (a whole cup of chopped iceberg has only 198 International Units of vitamin A, a mere 4 percent of the daily requirement).

Instead, try mixing different greens such as romaine, spinach, red leaf, watercress and beet or mustard greens. Spike it with parsley and chives and add tomato and cucumber for more color, taste and health value.

Keep in mind also that when you prepare greens such as kale, no law says you *must* cook them with pork. In fact, they're quite good—and much better for you—simply stir-fried with onions and mushrooms.

GOODNESS FROM GREENS

LEAFY GREENS	PORTION	VITAMIN A (IU)	VITAMIN C (mg)	FIBER (g)
Beet greens, cooked	1 cup	7,344	36	1.5
Chives, chopped	1 tbsp.	192	2	Trace
Collard greens, leaves and stems, cooked	1 cup	4,218	19	0.76
Dandelion greens, cooked	1 cup	12,285	19	1.4
Kale, cooked	1 cup	9,620	53	1
Lettuce, leaf	1 leaf	190	2	0.1
Lettuce, romaine	1 leaf	260	2	0.1
Mustard greens, cooked	1 cup	4,244	35	0.96
Spinach, chopped, raw	1 cup	3,760	16	0.5
Spinach, leaves, cooked	1 cup	14,742	18	1.6
Swiss chard, leaves and stems, cooked	1 cup	5,493	32	1.6
Turnip greens, cooked	1 cup	7,917	40	0.88
Watercress, raw	10 sprigs	1,180	11	0.2

beneficially on certain types of cancer such as breast and gastric. Second, eating cabbage or any vegetable will help us give up our dependence on fat by filling us up with complex carbohydrates. "The more vegetables you eat, the more you tend to push out fat from your diet," says Dr. Cohen.

MORE SPECIAL VEGGIES

It is possible that chlorophyll, found in many vegetables, may have protective properties. In fact, Chiu-Nan Lai, Ph.D., a researcher at the M.D. Anderson Hospital and Tumor Institute in Houston, believes that chlorophyll may be one of the key anticancer ingredients in vegetables.

"Brussels sprouts, broccoli, spinach and leafy lettuce are rich in chlorophyll," says Dr. Lai. "My laboratory research has demonstrated that extracts of chlorophyll from those vegetables have the power to inhibit the mutagenic activity of known cancer-causing agents. Those vegetables with the highest chlorophyll content have the most power against carcinogens."

Dr. Lai notes that vegetables that are high in chlorophyll also tend to be high in beta-carotene. "It's interesting that they are tied together," she says, "because in plants, the purpose of beta-carotene is to protect the structure of chlorophyll. Plants don't need carotene the way we do, but they do need chlorophyll for photosynthesis, and they apparently need carotene to protect the chlorophyll.

"People don't really absorb the chlorophyll they eat. In fact, the studies show that 95 percent of chlorophyll is still active in the colon, where it may help to protect against colon cancer."

Dr. Lai also notes that chlorophyll is destroyed by heat, so if you want to gain the benefits of this extra protection, concentrate on raw vegetables—spinach salad and broccoli florets with yogurt-and-fresh-herb dip.

Another vast vegetable kingdom we rarely consider is seaweed. These algae are rich in fiber, thiamine, and vitamins A, B_{12}, C and E. Experiments have shown that seaweeds may offer some special cancer prevention. One study in Japan, for example, showed that among rats who were subjected to a chemical treatment aimed at causing tumors, those who were fed sea algae showed a greatly reduced incidence of intestinal tumors.

William Fenical, Ph.D., professor of oceanography at Scripps Institution of Oceanography in La Jolla, California, says, "Look at societies that eat marine algae and ask yourself whether they are healthy or not, and I think you will find that generally they are healthy—probably healthier than Americans. No one has really looked at the nutritional content of seaweeds very deeply—even the Japanese, although they utilize seaweeds regularly in food. One has to view something like seaweeds as a great unexplored resource."

Family physician Michael Albert-Puleo adds, "I'd like to see the day when we have more data on different vegetables so we really understand their effect on people's health and can start making recommendations early. I try to get my patients to eat less meat and fat, to exercise more, to eat more vegetables and fiber. What's interesting is that 15 years ago, these were things the 'crazy' health food press was talking about—now the doctors are talking about them. I'm trying to start with people in their twenties and thirties—getting them to assume a better lifestyle now so I don't have to see them in the intensive care unit when they're 50 or 60, but of course, no matter how old you are, it's never too late to start."

CANCER PREVENTION PLAN: VEGETABLES

- Eat two servings of vegetables, two servings of fruit and one serving of whole grain cereal each day.
- Frequently eat vegetables containing the type of fiber called pentosans, which are found in such vegetables as cauliflower, onions, broccoli, endive, mushrooms, spinach, potatoes, eggplant, carrots, pumpkins or beans. Edible leaves like grape leaves and parsley are also good sources.
- For good amounts of vitamins A and C and fiber, frequently eat sweet potatoes, celery, green beans, broccoli, tomatoes and peppers, as well as zucchini, kale, lettuce and spinach. Eggplant, artichokes and collards and white potatoes are other sources.
- Put lots of cruciferous vegetables on the menu. These include Brussels sprouts, broccoli and cabbage.

Vitamin A

Save carrots in your gardens, and humbly praise God for them, as for a singular and great blessing.

Richard Gardiner, c. 1599

The scientific evidence is still far from conclusive, but that didn't stop the National Academy of Sciences from issuing an anticancer prescription in 1982 that sounded remarkably like something your mother once told you: Eat your vegetables.

Even some cancer researchers who won't be pinned down to anything more concrete than a "maybe" admit that they haven't waited for the final test results before changing their diet. "I've seen it in this business for the last seven years," says one whose work on vitamin A and skin cancer is still in its early stages. "What I—and all my colleagues—eat has changed. I used to be a typical junk-food eater. Now I eat a vegetable-based, high-fiber diet. Does it prevent cancer? My scientific answer is that the data is overwhelmingly suggestive that diet makes a difference. My scientific answer is that what I eat has certainly changed."

Even without the definitive proof in hand, the normally conservative scientific community has become the unabashed patron of the salad bar. What convinced them? A persuasive collection of studies from all over the world that suggests that people who heap their plates with green and yellow vegetables and fruit reduce their risk of cancer.

- A Japanese study—one of the biggest of its kind—found that people who ate green-yellow vegetables every day had a decreased risk of developing lung, stomach and other cancers. The 20-year-old, ongoing study also indicates that the damage wrought by bad habits—spurning vegetables or smoking, for instance—is reversible. Ex-smokers who had their daily dose of green-yellow vegetables also experienced a reduction in their risk of lung cancer, and there was a more than 25 percent reduction in the number of deaths from stomach cancer among those who increased their vegetable consumption.
- A Harvard University study of more than 1,200 elderly Massachusetts residents found that those who reported the highest consumption of carrots, squash, tomatoes, salads or leafy greens, dried fruits, fresh strawberries or melon, broccoli or Brussels sprouts had a decreased risk of cancer.
- A researcher comparing the diets of healthy people and those with gastrointestinal cancer in both the United States and Norway found that the healthy people ate more foods such as carrots, leafy green vegetables and fresh fruits.

What's in a carrot that seems to counteract cancer? Buoyed by this impressive data, the National Cancer Institute (NCI) is spending millions of dollars to find out.

Starting with the only thing they knew for sure—there's something about green-yellow vegetables that acts as a buffer against cancer—NCI scientists latched onto color as their first clue. What gives these vegetables their hue? A naturally occurring pigment called beta-carotene, now the subject of at least 14 studies funded by the NCI.

Of course, beta-carotene is more than just a pigment. It is one of the dietary chemicals the body converts into usable vitamin A. Because so little is known about it, researchers are grappling with several questions. Does beta-carotene inhibit cancer by its own unique mechanism, or simply because it is converted into vitamin A, which has been shown in laboratory studies to be a cancer preventive? If it has its own potency, and since it is the common dietary source of vitamin A, could some of the anticancer claims made for vitamin A be more rightly credited to beta-carotene?

What evidence there is suggests that beta-carotene provides its own form of protection against cancer. And one cancer researcher, Richard Peto of Oxford, England, believes it's a strong possibility that it could prevent about a third of the cancer deaths in the United States.

One thing scientists do know is that beta-carotene acts as what one researcher describes as a "shock absorber," protecting the valuable genetic blueprints inside each cell from the damage caused by reactive molecules known as free radicals. Theoretically, the havoc wrought by those excited molecules can turn a healthy cell into a cancerous one.

And beta-carotene has two major advantages over other forms of vitamin A. First, it has no known toxicity. Vitamin A taken in doses over 50,000 International Units daily can be dangerous. "With an overdose of beta-carotene, on the other hand, all you do is turn yellow," says Frank L. Meyskens Jr., M.D., of the cancer center division of the University of Arizona in Tucson.

The dietary sources of beta-carotene are unarguably healthful foods. For most people, the main sources of the other major form of dietary vitamin A—the retinoids—are milk and cheese. "Unless you go with skim milk and low-fat dairy products, that can mean a very high-fat diet," says Judith Wylie-Rosett, Ed.D.

CERVICAL CANCER LINK

Dr. Wylie-Rosett and her colleagues at Albert Einstein College of Medicine in New York City are a few of the handful of researchers who are adding to the growing body of knowledge about this nutrient-come-lately.

When they examined the diets of a group of healthy women and women with abnormal Pap smears, they found that women with a low vitamin A or beta-carotene intake had a threefold greater risk of developing cervical cancer or severe cervical dysplasia, a precancerous condition.

One of the reasons Dr. Wylie-Rosett and her associates looked at beta-carotene intake, aside from their interest in the nutrient, was extremely practical. "In our computer analysis, we have the ability to evaluate it," she says. "Not all nutrition surveys do, which is probably one reason why so little has been done on it. The interest in beta-carotene is relatively recent."

Interestingly, at almost the same time the American researchers were probing the connection between beta-carotene and cervical cancer, so were a group of doctors in Milan, Italy. Their findings were similar. Women who averaged a goodly amount of beta-carotene daily, as measured by their consumption of carrots and green vegetables, had a reduced risk of cervical cancer. Significantly, the researchers found no such association with the retinoids—measured by the consumption of milk, liver and meats—when they compared the diets of 191 women with cervical cancer and 191 healthy women in the same age-group.

Of course, asking someone to recall the amount of carrots or squash she ate over any given period doesn't give the kind of rock-solid results experimental scientists prefer. These so-called retrospective studies are often severely criticized. So, researchers at the British Columbia Cancer Research Center in Vancouver made sure they knew exactly how much beta-carotene and vitamin A their test subjects were taking. They administered capsules of each twice weekly to 40 rural Filipinos living on Luzon, the largest island in the Philippines, who were chosen because of their habit of quid chewing.

A quid is a concoction made from the areca nut, the betel leaf, lime produced from heating and crushing snail shells, and dried tobacco leaf. It is believed responsible for several hundred thousand oral cancer deaths each year in Asia. The Filipino tribesmen selected for the trial, ranging in age from 30 to 60, admitted to chewing from 4 to 15 quids a day.

Working with medical missionaries in this poor community, where the daily fare was usually potatoes and rice, the researchers made sure their volunteers got 100,000 International Units of vitamin A and 300,000 International Units of beta-carotene each week—well above U.S. recommended daily allowances. Because the study was so short (only three months), the scientists knew they wouldn't see cancers develop, so they looked for the earliest warning sign: cell damage inside the mouth.

Needless to say, among the quid chewers there were quite a few damaged cells in the tissue samples scraped from the insides of their cheeks at the beginning of the study. But at the end, 37 of the 40 had substantially fewer damaged cells than they did at the start. In fact, the number of damaged cells decreased dramatically—by about 40 percent a month. The remaining 3 had no increase in the amount of damage.

The researchers found their results so "striking" that they suggested that it may be possible for people at high risk of oral cancer to lessen their risk by simply adding vitamin A and/or beta-carotene to their diet.

A "MORNING-AFTER" PILL

Like the 20-year Japanese study, the Canadian research appears to indicate that we have a grace period, a time when dietary intervention will save us from the consequences of our bad health habits. Several important animal studies are providing clues to just how long it lasts.

Eli Seifter, Ph.D., professor of biochemistry and surgery, and his colleagues at the Albert Einstein College of Medicine found out more about that critical grace period. They discovered the earlier beta-carotene is given, the better. When they gave a hefty dose to rats at intervals ranging from two to nine weeks after exposure to a cancer-causing chemical, the researchers discovered the grace period lasted for five to six weeks. Rats given beta-carotene more than a month after their exposure to the carcinogen did not develop tumors.

While the results can't yet be translated into a human timetable, they still provide some valuable information. "What our study really shows," says Dr. Seifter, "is that beta-carotene is protective against either late stages of tumor development or early stages of tumor growth.

"That's very good, because it shows in a sense that it's a 'morning-after' pill. Even after exposure to cancer-producing doses of some toxic chemicals, beta-carotene still has its effect."

That's good news for recent converts to health-consciousness and those who still haven't kicked their bad habits. It's not too late.

Dr. Seifter believes a daily intake of five to ten milligrams of beta-carotene—the equivalent of 8,375 to 16,750 International Units of vitamin A—will provide good protection against some tumors. "People at high risk for developing cancer—smokers, for instance—would require twice that amount," he says.

Unless you're the strictly meat-and-potatoes type, shunting other vegetables to the corner of your plate, it's hard to avoid getting at least some beta-carotene in your diet. If you're taking your beta-carotene in its usual form (vegetables), you can even take more than five to ten milligrams. Just remember though, in excess amounts (pounds of carrots a day, instead of one or two), that golden glow of health you were after may be a little more golden than you bargained for.

CANCER PREVENTION PLAN: VITAMIN A

- Eat plenty of leafy green vegetables, fresh fruit and other foods high in beta-carotene.

Vitamin B

Go to the mirror, stick out your tongue and take a good look at it. Is it pearly pink and velvety smooth? Or is it rough with angry purple splotches? If there is a fuchsia hue, it may tell more about your health (or lack thereof) than any words that fall trippingly off your tongue. A purplish tongue, for example, can be one of the symptoms that indicates that you may need more of the B vitamin riboflavin. And, according to recent research, if you are not getting enough of this B vitamin in your diet, you may be more susceptible to a host of problems, from fatigue to cancer.

But that's looking at it from the glass-is-half-empty viewpoint. What the studies really mean is that, miraculous though it may seem, just a few nutrients can help shield you from cancer. And several members of the B family have been shown to do just that.

FOLATE HAS IMPRESSIVE POWER

Picture the following scenario: You go to the doctor for a Pap smear. A few days later, the doctor calls you in for more tests because he or she has seen something there that warrants further investigation. You panic. It's the big C for sure, you think. Not necessarily. It may be nothing or it may be simply a mild case of cervical dysplasia, which occasionally leads to cancer far down the road.

"Nobody knows what causes cervical dysplasia," says Joe Chu, M.D., of the Fred Hutchinson Cancer Research Center in Seattle, Washington. "It may be oral contraceptives or smoking or a viral infection or perhaps nutrition." A dysplasia is an abnormal change in the surface cells, Dr. Chu explains. As the dysplasia gets worse and worse, more and more of the surface cells become abnormal until finally the full thickness of the epithelial (surface) cells is abnormal. That is called carcinoma *in situ*—the most severe precancerous abnormality of the cervix. It's when those abnormal cells break through what is called a basement membrane, which separates the surface cells from the tissue underneath, that it becomes an invasive cancer.

"Not everyone who gets dysplasia gets cancer," says Dr. Chu. "In fact, most do not, either because they get a spontaneous regression or because they've been treated." In recent years, quite a few studies have shown that women with cervical cancer often have deficiencies of the B vitamin folate. Researchers tested the patients' blood and questioned them about their diets, then they tested blood and questioned women who did not have cancer and found that the cancer patients had noticeably lower folate levels than the cancer-free group. (They also had lower levels of vital nutrients such as beta-carotene and vitamin C.)

Dr. Chu is in the midst of a long-term study on the effects of folate on cervical dysplasia. In a previous study that piqued Dr. Chu's interest, C.E. Butterworth, M.D., of the University of Alabama, in Tuscaloosa, tested 47 young women who were taking birth control pills and who all had mild or moderate cervical dysplasia. Birth control pills are thought to be associated not only with cervical dysplasia but also with folate deficiencies. In Dr. Butterworth's study, half the women were given 10 milligrams of folate daily, many times the Recommended Dietary Allowance (RDA). The other half, a control group, were given a tiny amount of vitamin C as a placebo. Abnormalities among the folate group were found to disappear faster than among the control group. In fact, in the control group, the abnormalities worsened.

It is too soon for any results from Dr. Chu's corroborative study. So far all he can tell us is that there have been no side effects from the daily doses of folate. This finding is important, because when you're talking about disease prevention, you want something you can take safely all your life. (Of course, any supplement should be taken in large doses only under a doctor's guidance.)

PROTECTING CHROMOSOMES

Why does folate have an effect on precancerous cells? "Folate is very much involved in DNA synthesis," explains Dr. Chu. (DNA is a cellular molecule that carries genetic information.) "It could be that with extra folate, these little abnormalities that appear in the chromosomes are repaired faster. Some scientists believe that all chromosomes have different places called fragile sites, which are more sensitive to breakage. The theory is that folate is involved in building and repairing of DNA and that if people have extra folate, these fragile sites are repaired faster before they replicate and become abnormal."

"Many researchers believe that chromosome damage is an important part of the process that causes malignancy," adds Richard Branda, M.D., a professor of medicine at the University of Vermont, Burlington.

Dr. Branda has established a possible link between defects in the cells' use of folate, chromosome damage and cancer. The clue came from studying a family with a history of chromosome damage and serious blood disease, including leukemia. Their cells weren't absorbing and using folate normally. In one family member with aplastic anemia, cell levels of folate were extremely low and remained low even after he took supplemental folate.

Dr. Branda believes the folate defect may have been the cause of the chromosome damage, which in turn brought about the aplastic anemia. The case, though extremely rare, suggested to the researcher that it is folate that keeps the chromosomes from breaking.

"There just hasn't been enough work done on folate," says Dr. Chu. "There have been a lot of studies done on vitamin C and cancer, and most people don't realize that some of the same foods that contain high levels of C also contain high levels of folate—citrus fruits contain folate, for example. A lot of studies that show the preventive effects of vitamin C may actually be showing the preventive effects of folate, and the researchers don't even realize it. That's an interesting possibility, and may mean folate affects other cancers, not just cervical cancer."

DEFICIENCIES ARE NOT UNUSUAL

Folate deficiencies are common, particularly in people whose bodies are under stress. If you smoke, drink alcohol excessively, take oral contraceptives or certain other drugs, if you are pregnant or breastfeeding, if you are an infant or an adolescent whose cells are multiplying rapidly as you grow, if you are old, lonely, poor or sick, you may be particularly susceptible to folate deficiencies.

Estimates show that most people's diets provide considerably less than the RDA, which has been set at 400 micrograms for adults. Others, such as those people mentioned above, may need even more. If you are careful, you may be able to get all the folate you need just from the food you eat. Be aware, however, that processing foods (that includes cooking it right in your very own kitchen) can damage the folate content of foods. Oranges and orange juice are dependable sources. Other vegetables high in folate include asparagus, broccoli, lima beans and spinach. Among fruit, high levels can be found in lemons, bananas, strawberries and cantaloupes. Other good sources are liver, potatoes, eggs, whole wheat bread and peanut butter.

DISINTEGRATING CANCERS WITH B$_{12}$

John Pinto, Ph.D., is studying B vitamins at Memorial Sloan-Kettering Cancer Center in New York. His research indicates that folate and vitamin B$_{12}$ work hand in hand to prevent DNA damage. A deficiency of B$_{12}$ can cause a deficiency of folate, he says. He has also found that some people may have deficiencies of these vitamins in just one area of the body.

Vitamin B$_{12}$ and folate help produce red blood cells in bone marrow. Without B$_{12}$, the body's production of red cells slows down and pernicious anemia can result. Scientists believe that red cells are hit harder than other cells by a B$_{12}$ deficiency because B$_{12}$ is needed in the process that churns them out faster than other cells. Cancer cells are produced at the same quick pace, which is why doctors sometimes induce a B$_{12}$ (and folate) deficiency in certain cancer patients to slow the growth of a malignancy.

But there is also some recent evidence that B$_{12}$ in conjunction with vitamin C is effective against cancer in a different way. The clues have turned up in animal studies conducted by Sister M. Eymard Poydock, Ph.D., a researcher at Mercyhurst College in Erie, Pennsylvania.

Dr. Poydock and her associates have had remarkable results with supplemental B$_{12}$ and vitamin C in increasing the survival rate of mice with leukemia and several forms of malignant tumors, including one stubbornly resistant to other treatment. What is most remarkable is how fast the vitamins work. "Even in the early stages we see no increase of malignant cells," says Dr. Poydock. "After the seventh treatment, no tumor cells at all are present. The tumor cells just disintegrate. It's very exciting."

Although the cancer-conquering process is still a mystery, Dr. Poydock suspects the vitamins work because they may alter the membranes of malignant cells so that the T-lymphocytes, the body's disease-fighting "killer" cells, recognize them as foreign and attack them. In fact, fluid extracted from their experimental mice revealed a veritable battlefield littered with disintegrating tumor cells, lymphocytes and other disease-fighting cells.

The RDA of B$_{12}$ is quite small—three micrograms—and unless you are a vegetarian who eats no meat, eggs or dairy products, you should be able to get plenty of B_{12} simply from food. Food sources for vitamin B_{12} are meat, particularly liver, and oysters, tuna, milk, cheese and eggs.

NIACIN THWARTS PANCREATIC CANCER

Another B that has hit the charts for cancer prevention is a form of niacin called nicotinamide. Terrence Lawson, Ph.D., of the Eppley Institute for Research in Cancer at the University of Nebraska in Omaha has shown that nicotinamide can inhibit the development of pancreatic cancer. Dr. Lawson and his associates injected hamsters with a carcinogen they knew would bring about deadly pancreatic cancer and then treated them with nicotinamide and found that the nicotinamide actually inhibited the development of cancer. "When the study ended after a year, we noticed there were no pancreatic tumors at all," says Dr. Lawson.

What's more, Dr. Lawson and his team got these results with small doses of nicotinamide—just 7 percent of a lethal dose. "Of course," says Dr. Lawson, "if you were recommending doses for people, it would probably be even less than that, because you would advise them to take it over a long period." Also, Dr. Lawson reminds us again, you should always take vitamins under the auspices of a physician who can take into account your complete health status and your nutritional requirements. "I don't know how many people listen to that statement, but I think it's one you have to stress all the time," he says.

DAMAGED CELLS REPAIRED

Dr. Lawson believes that nicotinamide, like folate, does something to stimulate the repair of DNA damage. Other vitamins such as A, C and E—known as antioxidants—seem to prevent DNA damage by interfering with the carcinogens that cause the damage, explains Dr. Lawson. But nicotinamide seems to repair the damage *after* it has happened. "We showed in our study that it didn't have any effect on the metabolism of the carcinogen we were using, so up to the point when the carcinogen interacts with the DNA, there was no change at all. But from then on, it seemed to cause profound changes." This would seem to prove that we need foods rich in antioxidant vitamins *and* in the B vitamins.

It takes a long, long time for cancers to develop, says Dr. Lawson. That is why, in many cases, old people are more susceptible than young people. Dr. Lawson finds an interesting parallel between the growth of cancers and current theories of aging, which hold that cells, and consequently organs, and consequently whole people, age because of an accumulation of DNA damage. "An accumulation of DNA damage has been shown to reduce our immunological functions—we become less resistant to disease. Antioxidant vitamins inhibit this damage.

"If you feed an old animal (an old person?) a diet high in antioxidants, you can reduce the number of toxins that can damage the DNA. Then, if you give him something like nicotinamide, you could stimulate the repair of any damage that is done, and you might then actually be able to delay the aging process as well as the onset of cancer."

Intriguing thought—no?

Most Americans get plenty of niacin from their diets to satisfy the Recommended Dietary Allowance of 18 milligrams for men or 13 milligrams for women. In fact, under normal circumstances, you need not worry about your intake of niacin unless your diet is extremely low in protein. Your best food sources for niacin are beef liver and other meats and poultry, peanut butter, legumes, milk and eggs.

RIBOFLAVIN PROTECTS THE ESOPHAGUS

Very often, a researcher's first insight into just how specific foods affect our health comes from studies of population groups who have special diets—the Finns who eat high-fiber foods and have low rates for colon cancer, for example, or the Seventh-Day Adventists who are vegetarian and have low rates for cancer overall.

Some populations may have a high rate of certain cancers and that, too, intrigues scientists who may find clues to help prevent future outbreaks of the disease. In parts of China, scientists have found that rates of esophageal cancer are extremely high. In the county of Linxian (Henan Province) in Northern China, for example, researchers reported that 108 people in 100,000 are hit with this cancer every year. One report revealed that 66 percent of the people suffered from esophagitis, which is a possible precursor of esophageal cancer. Could their nutritional status possibly explain these horrendous statistics?

The researchers compared the diets of people in Linxian with diets of people in a neighboring province whose rates of esophageal cancer were much lower. They discovered that the one major difference, measured in sample blood tests, was the level of riboflavin in the blood. The low-risk community appeared to have more of this nutrient than did the people of Linxian. There was even some indication from the study that where riboflavin levels are lower, the risk of esophageal cancer is higher. In Scandinavia, studies have shown similar results—riboflavin deficiency also was associated with esophageal cancer.

The Recommended Dietary Allowance for riboflavin is 1.6 miligrams for men, and 1.2 milligrams for women. Riboflavin is easily found in many meats and vegetables. The best food sources for ribofla-

vin arc beef, liver, asparagus, broccoli, milk, cottage cheese, and cheddar cheese.

B_6: THE IMMUNITY BOOSTER

In various studies at Oregon State University in Corvallis, scientists
have found that a vitamin B_6 deficiency can weaken your immunity. In
the Oregon study, groups of animals were fed varying amounts of vitamin B_6, ranging from large amounts to downright deficient. They were
then exposed to a virus that often causes tumors, and, not surprisingly,
the B_6-deficient mice were unable to resist the virus and were significantly more susceptible.

Another experiment at the Oncology Research Laboratory of Win-
throp Hospital in Mineola, New York, has shown that large doses of
vitamin B_6 can inhibit the growth of melanoma cells (usually malignant) both in animals and in cells examined under a microscope. The
researchers suggest that the vitamin may be acting on the cell membrane—perhaps fortifying them to resist the carcinogens used in the
study. Results showed that when mice were treated with B_6 before the
melanoma cells were administered, the vitamin inhibited tumor growth
by 62 percent. When tumors had already been allowed to develop,
treatment with the vitamin rendered a 39 percent reduction in growth.

The researchers feel that, although they achieved fantastic results,
the high doses they used for their experiment could not be prescribed

---

CANCER PROTECTION PLAN: VITAMIN B

- If you have cervical dysplasia, you should get sufficient
  amounts of the B vitamin folate. The RDA is 400 micrograms for adults. People with increased needs should get
  between 800 and 1,000 micrograms.
- If you are under special stress or you are a vegetarian who
  eats no meat, eggs or dairy products, you should monitor
  your B_{12} intake carefully. The RDA is three micrograms.
- If you are at risk for the development of pancreatic cancer,
  you should monitor nicotinamide intake.
- If you are at risk for esophageal cancer, you should monitor riboflavin intake.
- If you have depressed immunity, you should monitor B_6
  intake. The RDA for B_6 is 2 milligrams; the therapeutic requirement is 2 to 2.5 milligrams.

for people. They do suggest, however that an effective vitamin B_6 ointment could be used to treat skin cancer. In fact, they are testing just such a cream and preliminary results indicate that it can be very effective.

Finally, in Freiburg, West Germany, H.A. Ladner, M.D., and his colleague report that, with vitamin B_6, they have actually been able to increase the survival rates of women with advanced cancers. Like other experts, Dr. Ladner believes that B_6 works by boosting the patient's immunity.

The RDA for B_6 is 2 milligrams for women and 2.2 milligrams for men. The therapeutic requirement is 2 to 2.5 milligrams a day. Your best food sources for vitamin B_6 are white meats (chicken and fish), liver, whole grain cereals and egg yolks. Aside from bananas, avocados and potatoes, there are few good fruit and vegetable sources.

C H A P T E R 67
Vitamin C

Imagine that you lived in a sun-drenched hacienda right in the middle of a citrus grove. A few times a day, you'd just reach out a window and pluck a sweet orange or a juicy grapefruit for a snack. Every cell in your body would be saturated with vitamin C. According to many nutritionists, that's just the way cells *should* be—if they're properly armed to ward off cancer.

The evidence is clear from studies around the world, says Sidney S. Mirvish, Ph.D., of the University of Nebraska Medical Center in Omaha, that people who eat fresh fruits daily (especially citrus fruits), have a lower incidence of cancers of the stomach, esophagus, mouth, larynx and cervix. Some studies indicate that vitamin C-rich fresh fruits may even help prevent colon cancer and lung cancer.

In this country, the powers of protection concealed in vitamin C became glaringly evident when scientists looked closely at the changing rate of stomach cancer, which had been a terrible scourge at the beginning of the century; in fact, it was the number one cause of cancer death in the 1930s. But in recent times, stomach cancer has plummeted to a negligible seventh place. Researchers realized that this extraordinary health trend wasn't due to any medical treatment. Rather, it was caused by the simple fact that foods are now refrigerated so people eat fewer salted and pickled foods and more fresh fruits and vegetables.

"I'm old enough to remember when we got our first home refrigerator in 1935," says John H. Weisburger, Ph.D., of the American Health Foundation in Valhalla, New York. "Before then, I remember distinctly that my mother had salt and saltpeter by the kitchen sink and whenever she bought fish or meat or even some vegetables, she would pickle and salt them because that was the only way to keep them for any length of time at room temperature.

"In those days, we had fruits and vegetables only when they were in season. In the winter, we had very little—some potatoes in the basement. Apples and oranges were very expensive, so we didn't eat them. Now, of course, with air transport that is efficient and cheap, you can run an air freighter from Mexico every day, and it doesn't cost any more than sticking fruits in refrigerated railroad cars. So, we have oranges, fruits and vegetables year-round. In fact, Brazil has become a big competitor to Florida and California as regards oranges.

"If you think of northern Japan, where stomach cancer is still high, mainly the same conditions prevail. That is, refrigerators were introduced there also, but 20 years after they became commonly used in America. In rural Japan, salted and pickled foods are still being used, not only for food preservation, but for the sake of tradition. The Japanese like soy sauce and pickled vegetables and salted fish—that hasn't changed even though they now have refrigerators. Also, fruits and vegetables are just not available.

"In parts of Iran, stomach cancer also was very high. There was no real explanation, except that people's nutrition was poor. They ate few vegetables and fruits. And in China, salting and pickling of foods and poor nutrition seem to have led to high rates of cancer of the esophagus."

What is it that makes salted and pickled foods so bad, and fresh fruits so good?

VITAMIN C—THE CARCINOGEN BLOCKER

Salted, pickled and smoked foods contain nitrites (as do preserved meats such as bacon and sausage). Nitrites combine with chemicals called amines in the stomach to form the cancer-causing substances nitrosamines. (See chapter 48, Nitrites and Nitrates.)

Actually, we shouldn't lay the blame for nitrites entirely on preserved foods. Most of the nitrites that end up in our stomachs come from perfectly good fresh foods. They start out as nitrates, a natural part of the environment that provides essential nitrogen for plants to grow. Bacteria in our saliva turn these natural nitrates into nitrites and, in the hydrochloric acid of the stomach, these nitrites also combine into dangerous nitrosamines.

And all this happens down in your belly without so much as a by-your-leave from you. In fact, it happens without your even being aware of it. It happens, *except* when you also have eaten something containing vitamin C.

"Back in 1972 we showed that vitamin C prevents the formation of nitrosamines," says Dr. Mirvish. "We showed that when you have a nitrite and an amine and you add vitamin C, the vitamin prevents the formation of nitrosamines. Our research was the main reason why the meat industry started adding vitamin C to all nitrite-preserved meats.

"We had previously shown that mice fed nitrites and amines developed tumors, which we think are due to the nitrosamines being formed in the acid conditions of the stomach. In other studies with animals, we included vitamin C in the diet and showed that the C inhibited the tumors. The reason is clear—it's that the nitrites react first with the vitamin C, and the amines just don't have a chance; there are just not enough nitrites left to combine with the amines to make nitrosamines."

The perfect thing about this whole chemical dance in the stomach, according to Dr. Mirvish, is that unlike other nitrite-reducing agents, vitamin C reacts best with nitrites just when we are eating, because the acidic range of stomach juices present then just happens to be C's most effective catalyst.

Furthermore, scientists now have proof that vitamin C combines with nitrites not only in the stomachs of laboratory mice but also in people's stomachs. At the Massachusetts Institute of Technology, in Cambridge, Massachusetts, a group of students were given a diet containing nitrate and proline, an amino acid. When urine samples were measured, researchers discovered that the students were excreting significantly more of the combined nitrosoprolines than before they began eating the special foods, proving that the nitrates were mating with the amino acids. When the students took vitamin C with their meals, their urine tests revealed that these excess nitrite compounds had been reduced by 81 percent. For two of the students, the vitamin C blocked 95 percent of these potential carcinogens.

In Great Britain, researchers measured the mutagenic activity in the gastric juice of volunteers before and after they received supplements of vitamin C (1,000 milligrams four times a day for one week). Mutagenic activity is a measure of the ability to cause a change in the genetic material of cells. The higher the mutagenic activity, the greater the chance that cancerous cells will emerge. The researchers found that supplementation with vitamin C cut mutagenic activity almost in half. But the acidity of the gastric juice was not changed significantly by the vitamin C.

"These results support the suggested role for vitamin C in the possible chemoprevention of gastric cancer and demonstrate for the first time the relation between [stomach vitamin C] levels, mutagenic activity and increased intake of vitamin C," say the researchers.

"What vitamin C does best," explains Dr. Mirvish, "is to prevent the formation of nitrosamines. But if people take in nitrosamines that are already formed—from cigarettes, chewing tobacco, snuff, pollution and some foods—and if those nitrosamines are already acting in the cells to produce cancer, vitamin C can inhibit the nitrosamines. But there's only a 50 percent reduction in activity, whereas in the nitrosamine formation stage, we see a 90 percent reduction."

Still, a 50 percent reduction is nothing to sneeze at, especially when you consider that vitamin C is not in there fighting the battle single-handedly. No indeed. Vitamin C is water-soluble, which means it does its best work in the watery regions of the stomach and in the liquid pool inside each cell. But each cell also has a fatty membrane around it, and there, vitamin E takes over the anticancer fight. Vitamin A and its precursor, beta-carotene, are also strong allies.

In fact, the number of possible cancer-blockers in fruits and vegetables are so numerous that most researchers today agree with Dr. Weisburger that, "It is clear from what we have learned in the last 30 years in medical research, that it is not the intake of certain vitamins but of more fruits and vegetables that contain these vitamins, that seems to have been so effective in reducing the risk of certain cancer types."

Dr. Mirvish adds, "The recommendation is to consume the *foods* rather than pure vitamin C. This recommendation is reasonable because scientific links have been established only for the natural foods and because these may contain protective substances other than vitamin C."

That's good advice. Certainly most of us could stand to increase the number and variety of fruits and vegetables in our diets. In fact, in a land of plenty, so many of us choose such lamentably poor diets that Paul Lachance, Ph.D., professor of food science and nutrition at Rutgers University in New Brunswick, New Jersey, says wryly, "Fortunately, there is some vitamin C in french fries." On the average, most of us get a mere 80 milligrams of C from our food. "That's way above the recommended daily requirement of 60 milligrams," says Dr. Lachance, "so no one is going to get scurvy, but if we're talking about cancer protection, it's way below what we need."

Let's look at some studies that support Dr. Lachance.

WHAT THE SCIENTISTS SAY

Researchers from Louisiana State University Medical School in New Orleans found significantly lower levels of vitamins E and C in patients with lung cancer than in a group of healthy people. The differences "did not appear to be the result of malnutrition associated with cancer," they say. "Vitamin A," adds researcher William D. Johnson, Ph.D., "was seen in earlier tests to be strongly associated with lung cancer. But in our study, decreased levels of vitamins E and C seemed to have the strongest association and may in fact be of more importance than vitamin A in predicting lung cancer."

At the University of Alabama in Birmingham, researchers found that 67 percent of those with untreated cervical cancer had one abnormal vitamin value, while 18 percent had three or more abnormal values. Folate, beta-carotene and vitamin C levels were those most often below normal, the researchers found. "In our study, we did not try to say whether these values were a cause or an effect of the disease," says James W. Orr, Jr., M.D. "We do know that poor nutrition can interfere in the treatment regimen, however. We have come to realize the importance of nutrition in this area and are starting to see that it really needs close investigation."

In another study on cervical abnormalities, Seymour Romney, M.D., found that a low dietary intake of vitamin C is related to cervical dysplasia—abnormal cell growth that sometimes leads to cancer. Of the 80 women in his study at Bronx Municipal Hospital Center who had Pap smears taken, 34 had normal results. Their dietary intake of vitamin C was relatively high. The remaining 46 women took in considerably less vitamin C in the diet, and their diagnoses ranged from mild cervical inflammation to cancer.

"A lot of people have been intrigued by the prospect that vitamin C may have antitumor properties and there are reasonable scientific studies that support that idea," explains Dr. Romney. The preliminary research here suggests that women may not be getting enough vitamin C to prevent cervical cancer. Why? Because, says Dr. Romney, "if there's a disorder in the cervix, that increases the demand for ascorbic acid [vitamin C]."

A number of scientists are now pursuing the possible connection between vitamin C and colon and rectal cancers. At the Royal Adelaide Hospital in Australia, a study compared 199 cases of rectal cancer to 396 people without the disease. The preliminary results show, according to the authors, that "high consumption of vitamin C is associated with a reduced risk."

Other researchers have found that people who eat the usual North American diet produce potential carcinogens in their feces which might be dangerous to the colon or rectum. These carcinogens disappear from the feces when 400 to 1,000 milligrams of vitamin C or 100 milligrams of vitamin C with 100 International Units of vitamin E and 10 grams of bran fiber are added to the daily diet. (Don't try this program without getting your doctor's okay.)

In another study, vitamin C in the diet was found to inhibit the recurrence of rectal polyps in four of five patients with familial polyposis—a genetic tendency to develop a large number of potentially malignant polyps, or growths, in the colon or rectum.

At Dartmouth Medical School, Robert Greenburg, Ph.D., is just launching a new large-scale study on the effects of different vitamins including C, E and A on colon polyps. The study will look at people who have had benign polyps removed. Normally, explains Dr. Greenburg, it is estimated that 10 to 20 percent a year will get recurring polyps. The study will then measure whether different vitamins will diminish the rate at which polyps return.

"The theory behind it has to do with the antioxidant properties of C and E," explains Dr. Greenburg. "And the idea is that first, the vitamins will prevent the formation of carcinogenic compounds in the bowel and, second, they may act within the cell as an antioxidant to trap or deactivate molecules in the cell. Oxygen can cause damage to the DNA in the cell which could eventually result in cancer."

In Japan, doctors have even used vitamin C effectively as a treatment for cancer. Noted scientist Fukumi Morishige, M.D., Ph.D., and his colleagues have been examining the healing potential of vitamin C for 30 years. Seven years ago, Dr. Morishige published data suggesting that large doses of the nutrient may increase the survival times of terminal cancer patients, and since then, he and his fellow researchers have been successfully treating cancer patients with combinations of C and other therapies. The latest news is that they may have just discovered how to make vitamin C more of a tumor killer than most researchers ever imagined.

Through a series of test-tube and animal studies, they found out that a mixture of vitamin C and a copper compound has surprisingly lethal effects on cancers—more lethal than either substance has alone. When they treated cancerous mice with this mixture, the animal life spans increased. And when they used it to treat a woman with terminal cancer, the results were astounding.

She was 34 years old and the victim of osteosarcoma, an incurable bone cancer completely resistant to chemotherapy. A tumor in her left arm was causing paralysis and so much pain that painkillers were worthless. Then she was injected regularly with the copper compound and large doses of vitamin C.

"Two months' treatment relieved the intolerable pain and paresis [paralysis] of the diseased left upper arm," Dr. Morishige reports. "From x-ray examinations the tumor lesion was found to be completely regressed [disappeared] and calcified within four months of treatment." Almost two years later the woman was still free of cancer.

HOW MUCH C DO YOU NEED?

In the ninth edition of the National Academy of Sciences' Recommended Dietary Allowances (RDAs) for vitamins, the RDA for vitamin C was set at 60 milligrams. Since then, says Dr. Weisburger, "there has been a real storm. The National Academy has refused to accept the recommendations of nutritionists and the tenth edition of the RDAs has never been published.

"The RDAs are set to prevent deficiency diseases, and nutritionists today feel that we really need to know more than what levels of certain vitamins would prevent deficiency disease. Scurvy (the vitamin C deficiency disease) doesn't exist in America, so now we are calling for a definition of the *optimal* amount of these micronutrients to promote health and wellness. There really are no sound data. But I'm reasonably sure that 60 milligrams of C is a bit too low."

Such organizations as the National Academy of Sciences and the National Cancer Institute (NCI) do not recommend vitamin supplements. They urge us instead to increase our vitamin intake by eating more vitamin-rich fruits and vegetables. Dr. Lachance has calculated just how much vitamin C you would be taking in if you followed these recommended diets. On the NCI diet, you would get 217 milligrams, on the Department of Agriculture diet, you would get 225 milligrams. "And that," says Dr. Lachance, "is 360 to 375 percent more than the RDA."

Remember to be extra sure to include vitamin C foods whenever you eat processed meats and pickled or smoked foods. Drink a big glass of fresh orange juice with your smoked salmon, for example. And, especially if you smoke or work in a polluted atmosphere, have a grapefruit for breakfast, add strawberries to your cereal, try a broccoli and pepper omelet for lunch, tomato juice at cocktail time and snap beans for dinner.

Vitamin C builds up in the fruit as it ripens, so vine- or tree-ripened fruits will contain more vitamin C than those picked green. Once fruits or vegetables are picked, they should be frozen immediately or refrigerated if they are to be eaten fresh. Frozen orange juice will probably contain more vitamin C than reconstituted juice. Buy small cans of frozen juice—the longer you let it sit around once it's thawed, the more C you lose.

But, of course, there's no better way to get your C than straight from the original container—the orange.

CANCER PREVENTION PLAN: VITAMIN C

- Eat plenty of foods high in vitamin C.
- If you are a smoker or if you have a depressed immune system, pay special attention to your vitamin C consumption.
- Remember to be extra sure to include vitamin C foods whenever you eat processed meats and pickled or smoked foods.
- Cook and store foods in the way that best preserves their vitamin C.

Vitamin D

Can you name the nutrient that is known for keeping your bones strong and healthy? If your answer is calcium, you're right. But did you know that calcium can't even *reach* your bones without help from vitamin D?

How does vitamin D help calcium do its good deeds? Imagine that the calcium in your diet has arrived in your small intestine. It can't get from there to your bloodstream unless it's absorbed through your intestinal wall. But it can't push its way through alone. It needs help.

At that point vitamin D comes to the rescue. When it arrives on the scene, it causes a calcium-binding protein to form in the cells lining your intestinal wall. This protein transports calcium through the wall to the other side and into your bloodstream. From there it's full speed ahead to your waiting skeleton, where vitamin D helps to stimulate the growth of new bone.

And that's not all. Now researchers believe that these two nutrients also may protect your colon from cancer. And that's a task of truly heroic proportions. Colon cancer has been estimated to be responsible for more than 50,000 deaths in a single year.

But no one even suspected that calcium and vitamin D were teaming up to protect us from this killer until 1976. It was late that year when two epidemiologists discovered that first clue, and since then scientists have been busy trying to solve the rest of the mystery.

It all began when Cedric Garland, Dr.P.H., and his brother, Frank Garland, Ph.D., were comparing rates of colon cancer and skin cancer in the United States. They followed these killers' "footprints" across the country and discovered an intriguing trail.

Colon cancer was attacking in the colder regions of the United States more often than it was in warmer climates. Skin cancer was doing just the opposite. Even we can understand why skin cancer preferred to strike in the south. The sun is its not-so-secret weapon. But why was colon cancer claiming more victims in the North?

Then the brothers had a bright idea. Suppose the sun wasn't *all* bad. If colon cancer, like most killers, did its best work in the dark, then maybe vitamin D from the sun was the bodyguard responsible for protecting the colon from cancer. And, since vitamin D is the sidekick of calcium, perhaps the two were working together, as usual, guarding the lining of the colon from the cancer-causing waste substances that pass through it.

"Vitamin D, we theorized, was binding with calcium," says Dr. Cedric Garland, assistant professor of community and family medicine at the University of California, San Diego, School of Medicine in La Jolla. "And calcium was reducing the rate of turnover of the cells lining the colon. You see, the cells that are turning over are the ones that can be attacked by cancer-causers. Cells that are *not* turning over are very resistant to carcinogens. Without calcium and vitamin D, the cells start to turn over extremely quickly. When they do that, any carcinogen that happens to be nearby may attack the cell and induce a cancer."

With this theory in mind, Dr. Garland set out to *prove* that the good guy was vitamin D. "We were able to speculate from the evidence we already had that the protective factor in sunlight was vitamin D. But it could have been some other factor in sunlight that was protecting people against colon cancer. The only way to be sure was to study *dietary* vitamin D to see if it had that same protective effect. The single factor that diet and sunlight have in common is vitamin D," says Dr. Garland.

In 1985 he published the results of his investigation. He and his colleagues had kept track of almost 2,000 Chicago men whose 28-day dietary histories had been obtained at the start of the study and again one year later. Twenty years had elapsed since the initial study of their eating habits. The results confirmed Dr. Garland's suspicions: The men whose diets contained the most vitamin D and calcium had only one-third the risk of developing colon cancer that those whose diets contained the least had!

The scientists concluded "that vitamin D and calcium may reduce the risk of colorectal cancer." While they cautioned that the evidence was not conclusive, Dr. Garland is still actively involved in the ongoing investigation.

FIGHTING BACK

But vitamin D may be more than just a partner for calcium. It may be an effective cancer-fighter all by itself. Scientists are exploring the possibility that one form of this vitamin may eventually become another treatment for cancer, helping us to fight back against the enemy *after* he sneaks in and starts his dirty work. If vitamin D can slow the turnover of *normal* cells, like those lining our colon, can it slow the growth of cancerous cells as well? Scientists are investigating this possibility, and the results of their work look promising.

In 1981 Researchers at the Stanford University School of Medicine found vitamin D receptors within cells from human melanoma tumors (a form of skin cancer). When they exposed these cells to the hormonal form of vitamin D in the laboratory, they discovered that the cells multiplied at a much slower rate.

And research from Japan has found that this same form of vitamin D suppresses leukemia cells as well, causing them to be turned into noncancerous cells. "Where this will go therapeutically isn't clear at this stage," says Hector DeLuca, Ph.D., professor and former chairman of biochemistry at the University of Wisconsin, Madision. "In the long run, someday we may be able to control some types of leukemia. This may also have application for controlling other types of malignancies."

HOW TO STOCK UP ON D

But the best way to deal with cancer is never having to deal with it at all. If vitamin D can help you stack the deck in your favor, then you want to be sure you play your cards right by getting your fair share.

The nice thing about vitamin D is that getting enough can be as much fun as spending a day at the beach. That's because you have a vitamin D factory in your skin, and it operates on solar power. The process begins when ultraviolet rays from the sun beam down on a substance in your skin, producing vitamin D_3. After submitting to further changes in your liver and kidneys, D_3 becomes active vitamin D, the substance that mobilizes calcium and hinders cancer cells.

Another source of vitamin D is your diet. But Mother Nature figured when she gave us the sun she was giving us more than enough of the big D, so she didn't include much of it in many of the foods we eat every day, like vegetables.

Do you remember the men in Dr. Garland's colon cancer study? Where do you think they got their D? We don't know for sure, but it's a pretty safe guess they got it from fortified milk. "Oily fish, such as sardines and anchovies also contain a healthy amount of this vitamin," according to Dr. Garland. "But except for a few anchovies on an occasional piece of pizza, most Americans quickly lose their taste for these strong-tasting fish." (Mackerel and salmon are also high in D.)

Other foods, like liver, butter, cheese, eggs and beef contain fair amounts, too. But, if you have some skim milk over a vitamin D-fortified cereal for breakfast, you'll get calcium along with your D and help keep the fat in your diet from getting out of hand. (High-fat diets have been implicated in colon cancer, too.)

But which is better, vitamin D from the sun or from your diet? Guess what: You *can* fool Mother Nature! Although the vitamin D in food is absorbed by your small intestine and the vitamin D from the sun gets in through your skin, by the time it reaches your liver your body doesn't know where it's coming from. So you can get your supply from whichever source you choose.

IN SEARCH OF THE D THIEVES

Getting your fair share sounds simple, doesn't it? Well, it would be if there weren't so many scoundrels trying to steal your D before and after it enters your body. By the time they're through taking their cuts, you'll be lucky to have much left, unless you do some careful planning. In fact, experts believe vitamin D deficiency, once thought as rare as bubonic plague, is a serious hidden problem, particularly for this nation's elderly.

The first real evidence of this suspected "epidemic" came in 1982 from John L. Ohdahl, Ph.D. and his colleagues at the University of New Mexico School of Medicine in Albuquerque. They conducted a five-year study to evaluate levels of vitamin D in nearly 300 elderly men and women.

At the beginning of the study, the researchers figured that if any group of elderly people had adequate levels of D, this one did. After all, their subjects had decent incomes, were free of major illness, and maintained a keen interest in their health. But the scientists were in for a surprise. Over half the group showed vitamin D intakes lower than 100 International Units (IU) per day (one-quarter of the U.S. Recommended Daily Allowance). Borderline vitamin D deficiency was present in 14 percent of the elderly. And this study was conducted in the Sun Belt! What about the elderly who live in the North?

A preliminary study by doctors at Massachusetts General Hospital in Boston recently reported that 40 percent of elderly patients entering that hospital with hip fractures had little or no vitamin D in their blood.

What's going on? Who are the D thieves, and how can we keep from becoming their next victims? To find out, just answer the following questions.

Did I vote for Herbert Hoover? No, your political persuasion is not the issue here—it's the number of candles of your last birthday cake. The truth is, as we get older, we become more vulnerable to D deficiency. Why?

In the first place, we may lose our place in the sun. We may avoid the sun by choice, or we may simply become less physically active (perhaps due to illness or disability) and thus spend less time outdoors. And when icy sidewalks try to give us the slip or we have to negotiate flights of stairs to reach the light of day, well, we may just decide the trip is not worth the effort.

If the sunny side of the street is easy to reach, problems may still arise. Our vitamin D metabolism may begin to malfunction, making it difficult for us to convert vitamin D into its active form. On top of that, our skin thins as we age, and this makes it a less efficient vitamin D factory.

Secondly, the D in our diets may disappear too. We may stop drinking milk because we have trouble digesting it, or simply because we think only growing children need it. But getting enough is only part of the problem. What D we do get from our diet may not move beyond our small intestines, due to faulty absorption.

Do I have trouble keeping in touch with the sun? The truth is, though the sun tries to reach out and touch you, it may have trouble making the connection. The tall buildings in large cities keep us in their shadows. Pollution decreases the amount of ultraviolet radiation (UVL) reaching the earth. And while a sunny window may raise your spirits it won't raise your levels of vitamin D. (Even clean glass filters our UVL).

When the low-lying sun of winter has to slant its rays through the ozone layer in the earth's atmosphere, our supply is further depleted. Subtract sunbeams lost to cloudier, shorter days and heavy winter clothing, and you'll begin to see why northerners get such dismal amounts of D on winter days.

In fact, Michael Holick, M.D., Ph.D., and Ann Webb, Ph.D., at the Vitamin D and Bone Metabolism Research Center at Tufts University in

Medford, Massachusetts, recently discovered that if you live in Boston, Massachusetts you can't expect to generate a single unit of vitamin D from the sun between the months of November and March. And that's probably true for the rest of us who live in cities in the northern part of the United States as well!

Does my skin block out the sun? It makes sense that keeping your skin in the dark by covering every square inch with heavy clothing blocks vitamin D production. But what if your skin is naturally dark? Heavily pigmented skin can actually stop as much as 95 percent of available UVL from reaching the deep dermal layers where D is made. And, believe it or not, the sun-blocking lotions we use to protect us from the skin-damaging rays of the sun can also limit vitamin D synthesis. Those with an SPF of 8 or more completely block out vitamin D (see chapter 61, Sunscreens).

Am I seeing my doctor for a current medical problem? Long-term use of anticonvulsants (drugs used to treat conditions like epilepsy) and some other drugs can add to your vitamin D losses. And chronic kidney problems or a malfunctioning thyroid gland can cause problems too. (But don't try to write your own vitamin D prescription if you have a medical problem or are taking medication. Ask your doctor.)

HOW MUCH IS ENOUGH?

Exactly how much vitamin D does the average person need? Although the Recommended Dietary Allowance for adults is 200 International Units, a report by a panel of experts convened by the National Institutes of Health warns that the amount of vitamin D your body needs to keep your bones healthy increases with age. If you are a woman who has seen menopause come and go, experts say you may need between 1,000 and 1,500 milligrams of calcium and 400 International Units of vitamin D daily to prevent bone deterioration.

And that's probably more than enough to protect your colon too. According to Dr. Garland, "We generally recommend people take in 200 International Units a day of vitamin D and 1,200 milligrams of calcium. Just don't shortchange your calcium intake or overdose on D. If there's not enough calcium in your diet, vitamin D will rob it from your bones."

YOUR PERSONALIZED PROTECTION PLAN

Now that you know all this, you have a decision to make: Shall I get my D from my diet, sunlight or supplements—or a combination of all three? It's really your choice.

If you opt for swallowing your D, we have a few suggestions, though, from the experts. "Drink four glasses of skim milk daily," says Dr. Holick, "or take a vitamin supplement. All you need is 400 International Units a day." (Four eight-ounce glasses of fortified milk provide this amount). But don't think that milk in your coffee will do the trick—it's just not enough.

Or if skim milk turns your taste buds upside down, and you choose to get your D from a supplement, you could do as Dr. Garland suggests and take a smaller dose with a single glass of low-fat (1 or 2 percent) milk. "It's reasonable to take fat-soluble vitamins [like vitamin D] with a small amount of fat, like that contained in a glass of low-fat milk," says Dr. Garland.

But what if you choose the sun? That's when the calculations get a bit tricky. If sunbeams wore labels saying "100 IU" we could prepare a prescription that included precisely the right amount. "Take two sunbeams, five times a week," we might say. But since sunlight can't be measured, even by the cup or by the pound, we'll just have to let the experts do the best they can.

When it comes to cancer prevention, the problem is getting the sun to work *for* you instead of *against* you. The solution to the problem is moderation.

"Young, healthy adults can synthesize all the D they need from the summer sun," says Dr. Holick. Using a formula containing what he calls "your personal sunburn factor," you can determine how much exposure you need. "If a half hour in the summer sun gives you a sunburn, then 10 to 15 minutes a day will be enough," according to Dr. Holick. "Sub-sunburning doses are what you're looking for."

But if you live in the North, summer doesn't last all year. And even though your body builds a "pool" of vitamin D, it will dry up before the winter thaw.

So what do we do while the snow falls? Some folks might say, "Let them drink milk!" But we have a solution that's even easier to swallow: head south. Doctors have found that a winter vacation to some sunny shore can raise your circulating D for up to four months!

CANCER PREVENTION PLAN: VITAMIN D
- Try to get at least the RDA of 200 IU of vitamin D daily.
- If you are a woman past menopause, you may need more.
- Drink fortified milk or eat oily fish such as sardines and anchovies.

Vitamin E

Suppose you have invented a crunchy new snack food. Suppose it's deep fried. You'd need to find some way to make sure it doesn't go bad on the supermarket shelves. Probably you'd add some sort of preservative, perhaps what food scientists call an "antioxidant"—a substance that stops the destructive mix of oxygen and oil that can make that fatty crunch turn rancid. You might choose the preservative alpha-tocopherol.

Oily snack foods are not the only perishables that need protection against the ravages of oxygen. Every cell in your body is surrounded by an oily membrane that can be just as susceptible as any corn chip, doughnut or french fry. Our cells can, in a sense, turn rancid. Oxidation pits and corrodes that protective oily membrane and makes it easier for bacteria, viruses or other harmful substances to enter the cell. Once there, they can damage the cell's genetic structure, leading to cancer.

Why can't you protect those precious cell membranes against oxidation the way you can a new snack food? You can. In fact, you already do. You even use the same preservative: alpha-tocopherol, which you probably know as vitamin E. New and ongoing studies show that vitamin E works not only as an antioxidant but also in several dramatic ways to protect us against cancer: by preventing the formation of cancer-causing substances; by actually changing newly formed cancer cells back to normal cells; and even by charging up the body's immune system to further ward off cancers. Let's look more closely at exactly how vitamin E does the job.

DOWN WITH FREE RADICALS

Perhaps you've heard about these rascals before: They're tiny molecular particles, compounds containing unpaired, highly charged electrons that are very unstable. Free radicals are super-oxidizers. And when they "rust" a cell, more free radicals are created in the process! What we need is something to put a damper on things. That's where antioxidants come in.

The big three antioxidants are vitamins E and C and selenium, but vitamin E plays an especially crucial role in protecting the cell. "The cell membrane is like a sandwich of fatty layers with vitamin E in the middle protecting the fats from oxidation," explains Jeffrey Bland, Ph.D., of the University of Puget Sound in Washington. "The vitamin E oxidizes instead, soaking up free radicals." In fact, Dr. Bland says, the free radicals prefer to latch onto vitamin E!

NUTRIENT PROTECTOR

Vitamin E not only protects the cell wall but, by soaking up free radicals, it leaves the work area clear for other vitamins and minerals that might otherwise be destroyed by oxidation. The trace metal selenium, for example, has proven to be an effective cancer blocker, especially with the back-up strength of vitamin E.

For a study in Finland, researchers took blood samples of a group of cancer patients and compared them to samples of another group of healthy people. The groups were evenly matched according to sex, age and smoking status. During the years that followed, the scientists found that patients who died of cancer had shown an average of 12 percent less selenium in their blood than had the people in the healthy group. Those who had had the lowest levels of selenium were 5 to 8 times more at risk than those with normal levels. Finally, those with both low selenium and low vitamin E concentrations in their blood had 11.4 times the risk.

The scientists noted that vitamin E did not seem to be associated with any particular cancer site and that, although by itself it was not shown to have much effect on the risk of cancer, it was strongly connected with the impact of selenium deficiency on cancer risk. "A selenium deficiency is associated with an increased risk of fatal cancer, and low vitamin E intake may enhance this effect," they concluded.

At Roswell Park Memorial Institute in Buffalo, New York, Clement Ip, Ph.D., came to a similar conclusion. "We supplemented vitamin E in the diet of animals that have been given a carcinogen to induce mammary tumors and what we found is that vitamin E by itself has no protective effect, but vitamin E is able to enhance the effect of selenium in inhibiting the development of mammary tumors," explains Dr. Ip. He and his colleagues are now studying why the two nutrients work together. "Is it because vitamin E is a very powerful antioxidant and selenium works better under conditions of lower oxidant stress?" he wonders.

NITRITES AND OTHER NASTIES

But scientists aren't wondering any longer about why vitamin E protects against nitrosamines. Studies have shown that when we eat foods containing nitrites (a common preservative in bacon and sausage), the nitrites combine with amines in the stomach to form nitrosamines, which can cause cancer. Vitamins C and E have been shown to block that process—they keep nitrites from hooking up with amines. Meat processors are responding to the scientific evidence and are now adding vitamins C and E to their nitrite-treated products. (For more information, see chapter 48, Nitrites and Nitrates.)

Sidney S. Mirvish, Ph.D., of the University of Nebraska Medical Center in Omaha, did some of the original research on the dangers of nitrites in processed meats. "We showed, back in 1972, that when you administered a nitrite and an amine, you could get tumors in mice. We think they are due to the nitrosamines being formed in the acid conditions of the stomach. We then did studies and showed that vitamins C and E in the diet inhibited the tumors. The reason is clear. It's just that the vitamins react with the nitrite and therefore compete with the amine for the nitrite.

"The reason you need vitamin E in addition to vitamin C in bacon," explains Dr. Mirvish, "is that when you fry bacon, you get small amounts of nitrosamines." Vitamin C deals with the nitrites in the lean parts of the meat, while vitamin E works better in the fatty parts. So you might want to check the list of ingredients on your bacon package to see if it includes alpha-tocopherol.

What happens if some nitrites escape the scavenging vitamins and turn into dangerous nitrosamines, or if your body is invaded by preformed nitrosamines or other carcinogens? Here, too, vitamin E can help. "In the experiments we reviewed," says Dr. Mirvish, "my impression is that both vitamins C and E work to inhibit the formation of tumors once the carcinogens are in the cells, but vitamin E seems to work even better." And Dr. Mirvish has discovered another way vitamin E helps protect you against cancer: by boosting your immune power.

BUILDING IMMUNITY

"Vitamin E may stimulate the immune system and so enhance immune surveillance of cancer development," he says. "We've done a couple of experiments where we've found that high levels of vitamin E in animals slightly enhanced some immune functions," adds Ronald Ross Watson, Ph.D., M.D., of the University of Nebraska Medical Center. "The animals were better able to destroy tumor cells with an enhanced immune system."

Jeffrey B. Blumberg, Ph.D., assistant director of the U.S. Department of Agriculture's Human Nutrition Research Center on Aging at Tufts University, Medford, Massachusetts, is studying whether vitamin E can prevent the usual decline in the immune response as people get older.

"In animal studies, we have found that vitamin E in relatively large doses is a potent stimulant of the immune system in very old mice," says Dr. Blumberg. "That would have a direct bearing on the body's ability to defeat cancer at rather early stages. And it's clearly known that a vigorous immune response is essential to any successful treatment of cancer. All other cancer treatments, including radiation, surgery and chemotherapy, require the help of a vigorous immune response to assist the medical interventions."

So much for theories about *how* vitamin E works to protect you against cancer. Now let's look at some of the studies in which vitamin E—or a lack of it—seemed to make the difference between health and disease.

WHAT THE EXPERIMENTS SHOW

According to some experts, vitamin E may ward off cancers linked to fatty diets, such as breast cancer. In one British experiment, for example, blood samples were taken from over 5,000 women. Vitamin E levels of women who subsequently developed breast cancer were compared with samples from similar women who did not develop cancer. Women with the lowest levels of vitamin E were found to have five times the risk of cancer than women with the highest levels.

R.S. London, M.D., director of the Division of Reproductive Medicine at North Charles General Hospital in Baltimore, did a study on 17 young women with mammary dysplasia (a condition that can lead to breast cancer). He treated the patients with supplements of vitamin E and found that 15 of the women showed remission from the disease. Dr. London and his colleagues recently reviewed additional research on vitamin E and breast tumors and concluded that "supplemental tocopherol may reduce a woman's risk for the development of breast cancer." The scientists recommend that large-scale, well-designed clinical trials be carried out to test this hypothesis.

Numerous experiments have shown that lung cancer is related to smokers' low levels of vitamin E. One study at the University of Kentucky in Lexington exposed guinea pigs to different kinds of smoke for five months. The scientists then measured levels of vitamin E in the animals' blood, kidneys, livers and lungs. They discovered that vitamin E levels in the lungs of animals who had been exposed to cigarette smoke was three times higher than levels in lungs exposed to a sham smoke. None of the other organs showed any difference.

The researchers concluded that the guinea pigs needed that extra vitamin E there to combat the toxic effects of cigarette smoke. "The increased levels of vitamin E in the lungs of chronically smoked guinea pigs suggest an adaptive response of the animals to protect against further injury."

In another study, Eric R. Pecht, M.D., and his colleagues in the Department of Medicine at Ohio State University in Columbus, checked the lungs of smokers and nonsmokers and found that nonsmokers had almost seven times more vitamin E in their lungs than did smokers. Even after the smokers were given supplements of vitamin E, their lung levels rose only slightly. The researchers explain that smokers used up their vitamin E in an attempt to overcome the pernicious effects of cigarette smoke.

At Johns Hopkins School of Hygiene and Public Health in Baltimore, researchers used blood samples collected 12 years earlier to assess nutrient levels in the blood of people who had subsequently developed lung cancer. They found that lung cancer victims had lower levels of vitamin E than did a group of healthy people. People with the lowest levels of vitamin E were 2.5 times more likely to contract cancer than people with the highest levels of E. "It is important to note, though," the researchers conclude, "that the magnitude of lung cancer risk associated with cigarette smoking is substantially greater than that associated with low levels of serum vitamin E."

At Harvard, several studies with hamsters have shown that vitamin E has an inhibiting effect on artificially induced tumors in hamsters. In one study, the scientists exposed two groups of hamsters to cancer-causing chemicals, giving one group vitamin E. After 22 weeks, all of

VITAMIN E FOR CANCER TREATMENT

Researchers at the University of Colorado's Health Sciences Center recently discovered that vitamin E may play an important role in the treatment of advanced cancer of the prostate, the second most common cancer among American men. The researchers found that the vitamin enhances the effectiveness of Adriamycin, a drug used to treat this cancer and a variety of other cancers.

In the laboratory, the researchers treated prostatic cancer cells with vitamin E or Adriamycin, and with both together. They found that both vitamin E and Adriamycin inhibited the growth of cancer cells but that when the two were used together, the results were far better than expected. They had a synergistic effect.

How vitamin E may inhibit cancer cell growth is not well understood, but several possible mechanisms have been suggested. Vitamin E may be toxic to the cancer cell, it may meddle with the division of the cell, or it may enhance immunity, enabling the body to mount a better attack on the cancer cells.

The levels of vitamin E achieved in the study could easily be attained in the human body, the researchers say, and the doses would not be harmful.

"The results of this study suggest that Adriamycin could be used more effectively at lower doses if given with vitamin E, reducing the side effects of the drug," says Mukta Webber, Ph.D., one of the researchers.

That's good news because, along with the hope of a cure, chemotherapy can bring some mean and nasty side effects. Some

the group without vitamin E had tumors of varying sizes, but the group who got vitamin E had no tumors at all.

All of these studies seem to show the tremendous promise of vitamin E and cancer prevention, or in the more cautious words of one researcher, Charles Hennekens, M.D., of Brigham and Women's Hospital in Boston, "There is some intriguing research about the potential of vitamin E, particularly since most cancers are epithelial [occurring in cells that line the surfaces of organs] and vitamin E may work well there." Perhaps that's why the National Cancer Institute has chosen vitamin E as one of the few nutrients in which it is willing to invest research funds. (A large-scale experiment on people and nutrients can cost up to $100 million.)

may even be life-threatening. Anticancer drugs like Adriamycin are highly toxic, not only to cancer cells. Because of this, doses must be limited, reducing the number of cancer cells that can be wiped out.

In past studies on animals, vitamin E protected against heart damage, the most serious side effect of Adriamycin. The heart is most likely damaged by free radicals created during the metabolism of the Adriamycin.

Other animal studies have shown that vitamin E can help heal skin damage from anticancer drugs. These drugs can cause ulcers if they accidentally leak from the blood vessel at the site of injection and into surrounding soft tissue. This can cause severe pain and sometimes requires the surgical removal of dead tissue and skin grafting.

Working with rats, researchers found that vitamin E could reduce the size of skin ulcers by up to 70 percent in two weeks when applied with dimethyl sulfoxide (DMSO) to carry the vitamin through the skin.

"There is no question, the potential for vitamin E to work with anticancer drugs is very high," says Kedar N. Prasad, Ph.D., president of the International Association for Vitamins and Nutritional Oncology. "The only evidence I have seen that vitamin E can reduce the side effects of chemotherapy has been very preliminary, but I think the experimental data looks promising."

THE RIGHT DOSE

The current Recommended Dietary Allowance for vitamin E is 30 International Units. But is that enough to prevent cancer? Some experts don't think so.

"There is really no vitamin E deficiency known," says John H. Weisburger, Ph.D., of the American Health Foundation in Valhalla, New York. "That's why the RDA is so low—because most people eat some food that contains vitamin E, we probably get enough so that there are no overt deficiencies. But, in the 1980s, we really need to ask further than what levels of certain vitamins would prevent deficiency disease. We want to promote health. And there are really no sound data. I'm reasonably sure that 10 International Units of vitamin E is probably a bit too low. My guess is that for vitamin E, we have to think not in terms of 8 or 10 Units a day, but more like 50 Units a day."

To get that much, you have to emphasize vitamin E-rich foods in your diet. Just one tablespoon of wheat germ has 37 International Units. Sprinkle that on a granola cereal loaded with sunflower seeds and almonds (nuts and seeds are good sources) and you've got even more E. Whole grains are also decent sources, as are polyunsaturated oils (particularly sunflower, safflower, soybean and peanut oils).

Dr. Weisburger advices those who want to take a vitamin E supplement to do so "with your main meal. Many people traditionally take their vitamin pills in the morning with breakfast. Now, if you eat a breakfast designed to help you prevent cancer you will keep it lean and low-fat. And if you have a low-fat breakfast, your fat-soluble vitamins— A, E, or D—will not be absorbed. I know any number of people who take vitamin E in the morning with orange juice, coffee and a piece of toast and those fat-soluble vitamins will not be absorbed." (Remember, however, to take nutritional supplements only with the approval and supervision of your doctor.)

Preventing cancer may be E-asier than you think.

CANCER PROTECTION PLAN: VITAMIN E

- If your immune system is suppressed, you may want to supplement your diet with small amounts of vitamin E.
- Do not freeze foods high in vitamin E.

Vitamin K

K. It can be an infamous letter. There's the KKK. And the shock of the KO. And then there's vitamin K, the little-known nutrient buried in the alphabet way behind the A-to-E group that gets all the good publicity. Fortunately, this vitamin is OK. Especially when it comes to cancer.

It was when cancer researchers at the UCLA School of Medicine were researching the effects of anticoagulant drugs on patients with advanced cancer that they began to discover the possibilities of vitamin K. The anticoagulants turned out to be very effective cancer cell killers, and the researchers thought that if they gave vitamin K *with* the anticoagulant, they could give more powerful doses of the drug. Then it turned out that vitamin K by itself was a potent cancer fighter.

Actually, a good deal of research over the last 20 years has shown the promise of vitamin K, but no one has really followed it up until recently. "Perhaps because it was a vitamin and up until a few years ago, there was always some sort of stigma associated with investigating vitamins for prevention or therapy," says Rowan T. Chlebowski, M.D., Ph.D. Now a growing number of scientists are studying K's remarkable abilities as a cancer killer.

In various experiments, Dr. Chlebowski and his colleagues at UCLA removed a variety of malignant tumors from patients—from the breast, colon, ovary, lung and other places—then subjected the tumors to vitamin K. And instead of continuing to grow, most of the tumors were stopped cold. "We found that in the lab, vitamin K will kill cancer cells to the same degree or maybe even more effectively than many conventional chemotherapeutic agents [chemicals used in chemotherapy]. We are now in the process of studying whether vitamin K will kill cancer cells and shrink tumors in people."

Perhaps the best thing about vitamin K as a cancer treatment drug, according to Dr. Chlebowski, is that it seems to be relatively nontoxic, at least in the doses he is giving patients—and those are the same doses that were killing cancer cells in the lab.

Nutritionists don't believe people need supplements of vitamin K. The National Research Council, which publishes the Recommended Dietary Allowances for most vitamins and minerals, has not been able to determine a level of K that would cause a deficiency—because no one has ever had one. It is synthesized in our bodies by intestinal bacteria and is plentiful in food, particularly dark green, leafy vegetables.

All in all, vitamin K has something of an aura of mystery about it, an aura scientists are eagerly working to dispel. "That a naturally occurring substance could have these tendencies to stop cancer development shows a lot of promise," says Dr. Chlebowski. "It's the kind of thing that's pointing the way to a new direction in cancer prevention and treatment strategies."

X-Rays

Several decades ago, people were exploring the potential of x-rays. The medical community used these high-energy waves to treat problems from tonsilitis to acne. And, in a try at preventive medicine, children were herded past x-ray machines on trailers in mass screenings for tuberculosis. Even outside the world of medicine, people came into contact with these invisible rays. Shoppers even wiggled their toes under x-ray machines to make sure their shoes fit.

However, the novelty of this miracle machine wore off when trouble reared its ugly head. When x-raying teeth first came into practice, for instance, dentists often used their hands to hold film in their patients' mouths. Many of these dentists developed skin cancer, which originated on their fingers. Several women who received repeated chest x-rays (to monitor their recovery from tuberculosis) developed breast cancer.

Nowadays, "To x-ray or not to x-ray?" is the question, and it has few clear answers. On one hand, the x-ray is an indispensable tool in diagnosis and treatment. We can use it to scan the skeleton for cracks, reveal a tumor before it gets very large and monitor the bloodstream to make sure it's running smoothly.

"In most cases, x-rays can lead to lifesaving or limb-saving medical efforts and are responsible for significant improvements in medical care," points out Daniel G. Miller, M.D., director of the Strang Clinic, New York, in *The American Cancer Society's Complete Book of Cancer.*

Furthermore, few studies have conclusively proven that occasional diagnostic x-rays cause cancer. The aforementioned cases of the dentists' hands and the women's breasts involved much higher doses of radiation than you'd get in a standard x-ray.

On the other hand, you can hardly say that x-rays are safe. Researchers are still trying to sort out the risks and benefits. Meanwhile, it's useful to be aware of some recommendations that may help your own risk/benefit analysis if you ever need x-rays.

UNDERSTANDING X-RAYS

Doctors had no way to take a picture of a living person's skeleton until 1895, when a scientist made an accidental discovery. Physicist Wilhelm Roentgen noticed that a cathode ray tube he was experimenting with emitted a mysterious form of radiation that penetrated cardboard, crossed his laboratory room and caused a specially painted screen to glow eerily. And when he placed his hand in front of the beam, there, on the screen, was a ghostly shadow: his bones.

Shortly afterward, these waves of electromagnetic energy, or "x-rays," as Roentgen called them, were enlisted to serve medicine. Here's how: A machine shoots x-rays through the body onto film. Since bones absorb the radiation more effectively than the soft tissues, the x-rays that hit the bones don't make it to the film.

"What you have is essentially a shadow picture, in which the bones come out light on the film and the organs come out dark," says Kenneth Mossman, Ph.D., associate professor of radiation medicine at Georgetown University, Washington, D.C.

It may sound strange that energy waves can enter one side of your body and emerge on the other side, but that's just what happens when you put your palm against a flashlight—you can see the light shining through your hand.

X-rays, like radio waves and visible light, are a type of electromagnetic radiation. However, x-rays are considered to be more dangerous, because they have enough energy to knock electrons out of atoms. This phenomenon is called ionization. Ionization can damage tissues by striking the genetic material in your body's cells or by striking a water molecule and producing highly reactive free radicals that attack vital molecules. Your body is capable of repairing such damage, so ionizing radiation is not always harmful. However, sometimes the genetic changes it has caused can eventually lead to cancer.

"We know that the type of radiation used in diagnostic x-rays can cause cancer and genetic defects," says Dr. Mossman. "But we know that primarily from studies that involved large doses of radiation. The atomic bomb and radiation therapy of benign diseases, for instance, are clear risks for cancer. But we have not been able to demonstrate excess cancer risk at the very, very low dose of radiation used in diagnostic x-rays."

Until recently, that is. A group of researchers at the Department of Environmental Science and Physiology at the Harvard School of Public Health, Boston, conducted the first study to estimate how risky x-rays are. They studied 75,000 people who had diagnostic x-rays in Maine, calculated their radiation doses and cancer rates, and compared them to cancer rates in the general population. And they estimated that about 1 percent of all cases of leukemia (bone marrow cancer) and less than 1 percent of all cases of breast cancer result from x-rays. A small risk, but it accounts for 267 excess cases of leukemia per year and 788 induced breast tumors per year in this country.

"We studied cancer of the breast and bone marrow, because that's what we had data for," says John S. Evans, Sc.D., who headed the research. "But it's certainly possible that x-rays can cause different types of cancer as well. What should you do about this? In one sense, don't be inordinately worried about x-rays. The risk is still small. Leukemia has a lifetime risk of 8.7 cases per 100,000 people, and breast cancer has a risk of 52 cases per 100,000 women. On the other hand, there's no benefit to getting more x-rays than you need."

In fact, it's been estimated that medical and dental x-rays are responsible for about 90 percent of man's exposure to man-made, low-level radiation. For that reason, members of the National Cancer Institute and the Environmental Protection Agency have stated that reducing the number of x-rays taken in doctors' offices may be the best way to reduce the total radiation burden on the population.

USING X-RAYS WISELY

"Even though the risk is very, very small, it is important to use x-rays judiciously," says Dr. Mossman.

In other words, you should try to limit your exposure to x-rays whenever possible, because there is some possibility that it could harm you. The alleged harm of x-rays is controversial, and there are no definitive answers, but here are some issues to consider next time a doctor or a dentist wants to photograph your insides.

AVOID ROUTINE SCREENINGS

In 1979, the director of Food and Drug Administration's (FDA) Bureau of Radiological Health (now called the Center for Devices and Radiological Health) estimated that up to 30 percent of the 278 million medical and dental diagnostic x-rays made yearly were unnecessary.

That percentage would probably hold true today, guesses Fred Rueter, D.S., medical physicist for the Center for Devices and Radiological Health (CDRH), Rockville, Maryland. "Most unnecessary x-rays are taken to defend doctors against malpractice suits, so they will have evidence to back up their decisions," says Dr. Rueter. "Also, some companies and hospitals require routine x-rays upon admission."

To avoid unnecessary radiation, you can merely ask what the purpose of the x-ray examination is. "If there is a clear benefit, then, by all means, they should be taken," says Dr. Mossman. "Since the risk is so small, a patient should not refuse a necessary x-ray."

How can you tell if the x-ray is really necessary? "You can try to establish the answer with a few general questions," says Donald Pizzarello, Ph.D., professor of radiology, New York University Medical Center. "Is the information the doctor is looking for in the x-ray new— something he doesn't already have at hand? Will it affect the treatment or the prognosis? If the answer to these questions is yes, and there is no safer way to get the information, then I think there's no question that the x-ray should be taken."

More and more radiologists and doctors are eliminating routine screenings—x-raying healthy people to screen for a possible disease— from their repertoire. In fact, the American College of Radiology (ACR) has urged that chest x-rays be eliminated as a routine procedure for hospital admissions, tuberculosis screening and as part of pre-employment physicals. The ACR found that most such x-ray sessions usually turn up very little, if anything, so it just isn't worth the cost and the risk.

You can refuse such unnecessary chest x-rays unless the doctor feels your health or medical history warrants having one, or if you are regularly exposed to chemicals or health hazards that could affect the lungs. Coal miners, for instance, have a high risk of black lung, so there's some justification to perform chest x-rays on them, according to Dr. Reuter.

Dental x-rays may be considered an exception to the "avoid screening" rule, since they're often taken in the absence of symptoms. However, they are extremely useful to dentists, since they can reveal tooth, gum and jaw diseases and abnormalities that could not otherwise be detected.

The guidelines as to how often these x-rays are needed are somewhat fuzzy. The American Dental Association has stated that x-rays should not be a routine part of every dental examination, but left up to the judgment of the dentist.

"Generally, a full mouth series (which consists of between 14 and 20 x-rays and includes the root portion of all teeth) is only necessary every two to five years, whereas the bitewing examinations (which consist of either 1 or 2 x-rays on each side of the mouth and shows only the crown portion of the teeth) depend on the individual needs of the individual patient," according to William Wege, M.D., professor of radiology, Medical College of Georgia School of Dentistry, Augusta.

Mammography, or breast x-ray, is also used in the absence of symptoms. The controversial question is whether it's more likely to *detect* breast cancer in its early stages and thus save a life, or to *cause* breast cancer and thus endanger life.

However, the danger has diminished since researchers first warned the public that mammography might cause cancer. "In the last 15 years, there have been tremendous advances made in mammography equipment so that the radiation dose has been reduced now by a factor of 10 or 100, depending on the equipment," reports Dr. Mossman.

Today, the National Cancer Institute recommends that routine mammography for women under 35 years of age should be limited to those women who have a personal history of breast cancer (see chapter 45, Mammograms).

KEEP A RECORD

It's a good idea to keep a record of all the x-rays you're exposed to at various doctors' and specialists' offices. After all, Doctor A probably won't know that Doctor B took the same routine x-rays two years ago— unless you tell him. The FDA's Center for Devices and Radiological Health supplies free cards which help you keep track of relevant x-ray information. You can request one by writing to: X-rays, Food and Drug Administration, Rockville, MD 20857. You can give this information to any new doctor you visit, and, the next time a doctor says you need an x-ray, ask him or her whether any previous x-rays can be used.

In addition, you may want to keep further records. "Charts and x-ray records are frequently destroyed after seven years, although this varies from state to state according to legal requirements," says Dr. Miller. "If this is the case in your state, ask the physician or hospital to send the x-rays (or at least the reports regarding them) to your home address. This may save unnecessary x-rays in the future."

PREGNANT WOMEN BEWARE

Perhaps most vulnerable of all is the unborn baby. In a landmark paper published in 1956, British physician Alice Stewart reported that diagnostic radiation delivered to the fetus provoked a significant increase in the frequency of childhood cancer. Many scientists have criticized the methods Dr. Stewart used, and some studies have appeared to disprove her findings, but other large studies have confirmed her results.

And even while the risk remains quite small, most doctors now recommend that pregnant women receive no x-rays at all, unless the doctor suspects a serious condition. And if the x-ray must be taken, the physician should be informed of the pregnancy, and should shield the pelvis if possible.

"It's tragic when a woman is two or three weeks pregnant, she doesn't know it yet, and she comes in for an x-ray examination of the lower abdomen," says Dr. Mossman. "Even though the radiation dose is small, the anxiety generated in the parents is extremely severe."

For that reason, a woman might ask the doctor if the examination can wait until she gets her menstrual period. Some doctors, especially in England, obey the "ten-day rule," a recommendation that an x-ray examination of a woman's abdomen be done only during the ten-day interval between the onset of the patient's menstrual period and the tenth day thereafter, according to Jacob I. Fabrikant, M.D., Ph.D., adjunct professor of radiology, University of California School of Medicine at San Francisco. It's based on the assumption that a woman won't be pregnant during that time, since she probably hasn't ovulated yet.

MAKE SURE THEY USE LEAD SHIELD

"If the doctor or dentist does not put a lead apron over areas of the body which are not being x-rayed, the patient should insist on having one," says Dr. Mossman. "Even though the x-rays are aimed at a particular area of the body, other parts of the body may be exposed to scattered radiation. Lead absorbs radiation so your body doesn't have to. It's especially important to shield the genital area if possible, to protect the sex glands from producing genetic defects in offspring."

LOOK FOR A QUALITY FACILITY

"Although diagnostic x-rays must be ordered by a physician, the taking of x-rays is not always supervised by a radiologist," says Dr. Miller in *The American Cancer Society's Complete Book of Cancer.* "In fact, in one survey, only 60 percent of diagnostic studies were supervised by radiologists. In 1978, 11,700 x-ray systems were installed, but only 3,152 safety tests were carried out. In seven states there was no safety-compliance testing at all."

Those figures can add up to higher risk. One way to avoid problems is to seek out a facility that has a certified x-ray technician or a full-time radiologist, suggest some doctors. Poorly trained or untrained technologists may tend to take too many films per examination and too many examinations per patient. They also may have too little knowledge of the hazards of radiation and the importance of proper shielding, reported Herbert L. Abrams, M.D., of Harvard Medical School, Boston, in the *New England Journal of Medicine*.

ASK ABOUT ALTERNATIVES

Whereas more and more radiation-conscious people are trying to limit their x-ray exposure, other people actually request an x-ray examination that might not be recommended. A common practice, for instance, is to x-ray a sore ankle because the patient expects it, even though the doctor's examination is usually all that's required to indicate a sprain.

This kind of thinking (the patient probably expects an x-ray, so we'd better do one) is one reason to ask your doctor whether there are less hazardous tests that would yield similar results.

Ultrasound is one x-ray substitute and is often used to monitor the development of a fetus. "We don't know as much about ultrasound's effects as we do about x-ray effects, but in my opinion, ultrasound doesn't pose as much risk," says Dr. Mossman.

"Ultrasound is a safe x-ray substitute in some cases," agrees Dr. Pizzarello. "It can image soft tissues, but for bones, x-rays are much better."

Another possible alternative is magnetic resonance imaging. "Magnetic resonance imaging is a relatively new technique that is used to make images of the head," explains Dr. Pizzarello. "It's still not in general clinical use, and there are certain conditions where x-rays remain superior. But they are being used increasingly as an x-ray substitute."

CANCER PREVENTION PLAN: X-RAYS

- Ask your doctor why you need an x-ray.
- Ask if a previous x-ray can be used.
- Ask if there are safer ways to get the information.
- When you are x-rayed, be sure a shield covers the gonads.
- Use an x-ray facility that has a full-time radiologist.
- Ask if the x-ray can be postponed until after your menstrual period.
- Tell the doctor if you're pregnant or think you may be.

Although science has yet to invent a machine that performs all functions of an x-ray machine without radiation, we have progressed from the days in which it took 25 minutes of exposure to x-rays to produce an image of the teeth and jawbones.

"Throughout the years, the ability to make a film of quality that facilitates a good diagnosis with a small radiation dose has improved," says Dr. Pizzarello.

Today, the risk of dying of cancer from a chest x-ray examination is small—about the same as that encountered in smoking about six cigarettes, according to Joel E. Gray, Ph.D., diagnostic radiology, Mayo Clinic, Rochester, Minnesota.

"It's good to be cautious of excess exposure to x-rays, but it's equally important to be aware of the benefits," concludes Dr. Mossman.

Yogurt

Remember when yogurt was something only a health nut would touch? These days, Americans are simply lapping it up. And that's good, because it's good for our health. In fact, it may even help protect us against cancer.

The key to yogurt's protective power is a little organism with a big name: *Lactobacillus acidophilus*. This friendly digestive bacteria is found naturally in your intestines (along with hundreds of other varieties) *and* in certain brands of yogurt and milk products. It has a special ability: It can block the activity of an enzyme that can change harmless substances into cancer-causers, or carcinogens. After researchers discovered this fact, an experiment was conducted at Tufts University in Medford, Massachusetts, to see if *increasing* the amount of *Lactobacillus acidophilus* in the body could decrease the activities of those nasty enzymes.

Well, it worked. As measured in the feces of both laboratory animals and people, the doses of acidophilus reduced the number of carcinogenic compounds produced by these enzymes. "Acidophilus reduced the three fecal enzymes that have the capability of generating carcinogens," says researcher Barry R. Goldin, Ph.D., associate professor of medicine at Tufts University Medical School.

In another study that Dr. Goldin conducted a few years ago, he discovered that when he gave animals acidophilus together with a carcinogen known to cause colon cancer, the acidophilus cut the number of colon tumors in half. "The acidophilus seemed to be slowing the growth of tumors rather than preventing them completely," he explained.

Dr. Goldin is quick to point out that these findings don't prove that yogurt helps prevent colon cancer. For one thing, those three enzymes have never been linked to colon cancer itself—only to an increase in carcinogens. Also, both studies are preliminary—clues that need much more evidence before a solid case could be made for yogurt. But Dr. Goldin is intrigued. And so are other researchers.

Through hundreds of experiments, Khem Shahani, Ph.D., professor of food science at the University of Nebraska in Lincoln, has found that yogurt inhibits the growth of tumor cells. "There is tremendous potential in this kind of nutritional therapy," says Dr. Shahani.

A RARE CULTURE

But don't rush out to your supermarket and buy a month's supply of yogurt—at least not before you read the labels. Most yogurts are made with *Lactobacillus bulgaricus* and *Streptococcus thermophilus*. These two strains did not have the same effect as acidophilus in Dr. Goldin's enzyme experiments. However, you could opt for acidophilus milk, or check carefully for a yogurt that *does* use acidophilus (an exclusive club that includes a few national and local brands) or make it yourself using acidophilus culture.

If you make the effort, you'll be an elite eater. "There are few acidophilus eaters in the world," says Dr. Goldin. But in some areas where people do eat a lot of acidophilus foods, colon cancer rates are lower. "In Finland, they have as high a fat consumption as we do [high-fat diets have been linked with colon cancer risk], but their colon cancer rate is half what ours is," points out Dr. Goldin. "They are big dairy eaters—much more yogurt, kefir and other products that are fermented using various bacteria, including acidophilus products. Some people say their low colon cancer rate is due to a higher fiber content in their bread and crackers."

Well, there's *something* about their diet that's protecting them from colon cancer. Maybe it's fiber, maybe it's the various yogurt cultures, maybe it's a combination.

But we may never know. "As far as yogurt preventing cancer—I don't know how we can *prove* that. It is unlikely that anyone would fund a controlled study of yogurt-eating and colon cancer; it would cost $100 to $200 million." But statistics comparing disease patterns to eating patterns may show us something.

"People in America have only been eating yogurt in large quantities for the last ten years. Before that, it was difficult to see any effects yogurt might have had on people's health, because there just weren't enough people eating it. Now there are, so maybe scientists looking at the data will find that yogurt eaters have lower colon cancer rates."

Dr. Goldin doesn't think this means you should ignore yogurt until scientists give it their seal of approval. "In good conscience, I can recommend yogurt because it's good for you, provided you don't eat the high-fat varieties. Stay with the low-fat and no-fat kinds. Yogurt is an excellent calcium source; it may even help lower blood pressure."

In other words, "milk" yogurt for all it's worth.

CANCER PREVENTION PLAN: YOGURT

- Eat yogurt cultured with the acidophilus bacteria.
- Use other acidophilus products such as acidophilus milk and kefir.
- Eat low-fat or no-fat yogurt.

Cancer-Fighting Recipes

PART THREE

Menus that Protect Your Health

Over the past 10 or 20 years, we have greatly changed our attitude about our health. Most people once felt helpless, for example, when confronted with a formidable foe like cancer. Today, we are beginning to feel as if we have some control. While there's no cure yet, there is prevention. Through research, health professionals have come to realize that there really are things that we can do to lower the risks of developing cancer, and they have been spreading the word.

If we protect ourselves from the sun, we can almost eliminate the risk of skin cancer. If we practice self-examination, we may be able to detect breast cancer or testicular cancer early enough to treat it successfully. If we don't smoke, we can greatly minimize our risk of many types of cancer, with lung, bladder, kidney and pancreatic cancer among them. And if we change the way we eat, we can increase our chances of avoiding a long list of cancers, including colorectal, prostate and breast cancer. That's because one of the discoveries researchers have made in the last few years is the role of diet in preventing (or promoting) cancer.

Now that this knowledge has become widely accepted, we see ads everywhere for high-fiber this, high-vitamin that, and all-natural everything else. However, as encouraging as this food trend may be, experts are finding that the best foods are those that are *really* natural, like vegetables and fruits, whole grains, lean meats and fish. These are the kinds of foods that give us optimum amounts of the cancer-fighting nutrients they contain and help us reduce our intake of fat, sugar, salt and additives. Some of these cancer fighters, which are described in more detail elsewhere in this book, are:

- Fiber, which speeds up digestion and may help protect against colon cancer by diluting potential cancer-causing substances and flushing them out of the body.
- Vitamin E, which may have protective effects against several types of cancer. It is an antioxidant that prevents the formation of harmful free radicals, it blocks the formation of nitrosamines and it strengthens the immune system.
- Vitamin C, which has the same benefits as vitamin E.
- Calcium, which may protect against colon cancer by reducing the effects of harmful substances in the colon.
- Beta-carotene, which may inhibit the growth and spread of cancer cells, as well as boost the immune system.

In this section of the book there are more than 50 recipes that will help make your anticancer diet appetizing and easy. There are ideas for breakfasts, lunches, dinners, snacks and desserts that supply beneficial amounts of cancer-fighting nutrients, with a bonus—great taste. All of the recipes were developed by the Rodale Food Center specifically for their health-boosting ability. But just knowing you're eating something that's good for you isn't enough—the dish also has to taste good, or you're not going to eat it very often. These recipes were tested for taste appeal, and they all passed with high marks.

Use these recipes to plan a whole day's menu that will provide several of the most important cancer fighters. You can, for example, begin the day with Mixed Grain Griddle Cakes, which supply vitamin E. For lunch, you can add a generous, tasty helping of vitamin C, fiber, calcium and beta-carotene with the Spinach, Mushroom and Cheese Panino. And for the evening meal, consider tangy Chicken Tangiers, a low-fat source of fiber, vitamin C and beta-carotene, followed by luscious Prune-Apple Crunch, for additional vitamin E.

With the nutrient information provided elsewhere in the book and these taste-tempting recipes, you can take a big step on the road to health, which, it seems, is paved with good food.

Powerfully Protective Breakfast Dishes

Apples and Oats

You get a double boost of fiber from this cereal—about 10 grams per serving. Besides the fiber found in apples, oat bran contains water-soluble fiber. Both, scientists believe, can prevent colon cancer. What's more, it's delicious.

4 cups water
1⅓ cups oat bran
½ cup raisins or currants
1 apple, shredded
1 tablespoon maple syrup
½ teaspoon ground cinnamon
½ teaspoon ground caraway seeds (optional)

Combine water and oat bran in a 2-quart saucepan. Bring to a vigorous boil, stirring constantly. Reduce heat to low and cook, stirring frequently, for 2 minutes, or until thick.

Remove from heat and stir in raisins or currants, apples, syrup, cinnamon and caraway (if used). Let stand 5 minutes before serving. Serve with milk, if desired.

Yield: 4 servings

NOTE: *You may cook this cereal ahead and reheat it in the microwave. Cover cereal with plastic wrap, then microwave on high setting for 2 minutes.*

VARIATION: *Use this cereal to stuff baked apples. Core baking apples, such as Granny Smiths, and fill them with cereal mixture. Bake at 400°F for 20 minutes. If desired, bake the apples ahead of time and reheat in the microwave. Cover and microwave each apple on high setting for 2 minutes.*

Apple-Bran Muffins

Fiber, fiber everywhere—a luscious bite to eat.

1 cup wheat bran
1 cup buttermilk
1½ cups whole wheat flour
2 teaspoons baking powder
1 medium unpeeled apple, grated
½ cup raisins
1 egg
2 tablespoons vegetable oil
⅓ cup molasses
1½ teaspoons vanilla extract

Preheat oven to 375°F. Coat a 12-cup muffin tin with vegetable spray.

In a medium-size bowl, soak bran in buttermilk for 10 minutes. Meanwhile, sift together flour and baking powder into a medium-size bowl, then mix in apples and raisins. In a small bowl, combine egg, oil, molasses and vanilla.

Add bran mixture to flour mixture. Then add wet ingredients to dry ingredients, combining gently and quickly.

Fill prepared muffin tin three-quarters full. Bake for 20 to 25 minutes. Cool on wire rack.

Yield: 12 muffins

VARIATION: *Substitute ⅔ cup chopped dried fruit for the grated apple.*

Baked Bananas with Apricot Breakfast Cheese

A different breakfast idea that supplies plenty of vitamin C and beta-carotene.

Apricot Breakfast Cheese
½ cup dried apricot halves
½ cup apple or orange juice
2 tablespoons maple syrup
   or honey
⅛ teaspoon ground nutmeg
   dash of ground cardamom
½ cup low-fat cottage cheese
Bananas
4 bananas, cut in half
   lengthwise, then
   crosswise
1 tablespoon lemon juice

To make Apricot Breakfast Cheese: In a small saucepan, combine the first five ingredients. Bring to a boil over medium heat. Reduce heat to low, cover and simmer 20 minutes, or until apricots are very soft.

With a slotted spoon, transfer apricots to a food processor or blender and let cool. Reserve cooking liquid. Process until apricots are finely chopped. Add cottage cheese and process again until mixture is smooth.

To make bananas: Preheat oven to 400°F. Place bananas in a baking dish. Brush with lemon juice, then with reserved apricot cooking liquid. Bake 6 to 8 minutes, or until bananas are soft. Gently remove to a serving dish and top with Apricot Breakfast Cheese.

Yield: 4 servings

VARIATION: *Use Apricot Breakfast Cheese as a spread on whole grain bread, pancakes or waffles or as a topping for fresh fruit.*

Breakfast Pilaf with Maple Yogurt

Flaked grains are conveniently quick to cook, but offer the long-term benefits of fiber.

Pilaf
1 teaspoon safflower oil
½ cup rolled oats
¼ cup barley flakes
¼ cup wheat flakes
¼ cup rye flakes
¼ cup brown rice flakes
1 tablespoon wheat germ
3½ cups apricot-apple juice
3 tablespoons chopped
   dried apricots
2 tablespoons golden
   raisins
½ teaspoon ground
   cinnamon
   dash of ground nutmeg
Maple Yogurt
½ cup low-fat yogurt
1 tablespoon maple syrup
½ teaspoon vanilla extract

To make pilaf: In a nonstick 3-quart saucepan, heat oil over low heat. Add oats, barley, wheat, rye and brown rice flakes and wheat germ. Toast, stirring constantly, for about 2 minutes. Remove from heat.

In a 2-quart saucepan, bring juice to a boil. Add apricots and raisins. Add toasted grains, then reduce heat to very low, cover and simmer for about 15 minutes, or until juice is absorbed. Remove from heat and stir in cinnamon and nutmeg.

To make Maple Yogurt: Combine ingredients in small bowl. Serve with pilaf.

Yield: 6 servings

Carrot-Pineapple Muffins

These tasty, colorful muffins are high in both fiber and beta-carotene.

2 cups whole wheat flour
3 teaspoons baking powder
½ teaspoon baking soda
½ teaspoon ground ginger,
     nutmeg or cinnamon
1 cup bran cereal
2 eggs, well beaten
½ cup milk
3 tablespoons corn oil
¼ cup honey
½ cup orange juice
1 cup shredded carrots
½ cup crushed pineapple,
     drained

Preheat oven to 350°F. Butter muffin tins or line with paper muffin cups.

In a medium-size bowl, mix flour, baking powder, baking soda, spice and bran cereal. In a small bowl, mix eggs, milk, oil, honey, orange juice, carrots and pineapple. Add wet ingredients to dry ingredients and stir just until dry ingredients are moistened.

Fill prepared muffin tins three-quarters full. Bake for 12 to 15 minutes, or until golden. Cool on wire rack.

Yield: 18 muffins

Creamy Blueberry Breakfast Pudding

More than simply delicious, this breakfast starts your day right with fiber and calcium.

1   cup long grain brown
       rice
4   cups skim milk
¾   cup raisins or currants
1   vanilla bean or ½
       teaspoon vanilla
       extract
1   stick cinnamon, 3 inches
       long
1–2 tablespoons maple syrup
       or honey, to taste
1½   cups fresh blueberries

Grind rice in a food processor or blender until kernels are half their original size. Combine with milk in a medium-size saucepan and bring to a boil over medium heat. Reduce heat to low, then add raisins or currants, vanilla and cinnamon. Cover and simmer for 15 to 20 minutes, or until rice is tender and milk is almost completely absorbed. Stir in syrup or honey and blueberries.

Yield: 4 servings

VARIATION: *Use your choice of seasonal fruits like raspberries, blackberries, chopped peaches or apricots, and halved strawberries in place of blueberries.*

Fruit Compote

Make this ahead of time and serve warm or cold for a breakfast
that provides more than 5 grams of dietary fiber per serving.

1   cup applesauce
1   cup apple juice
    juice and grated rind of 1
      lemon
1   tablespoon vanilla extract
½   teaspoon ground
      cinnamon
¼   teaspoon ground ginger
¼   teaspoon grated whole
      nutmeg
½   cup dried apricot halves
¼   cup pitted prunes
6   dried figs, halved
¼   cup dried currants
1   pear, thinly sliced

Preheat oven to 300°F.

In a 2-quart ovenproof casserole, combine applesauce, apple juice, lemon juice and rind, vanilla, cinnamon, ginger and nutmeg.

Stir in apricots, prunes, figs, currants and pears. Cover and bake for 1½ hours.

Yield: 4 servings

Golden Aura Waffles

The pumpkin does more than add flavor. It accounts for
goodly amounts of vitamin A.

1¼   cups whole wheat flour
1½   teaspoons baking powder
½   teaspoon pumpkin pie
      spice
1   egg, slightly beaten
¾   cup pumpkin puree
¾   cup skim milk
2   tablespoons safflower oil
1   tablespoon maple syrup
1   teaspoon vanilla

In a large bowl, sift together flour, baking powder and spice. In a medium-size bowl, beat together egg, pumpkin, milk, oil, syrup and vanilla. Add wet ingredients to dry ingredients and stir just to blend.

Heat waffle iron and brush lightly with oil, if necessary, then pour on batter and bake until steaming stops. Serve with maple syrup or applesauce.

Yield: 4 servings

VARIATION: *Add 2 tablespoons currants or chopped raisins to the batter.*

Mixed Grain Griddle Cakes

Hearty and wholesome, these hot-off-the-griddle cakes were developed to contain substantial amounts of vitamin E.

½ cup whole wheat pastry
    flour
¼ cup rolled oats
¼ cup cornmeal
1 teaspoon baking soda
1 tablespoon wheat germ
1 tablespoon finely chopped
    sunflower seeds
2 teaspoons sunflower oil
1 cup buttermilk
1 egg

In a large bowl, stir together flour, oats, cornmeal, baking soda, wheat germ and sunflower seeds. In a small bowl, beat together oil, buttermilk and egg. Add wet ingredients to dry ingredients, stirring just until combined.

Coat a nonstick skillet with vegetable spray and heat the skillet over low heat. Pour batter onto the hot skillet, using about 1½ tablespoons per griddle cake. Cook griddle cakes until golden on both sides. Serve with maple syrup or a topping made of yogurt or sieved low-fat cottage cheese, crushed berries, applesauce and honey or maple syrup.

Yield: 4 servings

VARIATIONS:
• *Stir ⅓ cup wild blackberries into the batter.*
• *Add ¼ cup grated raw carrots or sweet potato to the batter to boost your intake of beta-carotene.*

Raisin and Sweet Potato Scones

Enjoy these fiber-rich scones warm with Prune Butter (page 453) or orange marmalade.

½ cup unbleached flour
½ cup whole wheat flour
¼ cup corn bran
½ cup raisins, chopped
½ cup shredded sweet
    potato
1 teaspoon cream of tartar
½ teaspoon baking soda
    pinch of ground
      cinnamon
    pinch of grated nutmeg
⅓ cup plus 1 tablespoon
      buttermilk
2 tablespoons oil

In a large bowl, mix the unbleached flour, whole wheat flour, corn bran, raisins, sweet potato, cream of tartar, baking soda, cinnamon and nutmeg. Stir in the buttermilk and oil, until blended. With floured hands, knead the mixture for about 2 minutes.

Preheat oven to 475°F. On a lightly floured surface, roll out the dough to a generous ¼ inch thick. Cut out 2½-inch rounds, transferring each to a lightly oiled cookie sheet as you go. Use all the dough by rerolling leftovers. Bake for 6 to 8 minutes. Serve warm.

Yield: about 18 scones

Healthy Lunchtime Meals

Ambrosia Lobster Salad

This elegant and unusual salad holds two nutrients essential in the fight against cancer—vitamin C and beta-carotene.

⅓ cup orange juice
1 teaspoon grated orange rind
1 teaspoon minced, peeled ginger root
1½ tablespoons red wine vinegar
1 teaspoon French-style mustard
1 small cantaloupe
1 papaya or mango, diced
2 plum tomatoes, diced
1½ cups coarsely chopped cooked lobster
1½ teaspoons minced fresh dill or ½ teaspoon dillweed
1½ teaspoons minced chives or scallions
   watercress or other salad greens

In a small bowl, whisk together orange juice and rind, ginger, vinegar and mustard.

Cut cantaloupe into balls with a melon ball cutter. In a medium-size bowl, combine cantaloupe, papaya or mango, tomatoes, lobster, dill and chives or scallions. Cover and chill 1 hour.

Arrange greens on a salad plate and spoon lobster mixture onto greens. Spoon orange juice mixture over salad and serve immediately.

Yield: 4 servings

Brilliant Sweet Potato Soup

To be sure this soup is brimming with beta-carotene, use
yellow or orange sweet potatoes, not white ones.

1 tablespoon olive oil
1 medium onion, minced
½ cup minced celery
½ cup minced red or green
   pepper
1 clove garlic, minced
1 cup canned tomatoes,
   drained and finely
   chopped
½ teaspoon dried thyme
   freshly ground black
   pepper, to taste
4 cups Chicken Stock
   (page 452)
4 cups peeled, diced sweet
   potatoes (about 5
   medium)
1 cup corn
1 small zucchini, diced

In a Dutch oven or large saucepan, heat
oil over low heat. Add onions, celery, peppers and garlic. Cook until vegetables are
wilted but not browned, about 5 minutes.
Add tomatoes, thyme and pepper. Cover
and cook 5 minutes, then uncover and cook
about 7 minutes, or until moisture has evaporated and mixture is thick.

Add stock and bring to a boil. Add potatoes. Reduce heat to low, cover and simmer
5 minutes. Add corn and zucchini and simmer 10 to 15 minutes, or until vegetables are
tender.

Yield: 8 to 10 servings

VARIATIONS:
● *Add cooked, diced chicken.*
● *Add diced turnips, peas, okra or other veg-
etables.*

Bulgur Salad with Apples and Grapes

This truly satisfying salad provides a good amount of fiber.

½ cup bulgur
⅓ cup water
3 tablespoons apple juice
3 tablespoons lemon juice
¼ teaspoon finely grated
   lemon rind
1 stalk celery
1 large red apple, diced
½ carrot, grated
1 cup red seedless grapes
1½ teaspoons fresh mint

Place bulgur, water, apple juice, lemon
juice and lemon rind in a small bowl and let
soak until liquid is absorbed, between 30
and 60 minutes.

Cut off the top half of the celery stalk,
then cut the base in two lengthwise. Cut top
and base into thin slices on the diagonal.

Place bulgur mixture, celery, apples,
carrots, grapes and mint in a serving bowl
and toss until combined. Chill before serving, if desired.

Yield: 6 servings

Citrus and Chicken Salad with Fennel Dressing

A perfect summer meal, this salad contains plenty of vitamin C.

1   pound boneless, skinless chicken breasts
2   large, seedless pink grapefruits
2   large navel oranges
1   large green pepper, cut into fine julienne strips
½   cup pink grapefruit juice
2   teaspoons olive oil
2   teaspoons lime juice
½   teaspoon grated lime rind
2   teaspoons honey
¼   teaspoon crushed fennel seeds
  romaine lettuce leaves, torn into small pieces
2   teaspoons lightly toasted pine nuts

Preheat oven to 350°F. Place chicken on a baking sheet and cover with foil. Bake for 25 minutes or until chicken is cooked through but still moist. Let cool. Cut into thin slices and set aside.

Peel grapefruits and oranges, removing all the white pith, and separate into sections.

In a medium bowl, combine grapefuit sections, orange sections and peppers.

In a small bowl, whisk together grapefuit juice, oil, lime juice and rind, honey and fennel seeds.

Arrange romaine on a salad plate. Arrange chicken in center and spoon fruit mixture around chicken. Pour dressing over salad and sprinkle with pine nuts.

Yield: 4 servings

Cornbread with Cheese, Chilies and Beans

Serve as an entrée with soup or salad. It offers good amounts of calcium and fiber.

1⅓   cups yellow cornmeal
⅔   cup whole wheat flour
2   teaspoons baking powder
½   cup nonfat dry milk
2   tablespoons well-drained, finely chopped, canned chili peppers (mild or hot)
2½   teaspoons minced scallions (green part only)
1   cup well-drained, canned pinto beans
½   cup grated sharp cheddar cheese
2   eggs, beaten
1   cup skim milk
3   tablespoons oil or melted butter

Preheat oven to 400°F (if using a glass pan, preheat to 375°F). Butter a 9-inch pie plate or 8-inch square pan.

In a large bowl, sift together cornmeal, flour, baking powder and dry milk. Stir in peppers, scallions, beans and cheese, reserving a few beans and 1 tablespoon of cheese.

Place the prepared pan in oven for 3 or 4 minutes to heat.

In a medium-size bowl, beat together eggs, milk and oil or butter. Make a well in center of dry ingredients and pour in wet ingredients. Stir briefly to combine.

Pour batter into pan. Arrange reserved beans on top of batter, pushing them in slightly, then sprinkle with reserved cheese. Bake for 25 to 30 minutes, or until bread tests done. Cool slightly in pan. Serve warm.

Yield: 6 to 8 servings

Lentils in the Round

What a wonderful surprise this loaf is—it's stuffed with a fragrant lentil mixture. Use a loaf that's crusty and large enough to be stuffed. Whole wheat is nice, as are rye, pumpernickel and corn-rye. The bread, lentils, carrots, celery and onions provide lots of healthful fiber.

1	crusty loaf of bread, 9 inches round
2	cups apple cider
1	cup lentils
2	carrots, finely chopped
1	bay leaf
2	stalks celery, finely chopped
1	large onion, finely chopped
1	green pepper, finely chopped
2	cloves garlic, minced
1	tablespoon oil
1	cup shredded cheddar cheese
⅓	cup minced fresh parsley
1	egg, lightly beaten
1	teaspoon dried thyme

Using a serrated knife, horizontally cut the top quarter from the loaf. Wrap the top in foil and set aside.

Being careful not to puncture the sides or bottom, scoop out the soft interior of the loaf, leaving a shell ¾ to 1 inch thick. Set aside the hollow loaf.

In a 3-quart saucepan, combine the apple cider, lentils, carrots and bay leaf. Bring to a boil, then reduce heat and simmer, partly covered, for 35 to 40 minutes, or until lentils are tender and all liquid has been absorbed. Stir occasionally during cooking to prevent sticking. Remove bay leaf.

In a large nonstick skillet, sauté the celery, onions, peppers and garlic in the oil until vegetables are softened. Add to the lentil mixture. Stir in the cheese, parsley, egg and thyme.

Preheat oven to 350°F.

Spoon the lentil mixture into the hollow loaf. (If there are any lentils left over, they can be used in other ways—as a topping for baked potatoes, for example.) Wrap the loaf in foil and place on a baking sheet. Bake for 1 hour. Add the foil-wrapped top to the oven and bake for 5 minutes.

Unwrap the filled loaf and place it on a large serving platter. Unwrap the top and put it in place. To serve, scoop out the lentil mixture, then cut the bread with a serrated knife.

Yield: 6 to 8 servings

Pizza Niçoise

Here's a taste of the French Riviera that provides lots of calcium.

Dough
½ cup plus 2 tablespoons unbleached flour
½ cup plus 2 tablespoons whole wheat pastry flour
½ teaspoon dry yeast
½ cup skim milk
1 teaspoon olive oil
½ teaspoon honey

Topping
⅓ cup thick tomato sauce
½ cup red onion slices
1 teaspoon dried basil
1 clove garlic, minced
1 can (3¾ ounces) low-sodium, water-packed sardines
1 cup shredded part-skim mozzarella cheese

To make dough: In a medium-size bowl, combine flours, yeast, milk, oil and honey. Knead for 5 minutes. Cover and let rest about 10 minutes.

Preheat oven to 500°F.

Coat a pizza pan or baking sheet with vegetable spray. Press dough in pan to form a 12-inch round with raised edges. Bake for 5 minutes, or until light brown.

To make topping: In a medium-size bowl, combine the tomato sauce, onions, basil and garlic. Spread on baked pizza shell. Arrange sardines over sauce, then sprinkle with mozzarella. Bake for 5 minutes, or until cheese is golden and bubbly.

Yield: 4 servings

Smiling Tofu

This marinated tofu makes a face when you stuff it with savory shrimp filling. It smiles because it's high in calcium.

Marinade
- ⅓ cup Vegetable Stock (page 452)
- 1 tablespoon reduced-sodium soy sauce
- 1 tablespoon mirin (sweet rice vinegar)
- 1 teaspoon sesame oil
- 2 slices peeled ginger root, minced
- 1 clove garlic, minced

Filling
- 3 ounces shelled, deveined shrimp (7 or 8 medium)
- 3 scallions, chopped
- 2 slices peeled ginger root, chopped
- ¼ cup sliced water chestnuts
- 1 clove garlic, chopped
- 1½ teaspoons cornstarch
- 1 tablespoon marinade (above)
- ½ teaspoon sesame oil

Assembly
- 1 16-ounce block of smooth, firm tofu
- ⅔ cup Vegetable Stock
- 2 scallions, chopped

To make marinade: In a shallow dish, combine the stock, soy sauce, mirin, sesame oil, ginger and garlic.

To make filling: In a food processor or blender, combine the shrimp, scallions, ginger, water chestnuts, garlic, cornstarch, marinade and sesame oil and process until well mixed. Set aside.

To assemble: Cut the tofu into 4 equal triangles by slicing an "X" through the block. Cut each triangle in half horizontally to make 8 equal triangles. Make a pocket in each triangle by slicing each piece as you would a hamburger roll, starting at the point and stopping ½ inch from the wide end. Place tofu in marinade. Soak for 10 minutes, then turn and soak another 10 minutes.

Divide the filling into 8 portions. Gently stuff the triangles, smoothing the filled edges with your fingers. (See the tofu smile?)

Coat a nonstick skillet with vegetable spray. Place 4 of the triangles in the pan, standing them on their filled edges. (The filling will not come out.) Cook for 1 minute on each edge. Then cook for 1 minute on each flat side. Add ⅓ cup stock and simmer for 3 minutes. Flip the triangles and simmer for 3 minutes more. Remove to a serving platter. Repeat with remaining triangles and stock.

Add marinade to pan and reduce by half. Pour marinade over tofu and sprinkle with scallions.

Yield: 4 servings

Spinach, Mushroom and Cheese Panino

This "new, improved" version of the grilled cheese sandwich guarantees fiber, calcium, beta-carotene and vitamin C—or your money back!

1   tablespoon Vegetable Stock (page 452)
1   small onion, cut into thin strips
1   small clove garlic, minced
½   small red pepper, cut into thin strips
¼   pound mushrooms, thinly sliced
¼   pound fresh spinach, cut into thin strips
⅛   teaspoon dried basil
4   slices Triple Wheat and Millet Bread (on opposite page) or other whole grain bread or rolls
4   thin slices part-skim mozzarella cheese, each cut in half
4   slices tomato

In a nonstick skillet, heat stock over low heat. Add onions, garlic and pepper and cook for 5 minutes, stirring frequently. Add mushrooms, spinach and basil. Cook for 3 minutes.

Preheat oven to 350°F.

On each slice of bread, layer a half slice of cheese, one-quarter of the spinach mixture, another half slice of cheese and a slice of tomato. Sprinkle with a little basil. Wrap each sandwich loosely in foil. Bake for 5 minutes, or until cheese melts and sandwich is hot.

Yield: 4 servings

VARIATIONS:
● *Add a layer of sliced cooked chicken or turkey, or flaked, water-packed tuna.*
● *Use spinach mixture as a topping for baked potatoes.*
● *Add spinach mixture to cooked rice or other grains.*
● *Use spinach mixture as a side dish with poultry or meats.*

Triple Wheat and Millet Bread

Use this bread to make sandwiches that pack extra amounts of fiber, calcium and vitamin E.

1   package dry yeast
½   cup warm skim milk
       (105°–115°F)
2   tablespoons honey
1   cup part-skim ricotta
       cheese, at room
       temperature
1   cup very warm water
       (120°–130°F)
¼   cup safflower oil
3   cups whole wheat flour
1   to 1½ cups bread flour
½   cup cooked millet*
⅓   cup wheat flakes or rolled
       oats
2   tablespoons wheat germ
       or bran
1   teaspoon salt
2   teaspoons sesame or
       poppy seeds

Stir yeast into milk. Set aside to proof.

In a medium-size bowl, whisk together honey, ricotta, water and oil.

In a large bowl, mix flours, millet, wheat flakes or rolled oats, wheat germ or bran and salt. Make a well in center of dry ingredients. Pour in ricotta mixture and yeast mixture and stir to form a soft dough.

Turn out onto a lightly floured surface. Knead for 15 to 20 minutes, or until dough is very elastic, adding more flour only if necessary.

Coat a large bowl with vegetable spray, then turn dough into the bowl, turning to coat the top. Cover bowl with plastic wrap. Put into a warm spot and let rise until doubled in bulk, about 1¼ hours.

Divide dough in half. Cover and let rest 15 minutes. Shape into loaves and place in two 8 × 4-inch loaf pans. Cover and let rise again in a warm spot until doubled in bulk, 35 to 45 minutes.

Preheat oven to 400°F.

Spray or brush loaves with cold water and sprinkle with seeds.

Bake for 10 minutes, then reduce heat to 325°F and continue baking for 45 to 50 minutes, or until loaves sound hollow when tapped. Turn out onto a rack and let cool completely before slicing.

Yield: 2 loaves

*To cook millet, first toast ½ cup millet in a nonstick skillet, stirring constantly, until light brown. Heat 1 cup water to boiling, then add toasted millet. Reduce heat to low, cover and cook for 10 minutes, or until water is absorbed. Any remaining millet can be eaten as a cereal or side dish or in casseroles.

VARIATION: *You can also make rolls from this recipe. Coat muffin tins with vegetable spray. After the first rising, divide dough into 30 even pieces and form into 1½-inch balls. Place dough in muffin tins and let rise until doubled in bulk, about 25 minutes. Preheat oven to 400°F then bake for 20 minutes, or until rolls sound hollow when tapped.*

Warm Spinach-Chicken Salad

The cancer-fighting ingredient in this delicious luncheon dish is the antioxidant vitamin E.

½ pound spinach
⅓ cup julienned carrots
⅓ cup julienned snow peas
⅓ cup bean sprouts
2 cups shredded, cooked
   chicken
1 tablespoon sunflower oil
1 teaspoon sesame oil
2 teaspoons rice vinegar or
   white wine vinegar
1 teaspoon lemon juice
½ teaspoon soy sauce
¼ teaspoon dried basil
⅛ teaspoon dried oregano
2 teaspoons sunflower seeds
1 teaspoon sesame seeds
   freshly ground black
      pepper, to taste

Wash spinach thoroughly and dry on paper towels. Tear into bite-size pieces.

In a large, glass salad bowl, combine spinach with carrots, snow peas, bean sprouts and chicken.

In a small saucepan, combine oils, vinegar, lemon juice, soy sauce, basil and oregano. Heat just until warm over low heat.

Pour dressing over salad. Sprinkle with seeds and pepper and serve immediately.

Yield: 4 servings

VARIATION: *Replace chicken with 6 ounces tofu, cubed.*

Dinner Recipes Designed to Protect Your Health

Antipasto with Baked Oysters

Not only is this entrée delicious, it's also high in calcium.

Oysters
- 8 oysters on the half shell
- ½ teaspoon French-style mustard
- ¼ teaspoon fennel seeds, crushed
- ¼ cup minced tomato, well drained
- 1½ tablespoons minced scallions

Sauce
- ¼ cup low-fat yogurt
- 1 tablespoon instant nonfat dry milk
- ¼ teaspoon French-style mustard
- ¼ teaspoon fennel seeds, crushed

Antipasto
- 15 leaves kale (purple and green)
- 1 cup steamed broccoli
- 1 can (6 ounces) salmon, drained and chunked
- 8 dried figs
- ½ cup part-skim ricotta cheese

To prepare oysters: Preheat oven to 450°F. In a 9-inch pie plate, arrange oysters in their shells. Combine the mustard and fennel seeds and spoon mixture over oysters. Bake for 10 minutes, or until oysters change color from gray to a whitish shade. Sprinkle with tomatoes and scallions.

To make sauce: Combine the yogurt, dry milk, mustard and fennel seeds in a small bowl.

To make antipasto: Line a serving platter with kale. Arrange broccoli, salmon and oysters on kale.

Slit the fat part of each fig with a sharp knife. Using a small spoon or a pastry bag fitted with a small tube, fill each fig with ricotta. Add to platter. Serve with yogurt sauce. Use the kale leaves to scoop up other ingredients.

Yield: 4 to 6 servings

Asparagus and Tomato Gratiné

This generous side dish provides vitamin E.

2 tablespoons sunflower oil
1 pound asparagus
1 tablespoon minced fresh parsley
½ teaspoon dried basil or 1 teaspoon minced fresh basil
¼ teaspoon dried marjoram or ½ teaspoon minced fresh marjoram
¼ cup minced onion
¼ cup minced celery
1 can (16 ounces) whole tomatoes, drained and chopped
1 tablespoon whole-grain bread crumbs
½ tablespoon wheat germ

Preheat oven to 375°F.

In a gratiné dish or shallow baking dish, heat the oil. Arrange asparagus in the dish and top with parsley, basil, marjoram, onions, celery and tomatoes. Cover dish with foil and bake 20 minutes, or until asparagus is just tender.

Combine bread crumbs with wheat germ and sprinkle over the top. Bake uncovered for 30 minutes.

Yield: 4 servings

Broccoli-Stuffed Flounder

The crunch of almonds sets off the silken texture of the fish in this vitamin E-rich entrée.

½ pound broccoli spears
2 tablespoons chopped fresh parsley
1 tablespoon minced onion
¼ teaspoon dried thyme
⅛ teaspoon freshly ground white pepper
2 egg whites, at room temperature
4 flounder fillets, 4 to 6 ounces each
1 tablespoon sliced, unblanched almonds
2 teaspoons safflower oil
1 tablespoon lemon juice
½ teaspoon French-style mustard

Place broccoli in an 8-inch square, microwave-safe, baking dish and add 1 tablespoon water. Cover with plastic wrap. Microwave on high setting for 4 to 5 minutes, or until tender. Drain, then place in a food processor or blender with parsley, onion, thyme, pepper and egg whites and process until very smooth.

Spread about 2 tablespoons of puree onto each fish fillet. Roll up and secure with toothpicks. Arrange fillets in the baking dish.

Microwave almonds for 45 seconds on high setting.

In a small bowl, stir together oil, lemon juice and mustard. Spoon over fish. Cover dish with plastic wrap and microwave on high setting for 6 to 8 minutes, or until fish flakes easily with a fork. Allow to stand 5 minutes before serving. Sprinkle with almonds before serving.

Yield: 4 servings

VARIATION: *To cook conventionally, steam broccoli until tender. Puree vegetables and prepare fish as instructed above. Preheat oven to 375° F. Toast almonds in oven for 1 minute. Prepare sauce as instructed above and spoon over fish. Bake for 15 minutes, or until fish flakes easily. Sprinkle with almonds before serving.*

Bulgur Curry

This is a delicious high-fiber accompaniment to baked chicken.

1 onion, minced
2 tablespoons butter or margarine
1 cup bulgur
1½–2 teaspoons curry powder
2 cups Chicken Stock (page 452)
⅓ cup raisins

In a heavy 2-quart saucepan, sauté onions in the butter or margarine until lightly browned. Stir in bulgur and curry powder, sauté briefly, then add stock and raisins. Cover and cook over low heat for 20 minutes, or until all stock is absorbed. Fluff with a fork before serving.

Yield: 4 servings

Chicken Tangiers

Not only is this dinner low in fat, it also has a good supply of
fiber and beta-carotene, as well as vitamin C.

6¼   cups Chicken Stock
      (page 452) or water
1   cup whole barley
1½   teaspoons minced fresh
      rosemary or ¾
      teaspoon crumbled
      dried rosemary
1   pound boneless, skinless
      chicken breasts, cut
      into 1-inch cubes
1   medium onion, chopped
4   carrots, cut into 1 × 1½-
      inch pieces
1   small red pepper, diced
2   small turnips, diced
1   small head cauliflower,
      broken into small
      florets
5   sprigs fresh parsley
⅛   teaspoon saffron threads,
      crushed, then
      dissolved in 2
      tablespoons warm
      water
1   cup drained, canned
      chick-peas
¾   teaspoon cinnamon
      minced fresh parsley or
      cilantro

In a medium-size saucepan, bring 4
cups stock or water to a boil over medium
heat. Slowly add barley and 1 teaspoon rosemary. Cover and simmer about 40 minutes,
or until stock is absorbed and barley is
tender.

Meanwhile, in a Dutch oven, heat ¼
cup stock or water over low heat. Add half
the chicken cubes and cook for 3 minutes.
Remove with a slotted spoon and set aside.
Cook remaining chicken and remove.

Cook onions in liquid remaining in pot
until soft, about 5 minutes. Add carrots, peppers, turnips, cauliflower, parsley sprigs, ½
teaspoon rosemary, saffron with water and 2
cups stock or water. Bring to a boil. Cover
and simmer 15 minutes. Stir in chick-peas,
cinnamon and cooked chicken. Cover and
simmer 10 minutes, or until vegetables and
chicken are tender. Remove parsley sprigs.

To serve, spoon barley onto a large serving platter, arrange chicken mixture on top
and sprinkle with minced parsley or
cilantro.

Yield: 6 servings

VARIATIONS:
- *Add raisins with chick-peas.*
- *Add one plantain (if available), peeled and cut into ¼-inch rounds, with carrots.*
- *Chopped turnip greens will increase beta-carotene and vitamin C content. Add with carrots.*
- *Substitute cubes of very lean cooked lamb for chicken.*
- *Serve over cooked brown rice, millet or couscous instead of barley.*

Confetti Brussels Sprouts

This colorful side dish provides fiber, beta-carotene and vitamin C.

1   pound medium Brussels
      sprouts
¼   cup minced red onion
¼   cup minced red pepper
¼   pound mushrooms, finely
      chopped
1   tablespoon minced fresh
      parsley
1   teaspoon mustard seed
1   teaspoon coarse, French-
      style mustard
1   tablespoon balsamic or
      red wine vinegar
      freshly ground black
      pepper, to taste

Place Brussels sprouts and 2 table-spoons water in a microwave-safe casserole. Cover and microwave on high setting for 4 to 6 minutes, or until just tender. Let stand 5 minutes, then drain. Cut Brussels sprouts in half.

Meanwhile, place onions, peppers and 1 tablespoon water in 1-quart microwave-safe casserole. Cover and microwave on high setting for 2 minutes. Add mushrooms and microwave 1 minute. Let stand 3 minutes, then add parsley, mustard seed, mustard, vinegar and pepper. Stir into Brussels sprouts and toss gently. Serve immediately or at room temperature.

Yield: 4 servings

VARIATION: *To cook conventionally, place Brussels sprouts in a steamer over boiling water and steam for 10 to 15 minutes, or until crisp-tender. Drain and cut Brussels sprouts in half.*

Meanwhile, in a medium-size skillet, sauté onions, peppers and mushrooms in 2 tablespoons water until mushrooms give up their liquid. Add parsley, mustard seed, mustard, vinegar and pepper and sauté for 5 minutes.

Stir mushroom mixture into Brussels sprouts and toss gently.

Equinox Salad

A salute to spring and beta-carotene.

2 cups young spinach
8 red radishes, thinly sliced
4 scallions, cut into julienne strips
½ cup peas
½ cup coarsely shredded daikon radish*
¼ cup enoki mushrooms*
1 tablespoon olive oil
2 teaspoons balsamic vinegar
½ teaspoon French-style mustard
  pinch of grated whole nutmeg

In a large bowl, combine the spinach, red radishes, scallions, peas, daikon radishes and mushrooms.

In a small bowl, whisk together the oil, vinegar, mustard and nutmeg. Add to vegetables and toss well.

Yield: 4 servings

*Daikon radishes and enoki mushrooms can commonly be found at oriental markets or well-stocked supermarkets.

NOTE: *When shredding the daikon radish, try to make long ribbons. Either use the coarsest side of a grater and push the radish lengthwise along it or use a potato peeler.*

Green-Thumb Torte

A dinner dish that's high in calcium.

2 teaspoons olive oil
2 cloves garlic, minced
⅔ cup minced onion
½ cup blanched, minced green kale
½ cup blanched, minced collards or turnip greens
2 cups bite-size broccoli florets, blanched
2 cups cooked rice
1 medium tomato, chopped
1 teaspoon dried basil
½ teaspoon dried thyme
2 eggs
2 egg whites
½ cup part-skim ricotta cheese
1 teaspoon French-style mustard
⅓ cup skim milk
2 tablespoons freshly grated Romano cheese
  paprika

In a medium-size skillet, sauté garlic and onion in oil for about 3 minutes. Transfer to a medium-size mixing bowl, along with the kale, collards or turnip greens, broccoli, rice, tomatoes, basil and thyme.

Preheat oven to 375°F.

In another bowl, combine eggs, egg whites, ricotta, mustard, milk and Romano. Add to the rice mixture and combine well.

Coat a 10-inch pie plate with vegetable spray. Scoop the mixture into the pan. Sprinkle with paprika and bake for 25 to 30 minutes, or until firm to the touch. Let cool slightly before slicing.

Yield: 8 servings

NOTE: *Blanch greens by putting them in a strainer and pouring boiling water over them for 3 to 5 seconds. Blanch broccoli by placing in boiling water for 2 minutes.*

Pasta with Broccoli Sauce

This dish is a cancer-fighting bonanza, containing lots of calcium, beta-carotene and vitamin C.

4   cups broccoli florets
1   clove garlic, quartered
¼   cup sunflower seeds, toasted
2   tablespoons olive oil
1   cup part-skim ricotta cheese
½   cup skim milk
      freshly ground black pepper, to taste
⅛   teaspoon ground whole nutmeg, or to taste
12   ounces cooked spaghetti
⅓   cup diced tomatoes

Steam broccoli until tender, about 8 minutes. Cool slightly. Reserve a few florets for garnish.

Place broccoli, garlic, sunflower seeds and oil in food processor or blender and process until smooth. Add ricotta and milk and process again until smooth. Add pepper and nutmeg.

Turn cooked spaghetti into a heated serving bowl. Add tomatoes to spaghetti and spoon on half of sauce. Toss to combine. Garnish with reserved broccoli. Serve with remaining sauce if desired.

Yield: 4 servings

Savory Turkey Scallop Normandy

With this main dish, you get the health benefits of lean meat.

1¼   pounds boneless turkey breast cutlets, ¼ inch thick
¼   teaspoon dried savory
¼   teaspoon dried marjoram
1   teaspoon dried thyme
2   tablespoons lemon juice
2   tablespoons minced shallots
1   cup apple juice
½   cup Chicken Stock (page 452)
1   Golden Delicious apple, cored and cut into ¼-inch slices
      ground mace
      watercress sprigs

If necessary, pound cutlets to ¼-inch thickness. In a small bowl, combine savory, marjoram, thyme and lemon juice. Rub over cutlets. Cover and refrigerate for 1 hour.

Preheat oven to 200°F.

Coat a large nonstick skillet heavily with vegetable spray and place over medium heat. Add half the cutlets. Cook until golden, about 2 minutes on each side. Remove from pan and keep warm in oven. Cook remaining cutlets and place in oven.

Add shallots to skillet and cook 2 minutes. Add apple juice and stock and bring to a boil over high heat. Boil briskly until liquid is reduced by half, then reduce heat to low. Add apples and sprinkle lightly with mace. Cook 2 minutes, or until apples are tender, turning once.

To serve, arrange turkey on a serving platter. Spoon apples and sauce over cutlets and garnish with watercress sprigs.

Yield: 4 servings

VARIATION: *Use sliced pears, raspberries or strawberries instead of apples.*

Soup of Two Greens

This rather continental appetizer is high in beta-carotene.
Whole grain cornbread is a delicious accompaniment.

Dumplings
- 1 small onion, finely chopped
- 3 tablespoons minced fresh parsley
- 8 ounces ground veal
- 1 egg
- 3 slices whole grain bread freshly ground black pepper, to taste

Soup
- 6 cups Vegetable Stock (page 452)
- 1 small carrot, finely chopped
- 1 clove garlic, minced
- 1 bay leaf
- 4 cups chopped kale
- 2 cups chopped spinach
- 1½ cups drained, cooked or canned white beans

To make dumplings: Coat a small non-stick skillet with vegetable spray, then heat the skillet over low heat. Add onions and parsley. Cover and cook, stirring occasionally, until vegetables are tender, about 7 minutes. Transfer to a medium-size bowl. Add veal and egg.

Soak bread in water for 3 minutes and squeeze dry. Add to veal mixture along with pepper and mix well. Refrigerate 30 minutes. Using about 2 teaspoons veal mixture per dumpling, roll between your hands. Place dumplings in skillet and brown on all sides. Remove and set aside.

To make soup: Combine stock, carrots, garlic and bay leaf in a 4-quart saucepan or Dutch oven. Bring to a simmer, then add kale and simmer 30 to 40 minutes, or until kale is tender. Remove bay leaf. Add spinach, beans and dumplings. Simmer 3 minutes. Serve immediately.

Yield: 4 servings

VARIATIONS:
- *Use collards, escarole, endive, Swiss chard and turnips or mustard greens instead of kale and spinach.*
- *Substitute black-eyed peas, lentils or cooked rice for beans.*

Sweet Potato and Orange Casserole

This luscious concoction offers lots of protective beta-carotene.

2   pounds sweet potatoes
3   navel oranges
1   tablespoon cornstarch
1   cup orange juice
3   tablespoons honey or
      maple syrup
⅛   teaspoon ground cloves
2   tablespoons slivered
      almonds
2   tablespoons unsweetened,
      shredded coconut

In a large saucepan, cook the sweet potatoes, with enough water to cover, until they are easily pierced with a fork. Drain and set aside until cool enough to handle. Peel, then cut into ¼-inch slices. Set aside.

Coat a 13 × 9-inch baking dish with vegetable spray.

Finely grate enough rind from the oranges to equal 2 teaspoons; set aside. Peel the oranges, removing all the white pith. Cut oranges crosswise into ¼-inch slices. Mix gently with the sweet potatoes, then transfer to prepared baking dish.

Preheat oven to 375°F.

In a 1-quart saucepan, mix the orange rind, cornstarch, juice, honey or maple syrup and cloves. Cook over medium heat, stirring constantly, until mixture thickens. Pour over sweet potatoes and oranges. Sprinkle with almonds and coconut and bake for 15 minutes, or until heated through.

Yield: 8 to 10 servings

Swiss Chard Packets
Nestled in a Bed of Vegetables

The ingredients in this elegant casserole combine to provide
plentiful amounts of beta-carotene.

12   leaves Swiss chard
½   cup minced onion
1   clove garlic, minced
½   pound very lean ground
      beef
1   cup cooked brown rice
3   tablespoons tomato paste
1   egg white
1   tablespoon lemon juice
½   teaspoon grated lemon
      rind
2   tablespoons minced
      fresh dill
2   tablespoons minced
      fresh parsley
1   tablespoon chopped,
      toasted pine nuts
1   carrot, cut into julienne
      strips
1   leek, cut into julienne
      strips (white part plus
      1 inch of green)
1½   cups Chicken Stock
      (page 452)
4   sprigs fresh dill

Cut stems off Swiss chard leaves and
trim back ribs. Set 4 leaves aside. Pour boiling water over remaining leaves and let
steep for 5 minutes. Drain and pat thoroughly dry.

Cook onions and garlic in a nonstick
skillet for 5 minutes. Add ground beef and
cook until browned. Transfer to a medium-
size bowl. Add rice, tomato paste, egg
white, lemon juice and rind, minced dill,
parsley and pine nuts.

Preheat oven to 375° F.

Place a chard leaf on a flat surface,
trimmed side up. Place 2 tablespoons of filling in center of leaf. Fold up bottom, then
fold sides in and roll up. Repeat procedure
with remaining leaves and filling.

Chop 4 reserved chard leaves. Scatter
chopped leaves, carrots and leeks over the
bottom of a 10-inch square ovenproof casserole or 13 × 9-inch pan. Arrange stuffed
packets seam side down on vegetables.
Pour stock over packets and top with dill
sprigs. Cover dish with foil and bake for 35
to 40 minutes, or until leaves are tender.

Yield: 4 servings

Veal Stew with Harvest Vegetables

This great family meal provides lots of cancer-fighting beta-carotene.

1 tablespoon olive oil
1 pound boneless veal shoulder, cut into 1-inch cubes
1 medium onion, chopped
1 stalk celery, chopped
2 cloves garlic, minced
1 can (14½ to 15 ounces) whole tomatoes
½ cup water or Vegetable Stock (page 452)
⅛ teaspoon freshly ground black pepper
½ teaspoon oregano
4 sprigs fresh parsley
4 medium carrots, cut into 1-inch chunks
2 pounds butternut squash, cut into 1-inch chunks
  minced fresh parsley

In a large skillet or Dutch oven, heat oil over medium heat. Add veal to skillet in batches and cook each batch until browned on all sides, removing onto a plate with a slotted spoon. Add onions, celery and garlic to the skillet and cook, stirring frequently, until vegetables are soft, about 5 minutes.

Return veal and liquid that has accumulated to the skillet. Add tomatoes, water or stock, pepper, oregano and parsley sprigs. Bring to a boil. Reduce heat to low, cover and simmer 1¼ hours. Add carrots and squash. Simmer for about 25 minutes, or until vegetables and veal are tender. Sprinkle with parsley before serving. Serve with rice or orzo (rice-shaped pasta).

Yield: 6 servings

VARIATION: *Add other chopped vegetables, such as parsnips, turnips or mushrooms.*

Totally Wholesome Desserts and Snacks

Apple-Prune Crunch

Put vitamin E and fiber on the menu with this snappy, spicy dessert.

3½	cups thinly sliced baking apples (4 medium)
½	cup pitted prunes, chopped
2	teaspoons lemon juice
1½	teaspoons ground cinnamon
¾	cup rolled oats
½	cup wheat germ
¼	teaspoon ground nutmeg
1	tablespoon safflower oil
¼	cup date sugar*
¼	cup hot apple juice or water

Preheat oven to 375°F.

Coat a 1½-quart ovenproof casserole with vegetable spray.

In a medium-size bowl, combine apples, prunes, lemon juice and 1 teaspoon cinnamon.

In another medium-size bowl, stir together oats, wheat germ, nutmeg, oil, date sugar and ½ teaspoon cinnamon.

Spoon one-third of oat mixture on the bottom of prepared casserole, then cover with half the fruit mixture. Repeat layers, ending with oat mixture. Pour apple juice over top. Cover with foil and bake for 3 minutes. Uncover and bake for 10 minutes longer, or until apples are tender and top is lightly browned.

Yield: 4 servings

*Date sugar can be found in most health food stores.

VARIATIONS:
- *Use ground ginger or allspice instead of nutmeg.*
- *Use other fruits instead of apples—peaches, pears or plums would all work well. (This substitution will affect the vitamin E content, since apples are a better source than other fruits.)*
- *Use dried apricots (a good source of beta-carotene) in place of some or all of the prunes.*

Chewy Fruit Snacks

Sink your teeth into something luscious and healthful and loaded with beta-carotene.

¾   cup coarsely chopped
        dried apricots
¼   cup coarsely chopped
        pitted prunes
¼   cup chopped raisins
3   tablespoons orange juice
¾   teaspoon grated orange
        rind
1   teaspoon ground
        cinnamon
¼   teaspoon ground nutmeg
1   cup lightly toasted rolled
        oats
1   tablespoon wheat germ
1   tablespoon finely chopped
        pecans
     ground nuts or sesame
        seeds (optional)

In a large bowl, combine apricots, prunes, raisins, orange juice and rind, cinnamon and nutmeg. Let stand 1 hour, stirring occasionally. Transfer mixture to a food processor and chop fine.

Combine fruit mixture, oats, wheat germ and pecans. Shape rounded teaspoonful of mixture into balls. If desired, roll in nuts or seeds. Store in an airtight container lined with wax paper.

Yield: 36 snacks

VARIATIONS:
● *Substitute apple juice for orange juice.*
● *Use other nuts like walnuts or almonds, or chopped sunflower seeds instead of pecans.*

Cranberry Pears

Pretty as a picture, this dessert brings elegance—and fiber—to the buffet table.

8   pears
1   tablespoon lime juice
2   cups cranberries
1   cup apple or pear juice
2   tablespoons honey, or to
        taste
½   teaspoon ground
        cinnamon
⅛   teaspoon ground cloves

Using a melon scoop, core the pears from the bottom. Leave stems intact. Brush pears with lime juice and arrange them upright in a shallow baking dish.

Preheat oven to 350°F.

In a 2-quart saucepan, combine the cranberries, apple or pear juice and any remaining lime juice. Cook over medium heat until cranberry skins pop. Stir in honey, cinnamon and cloves. Pour over pears.

Bake for 30 minutes, or until pears can be easily pierced with a knife but still hold their shape. Serve warm.

Yield: 8 servings

Cucumber Cups with Herbed Jalapeño Cheese

These zesty snacks are especially good sources of calcium.

3 medium cucumbers
1 package (7½ ounces) farmer cheese
2 tablespoons minced scallions
1 small clove garlic, minced
2 tablespoons minced canned jalapeño peppers, well drained
1 tablespoon minced fresh cilantro or flat-leaf parsley

Score cucumbers with tines of a fork, then cut crosswise into 1-inch pieces. Scoop out most of pulp and seeds with a small spoon or melon ball cutter. Place on paper towels and let drain for 30 minutes.

Place cheese in a food processor or blender and process until smooth. Spoon into a small bowl. Stir in scallions, garlic, peppers and cilantro or parsley.

Fill each cucumber cup with about 2 teaspoons of cheese mixture. Place on a serving plate and cover with plastic wrap. Chill thoroughly before serving.

Yield: about 24 snacks

VARIATION: *Use other vegetables instead of cucumbers—zucchini cups, hollowed-out cherry or plum tomatoes, mushroom caps, thick slices of red or green pepper. (By using tomatoes or peppers you will increase vitamin C.)*

Frozen Cherry Pops

Their secret nutrient is calcium.

1 tablespoon unflavored gelatin
1 cup white grape juice
1 pound soft tofu
1 cup pitted, fresh or thawed frozen sweet cherries
2 tablespoons safflower oil
⅓ cup honey
1 tablespoon frozen orange juice concentrate
1 tablespoon lime juice
⅛ teaspoon almond extract
1 teaspoon vanilla extract

In a small saucepan, dissolve gelatin in grape juice. Bring to a boil, then reduce heat and continue to heat and stir for about 1 minute. Set saucepan in the refrigerator.

Meanwhile, combine remaining ingredients in a blender or food processor and process until mixture is completely smooth and no flecks of tofu are visible. While processor is running, add gelatin mixture and combine.

Freeze in ice cube trays or popsicle molds. Or, to serve the mixture as a dessert, freeze it in an 8 × 8-inch glass dish and process in a food processor before serving.

Yield: 1½ pints fruit mixture

VARIATION: *Substitute peaches for the cherries and maple syrup for the honey.*

Harvest Pumpkin Roll

The real harvest from this delicious dessert is health-boosting beta-carotene.

Pumpkin Roll

1	cup whole wheat pastry flour
1	teaspoon baking powder
1	teaspoon baking soda
1½	teaspoons ground cinnamon
¼	teaspoon ground allspice
2	eggs, at room temperature
2	egg whites, at room temperature
½	cup honey
1	cup pumpkin puree

Filling

1½	cups dried apricots
1¾	cups water
⅓	cup honey
1	stick cinnamon, 3 inches long
1	teaspoon grated lemon rind
¼	teaspoon ground ginger
¼	teaspoon ground nutmeg

To make pumpkin roll: Preheat oven to 350°F.

Coat a 15½ × 10½-inch jelly roll pan with vegetable spray. Line with wax paper, then spray wax paper. Lightly flour paper, shaking out the excess.

Sift together flour, baking powder, baking soda, cinnamon and allspice. In a medium-size bowl, beat together eggs, egg whites and honey until very pale and thick, 5 to 7 minutes. Beat in pumpkin at low speed. Sift dry mixture over pumpkin mixture and beat at low speed 1 minute. Pour into prepared pan and smooth with a spatula. Bake for 10 to 15 minutes or until top springs back when lightly pressed with your finger and cake has shrunk from the sides of the pan. Cool on a wire rack 3 minutes.

Lay a sheet of wax paper on top of cake and lay a baking sheet on top of wax paper, then invert cake. Lift off jelly roll pan and peel away baking wax paper. Starting with a narrow end, roll cake around the clean wax paper. Set aside to cool thoroughly.

To make filling: In a small saucepan, combine apricots, water, honey, cinnamon, lemon rind, ginger and nutmeg. Bring to a boil over medium heat. Reduce heat to low, cover and simmer for 45 minutes, stirring occasionally. Strain, reserving juice. Place in a food processor or blender and process until smooth, adding juice if necessary.

To assemble: Unroll cake and remove wax paper. Spread filling to within ½ inch of edges, then reroll. Place cake roll on a serving platter, seam side down. With a serrated knife, trim off ends, cutting on the diagonal. Refrigerate until ready to serve.

Yield: 12 servings

VARIATIONS:
- *Instead of apricot filling, fill cake roll with sweetened yogurt cheese, plain or mixed with pumpkin puree or applesauce; sweetened whipped Neufchâtel cheese and sliced strawberries, other berries or sliced apricots or peaches; fruit butters such as apple or peach; or fruit preserves or jam.*

Light and Creamy Mango Mousse

Special enough for your most formal company dinner, this unusual—and beautiful—dessert offers plenty of beta-carotene, as well as calcium.

1   cup fresh strawberries, cut lengthwise into quarters
1   tablespoon orange juice
1   tablespoon unflavored gelatin
¼   cup cold water
1   mango, peeled and pitted
½   cup low-fat yogurt
2   egg whites, at room temperature
3   tablespoons honey
½   cup cold evaporated skim milk

In a small bowl, combine strawberries and orange juice. Refrigerate 1 hour.

In a small saucepan, sprinkle gelatin over water. Let stand 10 minutes to soften, then heat mixture over low heat to dissolve gelatin.

Place mango in food processor or blender and process until smooth. Pour into a medium-size bowl, stir in yogurt and fold in gelatin.

In a small bowl, beat egg whites until soft peaks form. Gradually beat in honey, and beat until stiff. Fold into mango mixture.

In a small chilled bowl, whip skim milk. Fold into mango mixture. Cover and chill until set, about 2 hours.

Spoon strawberries into parfait or dessert glasses. Spoon mousse over strawberries and serve immediately.

Yield: 4 servings

Nectarine Cheese Tart

A luscious dessert that provides health benefits in the form of beta-carotene.

1   tablespoon wheat germ
2   cups low-fat cottage cheese
5   tablespoons honey
2   eggs
1¼   teaspoons vanilla extract
2   teaspoons lemon juice
1   tablespoon cornstarch
¼   teaspoon grated whole nutmeg
3   tablespoons peach or apricot preserves
5   nectarines, peeled and thinly sliced

Preheat oven to 350°F.

Lightly coat a 9-inch ceramic quiche pan or pie plate with vegetable spray. Sprinkle wheat germ over bottom.

Combine cottage cheese, honey, eggs, vanilla, 1 teaspoon lemon juice, cornstarch and nutmeg in a food processor or blender and process until smooth. Pour into prepared pan and bake for 30 minutes. Cool on a wire rack.

In a small saucepan, melt preserves with 1 teaspoon lemon juice over low heat, stirring constantly. Force the mixture through a sieve into a small bowl.

Arrange the nectarines overlapping in concentric circles on the tart and brush with apricot glaze. Chill for 1 hour before serving.

Yield: 8 to 10 servings

Raspberry Bread Puddings with Sunshine Sauce

Tangy and sweet, this pudding is high in both fiber and vitamin C. Serve with Sunshine Sauce.

Bread puddings
¾ cup skim milk
½ teaspoon vanilla extract
4 slices lightly toasted whole wheat bread, cut into ½-inch chunks
¼ teaspoon ground cinnamon
dash of ground mace
1 cup fresh or thawed and drained frozen raspberries
3 egg whites, at room temperature
2 tablespoons maple syrup

Sunshine Sauce
1 peach or nectarine, peeled, pitted and sliced, or ½ cup frozen peach or nectarine slices, thawed
2 teaspoons maple syrup
½ teaspoon vanilla extract
dash of ground nutmeg
¼ cup low-fat yogurt

To make bread puddings: In a small saucepan, heat milk and vanilla until warm.

In a medium-size bowl, toss bread cubes with cinnamon and mace. Stir in milk mixture. Let stand 20 minutes, or until all milk is absorbed. Stir in raspberries.

Preheat oven to 375° F. Beat egg whites until soft peaks form. Drizzle in syrup and continue to beat until stiff peaks form. Fold egg whites into bread mixture. Spoon mixture into 4 (6-ounce) ungreased custard cups, then place them on a baking sheet. Bake for 15 minutes, or until puddings puff and a toothpick inserted in center comes out clean. Remove from oven and let cool slightly.

To make Sunshine Sauce: Place fruit slices in blender or food processor with syrup, vanilla and nutmeg and process until smooth. Blend in yogurt. Spoon over bread puddings before serving.

Yield: 4 servings

Strawberry Shake

Vitamin C and calcium pack power into this shake.

⅓ cup halved strawberries
2 tablespoons frozen apple juice concentrate
¾ cup skim milk
2 tablespoons nonfat dry milk
⅛ teaspoon vanilla extract
dash of ground cinnamon or nutmeg
2 ice cubes

Combine all ingredients in a food processor or blender and process until ice dissolves and mixture is well blended. Serve immediately.

Yield: 1 serving

NOTE: *If strawberries are not especially flavorful, add ½ teaspoon honey.*

VARIATION: *Substitute fresh or frozen blueberries, raspberries or peeled peaches for strawberries.*

Basic Recipes

Chicken Stock

6   pounds chicken backs and
    necks
8   quarts water
2   large onions
3   stalks celery with leaves,
    coarsely chopped
4   carrots, coarsely chopped
2   bay leaves
1   cup parsley sprigs
½   teaspoon dried thyme
½   teaspoon peppercorns
2   cloves garlic

Place chicken in a large stockpot. Cover with water and bring to a boil, skimming froth off surface. Reduce heat to low and simmer for 2 hours. Add remaining ingredients and bring to a boil. Reduce heat and simmer 2 hours longer. Strain through a cheesecloth-lined strainer into a large bowl or pot. Cool bowl or pot quickly in ice water. Pour stock into storage containers and refrigerate or freeze. Spoon off and discard fat before using.

Yield: 4 quarts

Vegetable Stock

4   cups coarsely chopped
    onions
4   medium carrots, coarsely
    chopped
4   stalks celery with leaves,
    coarsely chopped
1   cup chopped tomatoes
½   pound parsnips, coarsely
    chopped
5   cloves garlic
1   bunch fresh parsley
2   bay leaves
1   teaspoon peppercorns
½   teaspoon dried thyme

Combine all ingredients in an 8-quart stockpot with enough water to cover vegetables. Bring to a boil, skimming froth off surface. Reduce heat to low and simmer about 4 hours. Strain through a cheesecloth-lined strainer into a large pot or bowl, pressing down on vegetables. Cool pot or bowl quickly in cold water. Pour into quart containers and refrigerate or freeze.

Yield: About 3 quarts

Sauces and Spreads

Tangerine Raisin Butter

A delightfully different bread spread that offers both vitamin C and fiber.

¾   cup tangerine juice
1½ cups raisins
    pinch of ground
    cinnamon
    pinch of ground cloves

Combine all ingredients in a 1-quart saucepan. Simmer, uncovered, for 10 minutes. Process in a blender or food processor until smooth. Refrigerate.

Yield: 1¼ cups

Orange-Almond Cheese

Serve this as a breakfast cheese with warm muffins or toast. Or mix it into hot cereal. It will give a boost to your calcium levels.

4   cups low-fat yogurt
2   tablespoons raisins, minced
1   tablespoon slivered almonds, toasted and chopped
1½ teaspoons honey
1½ teaspoons frozen orange juice concentrate
    pinch of ground cinnamon

Spoon yogurt into a sieve lined with cheesecloth and allow to drain 8 hours or overnight in the sink. Transfer to a medium-size bowl. Mix in raisins, almonds, honey, orange juice concentrate and cinnamon. Store in a covered container in the refrigerator.

Yield: about 1¼ cups

Pesto Cheese

Serve with crudités, whole-grain crackers or baked potatoes for a wholesome, calcium-packed snack.

4   cups low-fat yogurt
⅓   cup tightly packed fresh basil
2   tablespoons sunflower seeds
1   teaspoon olive oil
1   teaspoon French-style mustard
1   clove garlic

Spoon yogurt into a sieve lined with cheesecloth and allow to drain 8 hours or overnight in the sink. Transfer to a medium-size bowl.

Place basil, sunflower seeds, oil, mustard and garlic in a food processor or blender and process for 10 to 15 seconds, or until paste forms. Add paste to yogurt, mixing with a spoon or wire whisk. Store in a covered container in the refrigerator.

Yield: 1¼ cups

Prune Butter

Prunes—veritable fiber champs with 1.5 grams per tablespoon—make a delicious spread. Serve with muffins, scones, pancakes or waffles. Prune butter also makes an excellent dip for apple slices.

2   cups pitted prunes (12 ounces)
1¾ cups apple juice
¼   cup raisins or 4 dried figs
1   vanilla bean
    pinch of grated orange rind

In a 2-quart saucepan, combine all ingredients. Bring to a simmer, then reduce heat to low and cook, stirring frequently, for 30 minutes.

Let the mixture cool slightly. Remove and discard vanilla bean. Transfer mixture to a food processor or blender and process until smooth. If mixture becomes too thick, thin with additional apple juice.

Yield: about 2 cups

Preventing a Recurrence

CHAPTER 74

Chemotherapy

The burden of having to deal with the problems of chemotherapy almost all the time depressed my emotional threshold. Frustrations stemming from situations beyond my control triggered outbursts of rage. These powerful drugs interfered with body functions which most people take for granted, making me feel as though I had surrendered bodily control to a group of external agents."

Not a pleasant situation. It's even more unsettling when you realize these comments describe the effects of the *cure*—not the disease itself. They come from a Boston surgeon who, on October 20, 1980, had the unwelcome opportunity to view cancer from the patient's perspective. On that day he learned that a mass on the left side of his neck was cancerous. One month later he began a 37-week course of curative treatments called chemotherapy, which called for a series of drugs to be injected into his body in the hope of eliminating the cancer that a surgical scalpel couldn't cut out. The drugs did their job. Yet despite his clinical expertise and the practical knowledge he'd gathered dealing with cancer patients over the years, he was unprepared for this treatment's cruel side.

"Chemotherapy did not become easier with each successive treatment, merely different. Because of the cumulative toxicity of many drugs, symptoms such as nausea and vomiting became worse rather than better." He considered terminating the treatments early because of the many unpleasant "surprises." "Each one made me feel as though the light at the end of the tunnel represented an oncoming train rather than daylight."

Some veterans of chemotherapy will tell you matter-of-factly that they would rather face a train head-on than coping with the side effects of the anticancer drugs. Part of the problem is that too many people just accept side effects as the price they must pay to cure cancer. "Some patients assume, 'If there's anything that could have been done, someone would have told me,' or 'I don't want to complain because the doctor is trying to cure my cancer,' " says Marilyn Dodd, R.N., Ph.D., professor of nursing, University of California, San Francisco.

When she began researching how cancer patients cope with chemotherapy, Dr. Dodd found they were generally well informed about why a side effect may occur, but not what to do about it. Consequently, many patients don't even report side effects to their physician, says Dr. Dodd, author of *Managing Side Effects of Chemotherapy and Radiation Therapy: A Guide for Nurses and Patients* (Appleton & Lang).

The proverbial bottom line is that the more you know about chemotherapy before opting for the treatments, the better you'll fare. And horror stories aside, there are ways to minimize the discomfort and inconvenience of the side effects.

WHY CHEMOTHERAPY?

Cancer has spread, in many cases, by the time an initial diagnosis is made. Once it has spread, neither surgery nor radiation alone works well enough to eliminate the cancer. Thus, the treatment calls for chemotherapeutic drugs, which travel through your bloodstream and lymph channels to pursue and destroy cancer cells that have spread.

Chemotherapy interferes with the division and reproduction of cancer cells. Once cells can't divide, they will fall apart, and the tumor will stop growing and begin to shrink.

The cells don't all divide at the same time or rate, and some even rest after division. If various chemotherapeutic drugs are combined and used simultaneously, cancer cells can be attacked at different stages during the division process. This combination chemotherapy, as it's referred to, produces a more devastating effect on cancer cells than single medications used separately. In some cases, because the number of cancer cells killed by combination chemotherapy is higher than with individual drugs, tumors shrink faster.

Combination chemotherapy is useful for another important reason: cancer's complexity and variety. Two patients may be diagnosed with the same type of cancer, but they may respond differently to the same treatment. The reason is that there may be two or more varieties of cancer cells within a tumor. One may respond to a certain chemical, while the other cells may be sensitive to a different drug. A combination of chemicals offers a better chance of eliminating the various cancer cells.

Chemotherapy can be used to eradicate a variety of different types of cancer, although there are several types that it's more commonly used to treat, according to Vincent Anku, M.D., in his book *What to Know about the Treatment of Cancer* (Madrona Publishers).

Breast cancer. If a biopsy shows a breast lump to be cancerous and the cancer has spread to the lymph nodes or beyond, chemotherapy is usually advised. One recent advance has been the pinpointing of breast tumors that are fueled by female hormones. Now women can take chemotherapeutic drugs in tablet form to neutralize these hormones.

Hodgkin's disease. This type of cancer affects the lymph glands, and the extent of the disease is important to treatment. In the beginning, when it is confined primarily to the lymph nodes, radiation is used. Once it spreads and affects vital organs, chemotherapy is the treatment.

Leukemia. Of the more than ten types of leukemia, the one that's most treatable and has the highest cure rate—especially when found in children—is acute lymphoblastic leukemia (ALL). Since the disease is throughout the body, there's no specific area that can be pinpointed for attack, so surgery and radiation are often ineffective.

Lung cancer. Among the four main types of lung cancer, only one—small cell—is usually treated with chemotherapy. This type of cancer is characterized by rapid cell growth and spreading. Unfortunately, the disease returns to most people who show a good, early response to chemotherapy. Only about 25 percent of those with small-cell cancer limited to one lung, and who show complete response, remain free of the disease more than two years.

Ovarian cancer. Success depends on how early the diagnosis is made. Surgery is usually the initial step, often followed by combination chemotherapy.

Testicular cancer. There are four main types of testicular cancer. One type responds well to radiation, but the other three aren't curable with either surgery or radiation alone. Survival rates improve with chemotherapy, though. Testicular cancer is unique in that the tumor cells produce certain chemicals in the blood. Doctors can perform tests to see if, following treatment, those chemicals are present or not. From the test they can tell whether the tumor is still active or whether it's been eliminated. The physician then decides if treatments should be continued.

HOW IT'S GIVEN

The timing of chemotherapy can make the difference between a cure, temporary control and no control at all. Generally, chemotherapy is begun two to three weeks after surgery. The time lapse gives the patient time to recuperate. Chemotherapy drugs are usually administered through the veins. With the intravenous (IV) push method, the drugs are injected directly into a vein. A small needle attached to three to five inches of tubing is inserted into a vein, with the other end of the tubing connected to a syringe containing the medication. The procedure takes five to ten minutes and is usually done in a doctor's office.

Some drugs are too concentrated to be pushed directly into the vein. Sometimes the chemicals burn or cause vein spasms when rapidly injected. In these cases, the drugs are dissolved in a bag of fluid and enter the veins slowly, a procedure known as the IV drip infusion method.

Another method is called intra-arterial perfusion. Here, under local anesthesia, a small incision is made and a flexible tube is placed in the major artery leading to the tumor. The drugs are then injected at a predetermined rate by a portable pump.

In rare cases, the drugs will be injected directly into muscles. Oral chemotherapy medication is also uncommon, since enzymes and chemicals in the digestive system render the chemicals useless.

GOOD AND BAD EFFECTS OF CHEMOTHERAPY

If all works according to plan, chemotherapy's benevolent side will eliminate the tumor and halt any spreading. The time required for a complete cure depends on the type of tumor. Chemotherapy may be able to cure Hodgkin's disease in only six to nine months, for example, but it may take three years of intensive treatment to cure some forms of acute lymphoblastic leukemia. In many cases, chemotherapy doesn't reduce the size of the tumor. Instead it prevents the cancer from spreading, so the tumor can be attacked in other ways.

Unfortunately, the benefits of chemotherapy can be overshadowed by unpleasant and sometimes agonizing side effects. In some cases, the fear of these side effects keeps cancer patients at bay, delaying what could be lifesaving treatments. Physicians will be the first to stress that the discomfort and inconvenience caused by most side effects is temporary. They also emphasize that everyone reacts differently to drugs, and that the *fear* of treatment may be worse than reality.

There are about 30 chemotherapeutic drugs commonly used, each with its own spectrum of typical side effects. It's the rare patient who experiences them all. In some cases, the severity of the side effects increases with time, though in other instances it diminishes. Because chemotherapy treatments are usually given in cycles, with days or weeks in between to let normal cells recover from the drugs' effects, you can be hit with another round of drug-induced illness just as you're beginning to feel normal again.

It's also difficult to predict which side effects will show themselves. Granted, some people are barely bothered by chemotherapy, but chances are that you'll face some of them. Listed below are the more common side effects and suggestions for coping, adapted from Dr. Dodd's book. Of course, discuss these coping techniques with your doctor before trying them.

Abdominal pain. Change position while lying down. Take your pain medicine (analgesic) about 30 minutes before you know the discomfort will be at its worst during your treatment. Experience will teach you when the pain peaks.

Try mental relaxation or stress-reduction techniques. Contact your physician if medication doesn't relieve the pain, or if there are sudden, severe pains unlike those you've experienced before. If there's pain where the injection is given or at the site of the tumor soon after chemotherapy drugs are injected, try taking your pain medication just before your treatment. Contact your physician if this pain continues long after treatment.

Anemia (fewer red blood cells). Rest as much as possible to save energy. Eat green, leafy vegetables, liver and cooked red meats. Change position slowly if you're dizzy, and when you first wake up, sit at the side of the bed for a minute before standing to help decrease dizziness.

Bleeding (decreased platelet count). If you start bleeding, apply pressure to the area with a bandage or clean piece of linen, then apply ice in a plastic bag once the bleeding stops. When shaving, use an electric razor to avoid cuts. Brush your teeth gently with a soft toothbrush or your fingers.

If you must have blood drawn or be given an intravenous injection, apply pressure to the needle site for at least five minutes after the needle has been removed to control bleeding. Avoid blowing your nose too hard or coughing too harshly.

Take prescribed steroid medications with milk, food or an antacid. Avoid drinking alcoholic beverages. Don't use tampons. Call your physician if there's blood in your vomit, stool (it may be red, black or tarry), urine or sputum, or if you are coughing, vomiting or tend to be constipated.

If you have a major injury or hemorrhage spontaneously, go immediately to a hosptial emergency room. Be sure to tell them about your chemotherapy treatments.

Constipation. Eat high-fiber foods, such as whole grain cereals, bran, raw fruits, vegetables, nuts, dried fruits and raisins. Gradually add bran to your diet, starting with two teaspoons daily. Increase this amount gradually to four to six teaspoons daily; too rapid an increase can cause diarrhea. If you have trouble chewing raw fruits and vegetables, try grating them.

Eat fruits like oranges, pears, peaches and prunes. Drink six to eight glasses of fluids a day. If able, exercise regularly. Walking is an effective, easy exercise. You should also try to walk around more during your daily routine. If confined to bed, you can exercise by contracting and relaxing different muscle groups. Take stool softeners or laxatives; if ineffective, try enemas and suppositories. (Be aware that some laxatives when used constantly can irritate your bowels, often making it hard to regain normal bowel habits once chemotherapy or pain medicines are halted.) Contact your physician if you have had no bowel movements for three to four days.

Decreased appetite. Eat about six small snacks a day of foods you tolerate best, even if you're not hungry. Eat high-protein foods, such as milk, eggs, cheese, peanut butter and nuts. If meat tastes bitter—another possible side effect—marinate it in soy sauce, sweet fruit juices or sweet wine (if your doctor says you can have alcohol). Using plastic instead of metal utensils may reduce the bitter taste. Eat a high-calorie diet if you are not overweight. Add nonfat dry milk and egg whites, excellent sources of nutrition, to your cooking and baking. Use high-protein, high-calorie sandwich fillings. Vary foods from meal to meal. A change in odor and consistency may to help increase your appetite.

Drink acidic beverages, such as lemonade, to help increase your appetite. If swallowing dry food or meat is difficult, chop it and mix it with gravy or broth; try salad dressings or mayonnaise on vegetables or meats to increase swallowing ease. Since seeing food can decrease your appetite, keep it out of sight except when eating; for instance, use non-see-through containers, and keep food in cupboards instead of on the counter.

Clean your mouth after each meal. A half hour before your meals, exercise 10 to 15 minutes. Perform muscle relaxation or other stress-reduction techniques before meals to help reduce tension over eating. Try to eat one-third of your daily protein and calorie requirement at breakfast if you can. Consult your physician if there's a major change in appetite, or if you lose weight rapidly, such as five pounds in a week.

Diarrhea. Consider taking an antidiarrheal such as Kaopectate. Drink plenty of room temperature fluids to replace what you've lost; avoid hot or cold drinks, because they increase intestinal contractions. Avoid food that contains roughage and bulk. Get more potassium in your diet—bananas, apricots, peach nectar and nonfat milk are good sources. The severity of diarrhea can be decreased by drinking boiled milk and eating cottage cheese, yogurt, applesauce, nutmeg on applesauce, rice or bananas. Once diarrhea diminishes, gradually add these foods to your regular diet. Consult your physician if you have more than five liquid stools in a day and nonprescription drugs don't help.

Fever. Consume two to three quarts of fluid a day, which can be in the form of water and fruit juices or even ice cream, Jell-O or watermelon. Lukewarm sponge baths may reduce fever and offer some comfort. Consult your physician if your oral temperature goes above 101.5°F and taking an aspirin substitute hasn't helped reduce it. (Avoid aspirin, because it lowers the platelet count, which makes clotting difficult and can cause problems with bleeding.)

Fluid retention. Elevate your feet as much as possible. Restrict the amount of salt you eat or the amount of fluid you drink if retention is severe. Take your diuretic if prescribed. Weigh yourself daily and check your ankles, feet, hands and the area at the base of your spinal column for fluid retention.

Change your body position every two hours to prevent the breakdown of skin in areas where there's fluid retention. Contact your physician if you experience a sudden or severe degree of retention.

Headache. Take analgesics (pain pills) as in the past, but don't take aspirin products (salicylates) if your platelet cell count is low. If in doubt, ask your doctor. Lying down for one to two hours after chemotherapy may help. Avoid noise and bright lights.

Heart problems. Some chemotherapy drugs, particularly Adriamycin, can cause heart problems. Studies on laboratory animals, however, suggest that vitamin E may have protective qualities. Apparently the vitamin neutralizes free radicals, heart-damaging chemical agents created when the body metabolizes Adriamycin. Ask your doctor about taking vitamin E.

High or low blood pressure (hypertension; hypotension). If your blood pressure is elevated, take your blood pressure medication. Take naps, do mild exercises, try deep breathing or yoga or meditation—whatever measures you've found help you relax, because they may help lower your blood pressure. Call your physician if you experience headaches, nosebleeds or vision problems.

If you have decreased blood pressure, take your time when changing positions, such as when moving from sitting to standing. Sit or lie down if dizzy or lightheaded, and contact your physician.

Infection (fewer white blood cells). Avoid crowds, and especially people with colds; try to schedule trips out when there are fewer people to encounter (for example, go shopping early on a weekday morning instead of on a Saturday afternoon). Use antiseptic mouthwashes daily, and, to prevent possible infection, have dental problems taken care of before starting chemotherapy.

Wear sunscreen and avoid sunburn. Use a cuticle cream and remover instead of picking or cutting nail cuticles. Use a deodorant rather than an antiperspirant, which blocks sweat glands and can promote infection. Use sanitary napkins instead of tampons to reduce risk of infection. Use an electric razor to avoid breaks in the skin. Avoid rectal temperature-taking and the use of suppositories. Contact your physician at the first sign of an infection, if your oral temperature is above 101.5°F or if you have shaking chills.

Kidney damage. Chemotherapy can damage the kidneys when the anticancer chemicals pass through these organs on the way out of the body. Symptoms of kidney damage are headache, puffiness or swelling, especially of the ankles, and pain in the side. If any of these symptoms develop, contact your physician immediately and you'll be put on a different chemotherapy drug. The headaches and puffiness will subside, but the time needed to repair the kidneys varies from person to person.

Leukemia. Some people undergoing chemotherapy to cure bone tumors or cancer of the ovaries develop leukemia. In most cases, their treatments usually last three or four years, or else they receive high doses of radiation along with chemotherapy. It's unclear whether chemotherapy is the sole cause of the leukemia or whether the person affected had a high likelihood of developing another kind of cancer regardless of the treatment used.

Liver damage. Some chemotherapy drugs can damage the liver when the organ breaks down the chemicals as they pass through the system. Contact your physician if you have any of these symptoms: a yellow tinge to your skin and the whites of your eyes, nausea, fatigue, or pain on the right side of your body. Another drug will be used, and the symptoms usually subside within two weeks. In the meantime, rest as much as possible to save energy.

Mouth problems. Drink lots of liquids to keep your mouth moist. Brush your teeth with a baby-soft toothbrush, or cleanse dentures after each meal to remove irritating food particles and to help prevent infection. Use dental floss daily, but be gentle. A Water Pik can be used, but only on a low setting. If you wear dentures, don't use gummy adhesives. If your dentures don't fit well, have your dentist adjust them. Don't wear dentures, partial plates or retainers if your mouth is sore.

Sometimes a special mouthwash containing medication will be prescribed to ease mouth discomfort and promote healing. Gargle 15 to

20 minutes before meals to make eating more comfortable. Don't use a toothbrush if your gums are bleeding. Instead, clean teeth with a piece of moistened gauze or a cotton swab. Avoid very hot or very cold foods because they can cause irritation.

Make your own nonirritating mouthrinse by mixing one teaspoon of baking soda with one cup of warm water. Keep the solution in your mouth for about a minute and repeat every four hours, while you're awake. Avoid commercial mouthwashes that contain a lot of salt or alcohol. Keep your lips moist by applying thin layers of petroleum jelly or mineral oil.

Eat bland and cool, soft foods, such as custards, Jell-O, yogurt, soups and eggs. Check your mouth and gums three times a day for sores. If your home is heated by dry heat, a humidifier or steam kettle may help. If you have trouble eating with a fork or spoon, drink soft food from a cup or through a straw.

If you have difficulty swallowing, chew food well. Try a pureed or full liquid diet with fruit-ades or nectars. Sip beverages between bites of food during meals. Avoid hot, spicy or acidic foods. Avoid lying down immediately after eating, and when you do lie down, keep your head elevated.

If your mouth is excessively dry, sugar-free chewing gum or fluids may help. Drink at least three quarts of fluids a day. Keep liquids at your bedside and use a humidifier at night. Avoid breathing through your mouth. Check your mouth each morning for white patches. Suck on ice chips or cubes.

Muscle pain. Take analgesics (pain medication) for muscle discomfort if your physician has said it's okay. Avoid aspirin products when your platelet count is low. Contact your doctor if the pain suddenly intensifies and doesn't diminish after taking over-the-counter pain pills.

Muscle weakness. Stand up slowly. Rest when weakness increases. A lack of calcium, potassium or both can cause muscle twitching, accompanied by feelings of thirst, drowsiness and periods of confusion. If so, consume more milk products since they are rich in calcium. Eat foods high in potassium, such as bananas, tomatoes, oranges and apricots. Consult your physician about prescribing calcium or potassium medication or supplements.

Nausea and vomiting. Your doctor may give you antinausea pills, suppositories or an injection before each treatment. Take an antacid after taking the antinausea medication and avoid unnecessary movement. Eat five to six small snacks a day. Sweet or salty foods may be tolerated. Since activity can aggravate nausea, rest after meals, making sure your head is at least four inches higher than your feet.

If you're able, drink liquids frequently, but not with meals. Ginger ale, colas and Gatorade are good choices because they contain salt and water, both of which are lost during excessive vomiting and must be replaced. Avoid hot foods because the odors can aggravate nausea. Try cold meat and fruit plates with cottage cheese, and small sandwiches of bland food. To prevent dry heaves, eat crackers or hard candy when nausea occurs. Take only fluids in the first several hours after your treatment. It may help to eat a light snack before your chemotherapy.

When you feel nauseated, distract yourself from the sensation by doing something you enjoy. Avoid greasy foods because they take longer to leave your stomach. Carbohydrates, such as noodles and rice, exit faster. The volume of food in your stomach can be reduced by avoiding liquids at mealtimes and by drinking them one hour before or after eating.

Talk with your physician about scheduling treatments late in the day. The effects of chemotherapy may cause you to lose your evening meal, but you may regain some appetite by morning. Keep track of your sickness patterns by recording the onset and duration. Most side effects don't last longer than 48 hours, so by knowing your pattern of sickness you can determine when it's best to use self-care measures.

Clean your mouth well before meals and brush teeth afterward. Rinse your mouth with a mouthwash after vomiting. If the smell of food cooking makes you nauseated, sit in another room or take a walk while the meal is being prepared. Eat slowly and chew food well.

Get fresh air by sitting near an open window or outdoors. Contact your physician if you've been vomiting for 24 hours, experience signs of dehydration or are bloated with pain or a swollen stomach before vomiting but the condition subsides after vomiting.

Numbness (tingling in hands or feet). Exercise the affected limb by alternately flexing and stretching the muscles four times a day for a few minutes. If you're able, short walks are good exercise for legs and feet. Contact your physician if you lose feeling in your hands or feet.

Pigmentation changes. If there's increased coloring of your skin, wear clothes that protect your hands and arms from the sun, because the darkening of your skin is permanent.

Red urine. This occurrence is to be expected, and the color should return to normal within 2 to 12 days. If there's pain when you urinate, or if you're not sure whether the red is from chemotherapy or is blood, contact your physician.

Ringing in your ears. Chemotherapy affects the eighth cranial nerve used for hearing, which causes a ringing sensation. Usually when this occurs the drug is changed, and the sensation subsides within a few days. In rare cases, a permanent hearing loss can occur.

Sexual dysfunction. Some men will experience enlargement of their breasts, decreased sexual drive and finer or sparser body hair. The greater the amount of drug you're taking, the worse these side effects can be. Usually these changes are temporary, and all returns to normal when treatment concludes. Impotence may occur and be either temporary or permanent. In any case, find other ways to express affection that are satisfying to both you and your partner.

Chemotherapy can also alter the menstrual cycle, which should return to normal once treatments are complete. Because anticancer drugs can damage a fetus, birth control measures must be taken during chemotherapy.

Sterility can be temporary or permanent for men. If you're planning to have children, ask your physician about freezing some of your sperm before treatments begin. Women usually return to normal patterns of ovulation after chemotherapy.

Skin problems. Some chemotherapy drugs can cause skin ulcers if they accidentally leak from the blood vessel during injection, leading to severe pain and sometimes requiring surgical removal of the dead skin and skin grafting. Research on laboratory animals has shown that skin ulcers can be reduced in size up to 70 percent in two weeks when treated with vitamin E and dimethyl sulfoxide, better known as DMSO, which is used to carry the vitamin through the skin.

For dermatitis, take lukewarm baths with ¼ cup baking soda. Don't use soap for bathing, or shampoo on your scalp if your skin is sensitive. Avoid scratching, and if you scratch while asleep, wear mittens at night. Avoid excessive exposure to direct sunlight. Try oil-in-water baths or lotions.

If there's redness and peeling around your fingers, apply lanolin to your hands and wear gloves when you sleep. Also wear gloves during other activities that could produce discomfort, such as gardening or washing dishes.

Stomach irritation and ulcers. Take an antacid to help control heartburn. Avoid aspirin, because it can increase stomach irritation and bleeding; use an aspirin substitute. Eat bland foods, and avoid spicy, hot or acidic foods. Contact your physician if there is a raw, gnawing stomach pain, or blood in stools or vomit.

Taste and smell changes. Look for alternative foods that are palatable and are equally good sources of protein, such as cottage cheese, yogurt, milk, ice cream and peanut butter. A vegetarian or Chinese cookbook can offer nonmeat, high-protein recipes.

Thinning or loss of hair. Keep your hair clean, and wash it gently with a pH-balanced shampoo. Cut your hair to a shorter length if possible. Use a soft bristle brush to remove tangles. Your brittle hair will fall out faster if you bleach, tease, curl, perm or spray it. Buy wigs, scarves, and false eyelashes.

With certain types of chemotherapy, your physician may be able to place a tourniquet around your scalp and neck during treatment or place an ice pack on your scalp to minimize hair loss.

(If you experience *increased* hair growth, tweeze or shave off excess hair with an electric razor, but don't use electrolysis.)

Urine retention. Drink two to three quarts of fluid a day to dilute the urine in your bladder, and try to urinate every four hours while awake and prior to bedtime. Avoid milk products, because they tend to form bladder stones in people on chemotherapy, and don't take calcium supplements. If you've been drinking fluids but are still unable to urinate in a ten-hour period, contact your doctor.

Weakening of bones (osteoporosis). The drugs used in chemotherapy can leach calcium from your bones, making your skeletal system weak and susceptible to breaks. Walk with support if necessary. Avoid sudden movements, like jerking or twisting. Prevent falls by making your environment safer. Take 1,500 to 2,000 milligrams of calcium carbonate each morning. If you fall or have a pain in a bone without having fallen, contact your physician.

MEDICINE AND NUTRITION

If you're taking additional medication that is unrelated to your chemotherapy, be aware that some of the most innocent drugs you've taken for years can affect the way anticancer chemicals work and may harm your health. Notify your physician if you take any of the following: antibiotics, anticoagulants or blood medications, anticonvulsant (seizure) pills, aspirin, barbiturates (Seconal, Nembutal), blood pressure pills, cough medications (including Robitussin), Darvon, diabetes pills, diuretics (water pills), hormone pills (including birth control pills), sleeping pills, tranquilizers or nerve pills (including Valium) or nasal sprays.

Alcoholic beverages also can interact with chemotherapy drugs. Check with your doctor if you have an occasional drink, or if you use alcohol in cooking.

As for drinking in the nonalcoholic sense, the more fluids passing through your body the better. Some anticancer drugs can affect your bladder or kidneys and must be flushed out to keep your kidneys working properly. This need for a volume of fluid is especially important on days when you undergo chemotherapy. Try to drink at least eight to ten 12-ounce glasses of water, juice, tea or broth on those days. You can substitute ice cream, sherbet, soup, ice sticks and gelatin.

A proper diet is essential while on chemotherapy. Eating well helps maintain strength, enables you to cope better and lets your body repair and build new tissue and cells. Try to include the four basic food groups in your daily meal planning, but pay special attention to foods that are high in protein, the principal body rebuilder. Menus may need adjustment during periods of nausea, vomiting, loss of appetite, diarrhea or constipation.

Some people find that exercise stimulates appetite and also helps them cope with the strains of chemotherapy. This is something you and your physician will have to judge. If you're enduring treatments with little or no harsh side effects and feel like exercising, your doctor will probably give the go-ahead. The Boston surgeon who suffered such severe side effects found that "exercise allowed me to maintain my physical condition and to rebound quickly from the side effects of chemotherapy most of the time. I nicknamed swimming hydrotherapy because it renewed my feelings of control over my body, promoted self-esteem and helped dissipate tension and anger."

If you do start a regular program of physical activity, some doctors advise against exercising before you're scheduled to take laboratory tests. Exercise changes your metabolism, and some conditions, such as white blood cell count, can produce misleading test results if altered.

It's also advisable to forgo your exercise routine on the days you have your regular chemotherapy treatment, a precaution based on evidence of increased risk of heart problems the first two to six hours after treatment.

Self-Help Groups

The example set by other members seemed to strengthen people—I saw that each one could take it and they existed each day and that's what turned my life around.

Cancer patient describing a self-help group

Cathy Horne is a survivor. Diagnosed as having breast cancer in 1960, she's still fighting her cancer—and winning—and she's helping a lot of other people along the way. But her experiences with cancer haven't been easy ones, and she hasn't always had the sense of community and the feeling that she was helping others that she has now.

"In 1960, cancer was such a taboo that the doctors wouldn't even tell me I had it. It was more like I woke up in the hospital one morning with my breast removed and no one, including the doctors, would even talk about it. They pretty much just waited until I was able to leave and sent me home." Horne, who lives in Queens, New York, was in her thirties, had just undergone major surgery that left her with a lot of doubts about her appearance, sexuality, and health, and didn't really

470

have any knowledgeable person to discuss the experience with. Her doctors didn't discuss reconstructive surgery; they didn't really talk about her future. The whole experience was shrouded in an oppressive silence.

CANCER: A CONSPIRACY OF SILENCE

In a way, Horne was part of the conspiracy of silence she encountered. While over the years she would occasionally have the chance to talk to someone who had also undergone a mastectomy, until recently she didn't usually tell anyone about her surgery. "Cancer is a big secret for most people. People shy away from you when they find out you have it," she says. Forced to resolve most of her problems by herself, she "felt very alone for years after that."

Then the silence ended. After years of dealing with doctors, insurance companies and many of the other difficult aspects of living that sometimes seem inescapable for people who've had cancer, Horne went to her first meeting of an organization of self-help groups for women who've had breast cancer. "I went to a rap session one night and told them my story. They invited me to be on the board of directors and it was such a great feeling of relief to finally talk about cancer."

That was 1984. For Horne, 24 long years separated the diagnosis that she had cancer and the great comfort she found with the other women who'd had similar experiences. But years of silence and misunderstanding don't need to be the lot of people who get cancer these days. No longer is the disease a topic that's only to be whispered about. Granted, some people still have great misunderstandings about cancer. And discrimination, bad advice and a myriad of other problems confront people who've been treated for cancer. But this is the decade of the self-help group. From California to Maine (and in other countries, too) there are thousands of specialized groups made up of people who've had specific cancers. And because they know what cancer is like, they can help you understand your disease better and accept your condition, and together you can make the most of your lives despite your illness.

A PRESCRIPTION FOR A BETTER LIFE

"Admitting that you have cancer reduces the emotional stress of having the disease," says Dennis T. Jaffe, Ph.D., author of *Healing from Within* (Simon & Schuster), who is both a professor of psychology and director of the Health Studies Program at the Saybrook Institute in San Francisco. "And stress, to put it very simply, dampens your immune system's capabilities. This has been proved. So prolonging your life or defending your body could be a possible by-product of self-help groups—but it's not a primary effect. No one should join a group look-ing for a cure, even though there is evidence it will help. You should join a group to improve your life."

The benefits of self-help groups on a person's life have been proven by David Spiegel, M.D., psychiatrist at Stanford University Medi-cal Center. "We don't have any evidence that self-help groups stop the course of the illness, but we do have evidence that self-help groups result in reduced anxiety and depression, less pain and stress, and gen-erally improve peoples lives," he says.

Dr. Spiegel has done extensive research into the benefits of sup-port groups for women with metastatic breast cancer. And there's plenty of evidence that the groups are a great help.

"It's sort of like standing on the edge of the Grand Canyon and looking down when you are afraid of heights," says one group member. "You know that if you fell it would be the end. You would be dead. But you feel better about yourself because you can look. That's the way I feel about this group."

According to Dr. Spiegel, the woman "had used the group to dis-cuss her fears about dying, about living with an illness associated with increasing pain, weakness and loss of control, about her strained rela-tionships with her children and about her difficulties in communicating with her children and her doctor. The group countered her personal sense of isolation, provided concrete advice and helped to ease some of her suffering and pain."

STUDY COUNTERS THE SKEPTICS

Dr. Spiegel and his colleagues at Stanford, "spurred by widespread skepticism in the medical community" about the effectiveness of psy-chological approaches to cancer treatment, did a year-long study of the usefulness of support groups for women with metastatic cancer. Based on physician referrals, they selected 86 women with the cancer and put some of them into a support group. All the women were tested for phobias, self-esteem, mood disturbances, coping strategies, understand-ing of their illness, their family relationships, pain and how they com-municated with their doctors. These tests were given when the women began the study and repeated every four months throughout the year. The results cast favorable light on support groups.

"In summary, we found that the treatment groups showed signifi-cantly less mood disturbance over the course of the year than the con-trol group. The treated patients were less fatigued, anxious, phobic and confused than their counterparts. In addition, we have evidence that they suffered less from pain than their randomly assigned counterparts in the study. The control patients [those who did not join a group] became more disturbed and suffered more pain during the course of the year. This downhill emotional course was on our measures arrested and even ameliorated by the support groups," says Dr. Spiegel.

"Thus, there is objective evidence that supportive group interventions help cancer patients," the researchers concluded.

THE MECHANISMS OF SUPPORT

The groups work for quite a few reasons. Dr. Spiegel calls the keys to the success of these groups "mechanisms of support." Some of them are:

A feeling of control over oneself. This is a key mechanism, says Dr. Spiegel. People with cancer are usually as worried about things that affect them in the present as they are about the possibility that their disease will get worse and they will die. They are concerned about how much influence they have over their own remaining lives, and how they can live in the face of sickness and, sometimes, death. Once you get cancer and are being treated, a large part of your daily experience is dominated by your lack of self-control. You have doctors, nurses, family members and others telling you what to do. Self-help groups can help show people how to regain control of their lives.

Mutual support and education. "Doctors don't know a lot of the tricks that people in self-help groups would be able to tell someone. For instance, a group of people who have had colostomies would know a lot more than a doctor about the best way to deal with cramps or other problems, because they are living with the problem. They are figuring out techniques on their own that will be in the medical journals in two or three years," says Gerald Goodman, Ph.D., psychology professor and co-director of the California Self-Help Center at the University of California in Los Angeles.

In Dr. Spiegel's breast cancer group, the women were able to share information about how to buy breast prostheses, cope with side effects of chemotherapy, deal with social obligations and other problems they faced.

"Sometimes your oncologist isn't best informed about the choices, and frequently he won't have the time to tell you about them. A self-help group will help you develop the skills that you need to make the right decisions about your cancer treatment and your future. The self-help groups may know many things the doctor won't," says Dr. Jaffe.

Reduction of the fear of death. While much cancer is now curable and there are many cancer survivors, the association between death and a cancer diagnosis is still strong in the minds of many people. Self-help groups can prod people to overcome that fear, or face it realistically when necessary.

A stronger feeling of purpose in life. Some group members will discover ways to make their lives more meaningful. One woman in the group that Dr. Spiegel studied had always wanted to write a book of poetry, and decided that she should do it immediately, or she might never do it. And she ended up publishing two books of poetry. "A lot of people will develop a wisdom about themselves once they're diagnosed as having cancer. They face their lives and often get rid of the trivial, the meaningless things that sometimes take up so much of a person's life. Some people have told me that they wish they'd known all of this 20 years ago, instead of waiting until they had cancer before they reflected on their lives," says Dr. Spiegel.

"This is very important, because cancer is really a meaningless thing, a purposeless tragedy for those who get it," says Dr. Spiegel. "There seems to be no reason behind the cancer, but when a person joins a group and starts helping others, the whole experience of cancer is suddenly made meaningful."

Help with friendships. People learn to cope with friendships that sometimes fade away once a person is diagnosed as having cancer. Group members can openly discuss things like what to do when a person avoids drinking from the same glass as you because he fears that he might get your cancer, or avoids using the word cancer in your presence even when you'd prefer that things were in the open.

It's a common experience for cancer patients to receive sympathy and concern when they are first diagnosed, only to later feel they've been abandoned by their friends. "It's understandable," says Dr. Goodman, who is himself a cancer survivor. "What is your friend going to say when you tell him you have cancer. 'Gee, I'm real sorry to hear that'?" But people in groups can talk about it, because they've all been through similar experiences.

Help dealing with doctors. "The groups let you compare your experiences with doctors," says one California social worker. "You get to ask, 'Did they do this to you?' And people will be able to answer you, or maybe suggest other treatments you could talk to your doctor about."

To illustrate how a group can help a cancer patient deal with their doctor, Dr. Spiegel tells the story of one woman with breast cancer who was having a recurrent nightmare in which she was lying on a table, surrounded by men in white coats who were passing a wire back and forth among themselves. In her nightmare she knew that if the wire went over her head, she would die. This nightmare tormented her over and over. Fortunately her support group came to the rescue. Through it she realized that the dreams were a sign that she felt that the oncologist who was treating her for cancer was "putting something over" on her.

The woman realized this interpretation was true, that she did have problems with her oncologist. Whenever she became upset in his office and showed signs of starting to cry, he would change the subject. What particularly bothered her was having to undergo chemotherapy. The lack of control she had over this situation was really upsetting her.

The group advised her to explain to her doctor that she may cry when speaking to him, but to please allow her to continue. And that while he could still make the decision about whether she needed chemotherapy during any given week, she was going to decide whether or not she wanted to have it. As soon as she expressed these thoughts to her doctor, the nightmares went away.

THE GROUP EXPERIENCE

Clearly then, self-help groups offer many benefits to cancer survivors. But what is the experience itself like? Not everybody feels like going to a self-help group. For some, the whole idea might be a little too reminiscent of self-improvement workshops of the 1960s and 1970s that got a little out of hand. The idea of sharing the experience of having cancer with other people might seem upsetting rather than helpful.

Dr. Goodman outlines some of the more common reasons people give for not wanting to go to a self-help group—and why the fears behind these reasons might be more powerful than they deserve to be.

They don't want to walk into a room full of strangers. "You'll discover that the people in self-help groups change from strangers to partners and friends in a matter of minutes or hours. There's often a kind of instant bonding because you all share a powerful, uncommon experience," says Dr. Goodman. "Imagine this: You walk up to someone at a party, and you tell them you have cancer. Now this person who doesn't have cancer isn't going to know what to say. He'll probably be pretty uncomfortable, or say something like, 'I know how you feel.' But you'll know they don't know the first thing about it. And really, why should they?

"The result is that you're a victim of cancer—you didn't cause it— and you're in a sense punished for being a victim by being isolated from and misunderstood by other people."

That's a common experience for many people who have cancer. But a self-help group is different. The people you see there have been through the same problems you have. As Dr. Goodman says, "In the rest of the world, people say 'I know how you feel' out of a sense of helplessness and politeness. But when people in one of these groups say, 'I know how you feel,' it's not a gesture. They demonstrate their understanding repeatedly. They really *do* know how you feel."

They don't want to get involved with some commercial, money-making operation. Actually, true self-help groups are self-governing, financed by the members, and usually aren't owned by hospitals, therapists or corporations. While they might be affiliated with a national organization, the groups are, in effect, owned by their members. "Typically, it will be just eight or ten people sitting around a living room," says Dr. Goodman.

They don't want to be analyzed. The truth is that self-help groups don't try—or want—to analyze you. Rather, members will help you more as knowledgeable, spontaneous friends.

They just want to be left alone, and the people at the self-help group will try to "force" them to talk. If you don't want to talk because you're depressed, tired, angry—for any reason—chances are the self-help group isn't going to be pushy about getting you to say something. It's a self-help group, after all, not a forced-help group. Most groups will wait until you're ready.

WALKING INTO THE ROOM

In spite of these common and understandable fears, many people do go to self-help groups. And the experience of walking into the first meeting is like few other things a person can experience. Dr.Goodman, who has had colon cancer and has participated in and run self-help groups, describes the scene this way: "You walk into a room in the basement of a church, or someone's living room, or the poker room of the Elks lodge, feeling the oppressive weight of the stigma of having cancer, the alienation, all the bad advice you've received from doctors and friends, all the bad feelings of being a freak, unusual, wanting to hide. All of a sudden that stigma turns into something else.

"A transformation takes place and the disease that has made you deviant, sick, weird and unusual is suddenly your badge of acceptance into this group. You have a great feeling of instant connection. You are accepted by these people, whether they say anything or not. Suddenly everything is okay in this respect.

"You find that people are more open than they are in regular life. Perhaps you've never heard people speak so openly about cancer before—not your nurses, your doctors, your family. Not anyone.

"The lack of pressure allows you to deal with your very private feelings about cancer. This wonderful freedom is created naturally by a cycle of experiences coming from the group's common bond."

THE CYCLE OF SELF-HELP

Dr. Goodman has observed a special psychology occurring in all self-help groups. It goes like this: First you bond with the group. Second, you experience enough trust within the group to disclose private feelings. Third, you get bombarded with empathetic understanding. Then you repeat this process, one, two, three (in various ways) each time you go to a self-help group, visit after visit.

This repetition of the urge to disclose and the comfort of being understood is the foundation of the vital psychological help people get. It's a form of help not available from individual therapy or group therapy, or even from a loving family.

"One way of looking at self-help groups is as substitute for the nuclear family of days gone by," says Dr. Goodman. This family might best be represented by a fictional family like television's "The Waltons." Most people have probably never seen a family support each other in the way that the Waltons do. But even this rare family doesn't have going for it the one thing any self-help group does: the shared experience.

If John Boy got cancer and wanted to talk about it, Sue Ellen, who had never had cancer, couldn't really be on his wavelength for long. But people in a self-help group could be. "The relationship between people in groups is a unique, deliberately made form of emotional intimacy that gives the group the power to help its members," says Dr. Goodman.

REAL FAMILY THERAPY

The family does play a very important role in helping a person survive or live with cancer, however. And there are self-help groups for family members that can nudge this process along. "It is critical to have the family attend some kind of meetings or the same meetings you go to," says Dr. Jaffe. "This recommendation is especially important for husbands of women who have breast cancer. But it's good for any family that has someone with cancer. Cancer doesn't affect just the person who gets it, but everyone around him, also."

Julie Sullivan, executive director of the Candlelighters Childhood Cancer Foundation, Washington, D.C., which is an organization of groups for parents of children who have cancer, says the self-help groups provide a lot of emotional and practical help, but are also useful as just good places for the parents to let off some steam when they're upset.

FINDING A GOOD GROUP

There are thousands of cancer self-help groups in the United States. One good way to find one in your area is to go to the white pages of the telephone book and look under self-help clearinghouses. "Chances are very good, maybe 80 percent, that you'll find one, especially in a major city," says Dr. Goodman. Or, you might ask other patients, or call the county health department or the social services department at a local hospital. And you can look at the list that follows for the names of national offices and clearinghouses that will give you the names of local cancer self-help groups. Dr. Jaffe offers these simple tips on what to avoid when it comes to choosing a self-help group. Avoid the group if:

- It promises to cure your cancer, or prescribes medical or psychological therapy.

- It emphasizes that you should "obey" the group leader, or seems to be a cult.
- It charges more than a minimum fee to cover expenses. True self-help groups are always member supported.

Here are the national offices of some support groups and referral centers that might be of help to you.

The American Cancer Society
National Headquarters
90 Park Avenue
New York, NY 10016
(212) 736-3030

The American Cancer Society sponsors several self-help organizations for people with cancer. The national office recommends that you contact your local office of the American Cancer Society (see white pages of your telephone book) for information about the local offices of the following groups:

Cancer Care. This organization provides professional counseling and guidance to help patients and relatives cope with the emotional, psychological and financial problems associated with cancer.

CanSurmount. A cancer patient support group based on the belief that no one is better at helping a cancer patient help himself than another cancer patient.

I Can Cope. An eight-week series of two-hour classes taught by health professionals on anatomy, the causes of cancer, how it develops, mental and physical side effects, and how cancer is treated.

The International Association of Laryngectomies. This group provides referrals to local clubs made up of people who have had laryngectomies. These clubs offer moral support and information.

Reach to Recovery. This group helps women who have breast cancer.

Candlelighters Childhood Cancer Foundation
Suite 1011
2025 Eye Street, NW
Washington, DC 20006
(202) 659-5136

This is the national office of Candlelighters, which is a communications link for more than 250 self-help groups for parents of children who have cancer. This office will refer people to local groups. They will also send out a newsletter which gives current information about treatments and other things having to do with cancer in children. A good source of information.

Leukemia Society of America
733 Third Avenue
New York, NY 10017
(212) 573-8484
The society can refer you to self-help groups for people with leukemia and related diseases, such as lymphoma or multiple myeloma, and their families.

United Cancer Council, Inc.
650 East Carmel Drive, Suite 340
Carmel, IN 46032
(317) 844-6627
This group can refer you to self-help groups for people with cancer and their families.

New York City Self-Help Clearinghouse
1012 Eighth Avenue
Brooklyn, New York 11215
(718) 788-8787
The clearinghouse will refer you to New York's self-help organizations for further information.

United Ostomy Association, Inc.
2001 West Beverly Boulevard
Los Angeles, CA 90057
(212) 413-5510
This group provides information, a magazine and referrals to self-help groups for people who have had colostomy, ileostomy, or similar surgery, because of cancer or other illnesses. There are more than 700 local chapters made up of ostomates that give each other rehabilitative support and share information.

Make Today Count
P.O. Box 222
Osage Beach, MO 65065
(314) 348-1619
This group will refer people to the more than 200 chapters around the country that try to help cancer patients and other people with life-threatening illnesses live their lives as fully as possible. The emphasis is on emotional self-help through group meetings.

Hormone
Therapy

Hormones. They're responsible for the manly growth of hair on the chin, the bulging biceps, the strong sex drive.

Hormones. They determine the monthly cycle, the growth of breasts, the flow of milk.

From puberty to old age, many functions of life and reproduction are controlled by hormones, substances produced in the body to promote cellular growth.

Because of their involvement in the growth of cells, it's not too surprising that certain types of tumors are affected by the presence of hormones. Likewise, it's not surprising that doctors have learned to treat certain cancers by manipulating the body's hormone supply.

The whole idea behind hormone therapy, says Jay Roth, Ph.D., professor of molecular and cell biology at the University of Wisconsin and author of *All about Cancer* (G.F. Stickley Co.), is "to rearrange the hormones so tumor cells regress." Sometimes rearranging means administering one hormone to counteract another hormone's effects.

Sometimes it means bombarding the body with ultra-high doses of hormones.

Either way, the technique is called hormone manipulation, and the treatment that's been receiving the most attention lately is the one that deprives the body of hormones. This method prevents certain cancer cells—most notably those of the breast and prostate—from getting an adequate hormone supply. Starved of their hormones, these tumors shrink and may eventually even die.

Until recently, two rather drastic measures have been used to achieve hormone deprivation: surgery or administering massive doses of sex hormones. In the first, the organs responsible for hormone production are removed. Women have their ovaries taken out to curtail estrogen production, while men have their testes removed to close down testosterone output. And since the adrenal glands produce steroid hormones and the pituitary gland controls other endocrine organs, these structures are frequently removed, too.

Needless to say, surgical castration has devastating physical and psychological effects and removal of the adrenals can cause a lifetime dependency on steroid replacement drugs.

The second common way to halt hormone production has been only slightly more acceptable. Substantial doses of sex hormones may eventually stop the tumor from growing, but not without a price—severe hot flashes, an increased risk of heart disease, men growing breasts and women growing facial hair are only a few of the side effects.

HAZARD-FREE HORMONE THERAPY FOR BREAST CANCER

Thanks to new drugs, treatment today can stem the hormone supply without serious side effects. "New forms of medical hormone therapy are less toxic and may even make surgical hormone therapy obsolete for treating certain spreading cancers," reports I. Craig Henderson, M.D., associate professor of medicine at Harvard Medical School, Boston, and medical coordinator of the Breast Evaluation Center, Dana-Farber Cancer Institute.

What has experts like Dr. Henderson particularly excited is a drug called tamoxifen (trade name Nolvadex), now being used to treat certain advanced breast cancers. Tamoxifen blocks the estrogen before it can get to the part of the cell that ushers it inside. Called receptor sites, these are protein substances which sit on the surface of certain cells (those of the breast and prostate, for example). They snatch hormones out of the bloodstream, taking them inside and using them in order to grow.

Tamoxifen beats estrogen to the receptor sites. "The drug then gets taken inside the cancer cell like a Trojan horse," explains Dr. Henderson. "Once inside, the tamoxifen kills the tumor." The best part about tamoxifen may be that it's much less toxic than the treatment previously used for advanced breast cancer. This latter treatment involved giving doses of DES to deprive the tumor of hormones.

Tamoxifen was put to the test in a 1981 study. Researchers at the Mayo Clinic in Rochester, Minnesota, randomly assigned women with spreading breast cancer to be treated either by tamoxifen or DES. The results? Tumors responded similarily to both treatments, but the difference was that the DES group experienced nausea, vomiting and swelling while the tamoxifen group most commonly complained only of hot flashes.

A TAILOR-MADE HORMONE TREATMENT FOR WOMEN

Tamoxifen is tailor-made for only certain women with certain cancers. According to a National Cancer Institute consensus panel, those

---

THE MANY WAYS HORMONES HALT TUMORS

The goal of all hormone therapy is basically the same: to stop tumor growth. The method used to achieve that goal varies according to the tumor being treated.

In some cases, one hormone is given to counteract another hormone's harmful effects. Some women, for example, have a condition called endometrial hyperplasia. The condition involves developing an overabundance of endometrial tissue. Sometimes it is caused by the normal stimulation of the hormone estrogen. One serious aspect of the condition is that it can lead to endometrial cancer. To correct the problem, women with hyperplasia may be given high doses of another female hormone, progesterone.

Progesterone also is used with chemotherapy to treat some advanced cases of endometrial cancer, adds George Richardson, M.D., assistant professor of surgery at Harvard Medical School, Boston. "High doses of this hormone can cause cancerous lesions to shrink or even disappear in 30 percent of the women with the recurrent, spreading kind of endometrial cancer," he says. The plus for progesterone is that it has virtually no side effects.

In other cases, hormone therapy involves administering large quantities of the same hormone that prompted the tumor to grow in the first place. Bombarded by the hormone, the body stops pro-

who respond best to tamoxifen are postmenopausal women whose cancers depend on hormones to grow.

How can you tell if a cancer is classified as hormone dependent? Fortunately, there is a test that detects the presence of estrogen receptors in the cells of a tumor. A "positive" test result means the cells have estrogen receptors, and that the cancer depends on hormones to grow. Such a cancer is very likely to shrink with hormone manipulation. "The more receptors the tumor has, the more dependent on hormones it is likely to be and the more easily it responds to hormone therapy," writes Penny Wise Budoff, M.D., clinical associate professor of family medicine at State University of New York in her book *No More Hot Flashes and Other Good News* (Putnam).

If the cancer recurs or does not respond to tamoxifen, treatment may call for an additional hormone deprivation drug, called aminogluthethimide. This drug shuts down the adrenal glands, another hormone production site. Like tamoxifen, it can spare you from surgery. What's more, even though you must replace steroids while taking the

ducing its own supply. This "negative feedback" method of hormone therapy is often used with patients who have thyroid cancer.

Apparently, the pituitary gland secretes a thyroid-stimulating hormone, which circulates in the bloodstream. When a patient with thyroid cancer is given a thyroid hormone, the body is fooled into believing that the hormone quota has been met, and the body no longer requires the "stimulating" hormone to make the thyroid produce more. As a result, thyroid production shuts down and the tumor eventually shrinks.

Still other forms of hormones called corticosteroids, produced by the adrenal glands, are given in doses much higher than the body usually produces. These steroids come in many synthetic and natural forms and may directly affect certain cancers such as lymphoma, or else alleviate symptoms. They may, for example, decrease the swelling around brain tumors and reduce headaches.

One possible problem is that patients can become dependent on these drugs. Why? Because when the adrenal glands stop producing their own steroids, the patient may permanently have to rely on replacement hormones. That hazard can be avoided by taking steroids in short courses over several days, with a few weeks between courses.

drug, your adrenal gland will once again take over this function when you discontinue drug therapy.

All in all, drugs like tamoxifen and aminogluthethimide are making the picture brighter for treating breast cancer patients with advanced tumors. Sums up Dr. Budoff: "These new drugs not only give women new avenues of therapy, but they avoid the need for further surgery and thus improve the quality of life."

HORMONES WORK FOR PROSTATE CANCER

Hormone drugs might hold promise for men, too, especially those with advanced stages of prostate cancer. And that may be especially important when you consider that 30 to 50 percent of all prostate cancer patients tumors have spread to the advanced stages by the time they are diagnosed.

What's more, the two leading ways to treat prostate cancer are drastic. One method is castration removal of the testes. Castration stops most production of the male hormone testosterone. The surgery has a profound physical and psychological impact. The second treatment involves giving men massive doses of the female hormone DES to block testosterone. DES can cause their breasts to enlarge and can increase the men's risk of heart disease.

Here's where the new hormone drugs come in. One drug is called leuprolide. It's a synthetic version of a hormone produced in the pituitary gland (called the luteinizing hormone-releasing hormone or LH-RH by scientists). This natural hormone regulates testosterone in the blood. Leuprolide, the synthetic hormone, acts the same way. After an initial rush of testosterone, leuprolide causes testosterone levels to plummet, starving the tumor. An additional bonus is that leuprolide's only major side effect appears to be hot flashes.

A SHORT-TERM SOLUTION

The hitch to this mode of hormone deprivation, say some doctors, is that the effects of leuprolide or any hormone treatment may not hold up over time. "After a year or two, the body may become immune to hormone suppression and the cancer could become resistant to the therapy," explains Robert Huben, M.D., chief of urologic oncology, Roswell Park Memorial Institute in Buffalo, New York.

"If there are one million prostate cancer cells and hormone therapy even halts 99 percent of them, the tumor may at first appear to regress," says Dr. Huben. "Eventually, though, the remaining 1 percent of tumor cells will emerge and progress."

Could the answer to wiping out testosterone in total be a combination of drugs? One Canadian physician who appears to think so is Fernand LaBrie, M.D., Ph.D., of the Department of Molecular Endocrinology at Laval University Medical Center in Quebec. Dr. LaBrie has combined a LH-RH drug with flutamide, a drug that blocks the action of testosterone. This combined blockage is necessary, he claims, to ensure a more complete deprivation of the male hormone.

But does this combination of drugs work? According to Dr. LaBrie's studies, 95 percent of prostate cancer patients responded to the combined hormone treatment after a year. After two years of treatment, he predicts, the probability of that response continuing would be 70 percent, compared to less than 10 percent by previous approaches.

The problem with Dr. LaBrie's studies, notes Dr. Huben, is that they did not compare the combination approach to either castration or DES. So it's "not yet known if this combined hormone therapy will effectively suppress testosterone over the long run." More recent studies have not shown the combination approach to be superior to single treatments. Still, he admits, LH-RH drug therapies may prove an effective alternative for men who cannot have surgery or take DES.

DO HORMONES PLAY A SUPPORTING ROLE?

Will other hormone therapies play as big a role in treating advanced cancers as tamoxifen does for breast cancers? At this point, no one knows. Yet, most experts agree they will play a very important *supporting* role.

"The real value of hormone therapy may prove to be in combination with other therapies—part of a regimen of controlling cancer," says Douglas Tormey, M.D., Ph.D., professor of human oncology and medicine, University of Wisconsin. Hormone therapy may be used before surgery, for example, to help shrink tumors so they can be removed with less extensive surgery. Or hormones may be used as a postoperative "mop-up," to control cells that have escaped the scalpel.

In other instances, hormone therapy may be used to stop cells and keep them in their place. "This holding pattern might be enough to curb some cancers," says Dr. Tormey. But others may require additional therapies—like chemotherapy—to finish the job. The bonus of hormone therapy is that perhaps less toxic doses of these powerful drugs may need to be administered.

In the future, echoes George Richardson, M.D., assistant professor of surgery at Harvard Medical School, hormones will likely be administered not so much as a single agent but as part of a treatment sequence. "Perhaps what hormones do best is provide a tool to help us learn about tumors. They help us see how cancer cells grow and what other treatments may be required to stop them."

PREPARE FOR SIDE EFFECTS

"It's important for patients to know that there are no hard and fast rules for hormone therapy," says Debra N. Pollack, R.N., M.S.N., coordinator, National Surgical Adjuvant Breast Project at the University of Pittsburgh. "Reactions resulting from hormone therapy are usually less life-threatening than those experienced from chemotherapy," she says. But that does not mean side effects should be dismissed. Often hormone therapy side effects can be more visible or require special psychological preparation.

That's especially true if you are taking certain sex hormones. Men who receive a female sex hormone like DES may develop softened skin or larger breasts, while women taking male sex hormones may develop a lowered voice. "Psychological counseling and relaxation techniques can help allay anxiety and promote a more positive body image," assures Pollack. "It's important to know that these side effects are reversible, and to get emotional support."

Hot flashes that often accompany sex hormone therapy are often easily relieved with a daily dose of vitamin E (400 International Units). Side effects caused by other types of hormone therapy may require a bit more rearranging of your lifestyle. If you take corticosteroids, for example, you may gain weight. If so, a low-sodium diet and a regular exercise program can help.

The most important thing you can do when taking hormone therapy is to become savvy about your side effects. "Monitoring your side effects can tell you how the treatment is working," says Pollack. If you experience bone pain, for instance, it can be a sign that hormones are effecting distant sites.

Whatever the side effects, report them. "Keeping your doctor appraised of your symptoms can provide important clues as to how your tumor is responding to treatment and what the next treatment step should be," she says.

Immunotherapy

When you think of cancer treatments, you probably think of destruction. The usual approach is to kill off cancer with poison, deadly rays or the knife. But these three traditional approaches to cancer (chemotherapy, radiation and surgery, respectively) can easily go beyond damaging cancerous cells and end up destroying healthy body tissue. Even though these traditional treatments have helped a lot of people, the experts are optimistic about a new class of cancer treatment called immunotherapy. They're looking forward to this treatment because it may turn out to be harmless to cells that aren't cancerous, but deadly to those that are.

In a sense, immunotherapy encourages the body to help itself. With almost all cancer, a person's immune system will try to control the disease. But it isn't always strong enough. Immunotherapy is focused on trying to overcome this weakness by enhancing the body's natural cancer-fighting abilities. In a variety of different processes, researchers are doing things like removing some of the cancer-fighting cells from a person's body, boosting their strength in the lab, then returning them to fight the cancer. While this may sound as simple as shoring up the foundation of a house with a few struts, it's really a very complicated and still-to-be-understood science.

HOW MANY IS 1,000,000,000?

To give an idea of how difficult the immune system is to work with, and thus how difficult it might be to control, consider how small cells are. They are so small that there is really no way to describe a single cell. It's easier to give an example of how big a billion cells would be—they'd be about the size of the tip of your little finger. That's right, 1,000,000,000—nine zeros—equals one little fingertip. There are about 70,000 billion (70,000,000,000,000) of these cells in a 155-pound person.

And cancer can start in just 1 of these cells, or 10, or 100, with changes so tiny they are hard to detect. In fact, by the time cancer becomes obvious enough for doctors to be able to detect it, it already affects billions of cells. And by that time, the body's natural immunities and defenses have been exhausted. Immunotherapy comes in when the immune system can't control the cancer.

While there are many types of immunotherapy now being researched, perhaps the three most promising and widely studied types are based on interferon, monoclonal antibodies and interleukin-2 (IL-2).

WHAT EVER HAPPENED TO INTERFERON? (A LOT!)

Interferon made the cover of *Time* magazine in the spring of 1980, and it's been trying to live up to its reputation as a miracle drug ever since. For a while it seemed as though interferon was being touted as a cure for everything from the common cold to cancer, and the only thing standing in its way was the fact that there wasn't enough of the stuff around to cure everybody. One way it could be made was in tiny amounts that were painstakingly distilled from human white blood cells in laboratories.

But now, thanks to modern genetic engineering, scientists can make interferon by the vat. There's plenty of interferon to conduct all the tests that are needed to prove its worth. Unfortunately, like an actor who receives too much advance praise and then flops on the stage, interferon hasn't lived up to its billing as a miracle drug. Fortunately, it still has a lot of inherent value. It won't cure the common cold or end all cancer or save the human race, but interferon is thought to be the best treatment for one rare form of leukemia.

Interferon, which is a protein made by human cells, helps them battle viral infections. There are three main types of interferon—alpha, beta and gamma—which are produced not only by the body but also in laboratories. Because alpha interferon was the first that could be engineered in laboratories, it's been more thoroughly studied. And for now we'll use the word interferon to refer only to alpha interferon, which is at the forefront of interferon therapy.

A CURE FOR ONE TYPE OF LEUKEMIA

Interferon is now a standard and highly valued treatment for a type of cancer called hairy cell leukemia (HCL). In fact, the Food and Drug Administration (FDA) approved interferon as a drug for HCL in May, 1986, making it the first drug of its type to be approved for general use. HCL usually grows slowly. It's a serious cancer that has traditionally been treated with surgical removal of the spleen and chemotherapy. Interferon offered great prospects for HCL right from the start. All seven people in the first study, done at the M.D. Anderson Hospital and Tumor Institute in Houston, showed great improvements after being treated with interferon.

Other tests confirmed these first results. Researchers at the University of Chicago Medical Center studied 64 people who had HCL, 61 of whom had undergone surgery to halt the cancer. HCL was totally eradicated in 3 of the people, 45 were partially cured, 9 showed minor improvement, 3 didn't improve, and 3 died.

Studies of the effects of interferon on other blood cancers haven't equaled the 90 percent response rate found for HCL, but researchers are optimistic about its possibilities. And it is used in combination with other treatments to treat some types of kidney cancer, melanoma and a few types of lymphoma.

ONE STRANGE SIDE EFFECT

Even when it is used for those cancers it is *known* to help, interferon can cause problems. Side effects include fever, fatigue, muscle pain—in general, symptoms that are similar to the flu. After long-term treatment, people can begin to suffer from confusion, poor concentration, hallucinations and even coma at very high doses. And one very strange side effect was found in two people—their eyelashes grew so quickly and thickly that they needed a trim twice a week.

Dosage also can be a real problem. Logic would say that the more interferon a person gets, the more quickly his cancer will disappear, but interferon doesn't follow this logic. Low doses can work well and cause fewer side effects than high doses. And sometimes it takes several weeks for interferon to start to work.

USING ANTIBODIES
LIKE HEAT-SEEKING MISSILES

Sherry Brown, M.D., a fellow in oncology working under the direction of Ronald Levy, M.D., at the Stanford University Medical Center in

Palo Alto, California, uses interferon in combination with another treatment that is on the cutting edge of immunotherapy: monoclonal antibodies.

Monoclonal antibodies are considered by some to be the most powerful of the immunotherapies. *Mono-* means single, and monoclonal antibodies are single antibodies that are produced naturally in the body and then reproduced in laboratory animals. The amazing thing about monoclonal antibodies is that they will seek out particular cancer cells in the body, like heat-seeking missiles going after a target. Many experimental treatments with monoclonal antibodies have produced very encouraging results.

"We custom-make the treatment for each patient," says Dr. Brown. "Right now we are only working with people who have non-Hodgkin's lymphoma. And studies we've done show that, in animals at least, interferon and monoclonal antibodies work better together against lymphomas than either would alone. We are now testing these results in people at Stanford, but all the trials we are doing won't be in and published for some time. Still, I am excited by what's happening. The results so far look very promising.

"It's important to remember that monoclonal antibodies aren't a miracle cure or anything like that. Even if we were to get wildly successful results right now, it will be years before the average person will be able to get the treatment," says Dr. Brown. "We use patients who are already at the medical center here, and they have to fit tight protocols for the studies. In fact, I don't know of any cancer for which monoclonal antibodies are now considered a standard treatment. It is still highly experimental."

Despite the experimental nature of the therapy, other studies done at Stanford have also pointed to a bright future for monoclonal antibodies used to treat cancer. Dr. Levy, in whose laboratory Dr. Brown works, used monoclonal antibodies to treat a 67-year-old man suffering from a type of lymphoma. The man had undergone a variety of treatments already, including interferon, bleomycin, cyclophosphamide, vincristine and prednisone, with only partial success. The man still had a lot of cancer in his body and suffered from fevers and night sweats.

SYMPTOMS DISAPPEAR

Dr. Levy removed a lymph node from the man and came up with a monoclonal antibody treatment in the laboratory. He treated the man with this solution twice a week, six hours a day, for four weeks. After four treatments, the man's fever and night sweats stopped. After five treatments, the man's tumor started to get smaller. After eight treatments, the cancer was in total remission.

"Dr. Levy's work with that one patient showed the great potential for monoclonal antibodies," says David Segal, Ph.D., senior investigator in immunology at the National Cancer Institute in Bethesda, Maryland. "We know that they work; now we have to figure out how best to use them."

TRANSPORTING DRUGS RIGHT TO THE TUMOR

Their ability to recognize tumor cells makes monoclonal antibodies handy carriers for anticancer drugs, too. "Just getting the monoclonal antibody to find the tumor cells that are 'hidden' in the body doesn't kill the tumor," says Dr. Segal. "You need an affector, whether it's man-made or from the immune system. The antibody will recognize the tumor. Then the immune system will recognize that the cell is covered with antibodies and will go and wipe out the cancerous cell—theoretically." In other words, the monoclonal antibody is like a scouting party going out to find an enemy position and calling in an air strike. "You can do this artificially or use the body's own cells. There are lots of ways to do it," says Dr. Segal.

"While this is all experimental, I'm optimistic that down the road we will see remarkable breakthroughs. In ten years, which really isn't too long, great things will happen. It's a long time to research something, and unfortunately a lot of people will get cancer during that time, but in the scope of things ten years won't seem so long once there is a breakthrough."

"Monoclonal antibodies still face a lot of technical obstacles, whether they're used to trigger the immune system or to carry drugs to tumorous cells," says John Lazlo, M.D., vice president for research at the national office of the American Cancer Society in New York. "You can send the antibody in to work on a tumor cell, and it might end up reacting badly with another cell, like a kidney cell, that you hadn't even considered. Or maybe if you are using the antibody to deliver a poison to the cancer cell, the poison will leach off into the body and be toxic instead of going to the cancer cell. These are just a few of the many possible problems that have to be worked out. There's a lot of research to be done on these, but there are also a lot of possibilities for treatment," says Dr. Lazlo, author of the book *Understanding Cancer.*

"MIRACLE CURE" STILL IN THE LAB

In December, 1985, Steven Rosenberg, M.D., Ph.D., and his colleagues at the National Cancer Institute and Clinical Center, released some data that prompted a frenzy of headlines and television news reports about a possible cure for cancer. While Dr. Rosenberg didn't claim to have a cure, the results of his study were exciting and perhaps people made too much of them. He and his colleagues took 215 patients who had advanced and spreading cancer that hadn't responded to traditional therapies and treated them with a combination of interleukin-2 and another immune therapy called lymphokine-activated killer (LAK) cells. One person's tumor completely disappeared after the treatment, and ten others had tumors that decreased in size by more than 50 percent.

Then, in December of 1986, Dr. Rosenberg and several other scientists published a study that showed that IL-2 alone reduced the size of tumors, at least temporarily, in some people. But while these studies did offer hope for IL-2, Dr. Rosenberg's results weren't greeted with unbridled enthusiasm by the experts.

"Dr. Rosenberg was very optimistic about these treatments," says Dr. Lazlo. "But we are still awaiting confirmation of the extent of the effectiveness of IL-2 alone or with LAK. In the future, perhaps it will prove to be of great benefit. It is still very much in the running as a treatment. But it was probably oversold, in my opinion."

Part of the reason it might seem to have been oversold is that IL-2 therapy is very toxic. The *Journal of the American Medical Association* published a description of the possible side effects of IL-2 in an editorial in the same issue that presented the findings of Dr. Rosenberg's second study.

"Treatment with high doses of IL-2 is an awesome experience," the article said. "It requires weeks of hospitalization, much of which must be spent in intensive care units if the patient is to survive the devastating toxic reactions. For most patients, these include anemia requiring multiple transfusions, severe thrombocytopenia [a decrease in blood platelets], rigors [chills], fever, marked hypotension [low blood pressure], gastritis, azotemia [excess urea in the blood], jaundice, skin eruptions, malaise and confusion. Many also experience ascites [accumulation of fluid in the abdominal cavity], agitation and respiratory insufficiency requiring intubation. The price in dollars for treatment and management of toxicity may reach six figures. Such high human and financial costs demand commensurate therapeutic benefit."

Clearly, the author of this editorial, Charles G. Moertel, M.D., of the Mayo Clinic in Rochester, Minnesota, didn't feel that the results of IL-2 therapy were worth the frightening after-effects—at least not at this stage of IL-2 development. Still Dr. Moertel did write, "On the positive side, however, these studies as well as many others have demonstrated that the lymphokines do have definite antineoplastic [anticancer] activity in human cancer." So, while IL-2 may offer a lot of possibilities for the future, it isn't a quick fix for cancer in the present.

PURCHASE YOUR OWN RESEARCH

The future in which immunotherapies like interleukin-2, monoclonal antibodies and other experimental treatments are widely used may not be too far off, if the instincts of Robert K. Oldham, M.D., are right. Dr. Oldham worked as a researcher at the National Cancer Institute for a time and then established the department of oncology at the Vanderbilt University Medical School in Nashville, Tennessee. In 1980, he started work for the NCI again, looking into biological treatments for cancer. All of his experience with traditional research institutions led him to believe that he could offer a better alternative. And now, in his opinion, he does.

He founded Biotherapeutics Incorporated, a research laboratory in Franklin, Tennessee, as a private, profit-making research group. People are referred to him by their doctors and, if they seem to have the kind of cancers that will respond to the therapies devised in Dr. Oldham's lab, he'll accept them. Then the patients, in effect, are required to fund their own research.

For a cost of anywhere between $2,750 and $35,000, the lab will outline a course of treatment, produce monoclonal antibodies or whatever is needed and refer the patient to a doctor who is qualified to treat him. At the moment, patients are referred to doctors associated with Dr. Oldham, because they've been trained to work with the biological treatments the lab often suggests. But Dr. Oldham says that soon he'll start training doctors around the country to administer the therapies.

For their money, people get the latest experimental therapies—the same ones being used in experiments at universities and government research centers like the National Cancer Institute. "When you come here, you get what you pay for. You don't pay to run a whole university or research center—you pay for research into your own cancer.

"Yes, the treatments are experimental," says Dr. Oldham, "but they're all being used in research centers around the country. What we do here is let people have access to the treatments at the same time that we are trying to figure out how best to use them. Yes, there's risk. But realistically, there is a risk in any cancer therapy."

The risk, and the possible benefits, are now available only to those who can fund their own research or those who have the luck to be accepted into a government- or university-funded research program. But according to Dr. Oldham, "these biological treatments will be available to the average person in the not-too-distant future. Each of these substances will gain more favor, or lose favor, depending on their effectiveness, and in the next several years the useful ones will pass into the realm of standard therapy."

Mind/Body Healing

Every week a dozen or so people come together in Boston, for one purpose: to learn how to make a contribution to their own recovery from cancer.

Here, there are no visible treatment tools—no radiation equipment, no surgical instruments. Rather, the treatment tools these people are using are methods that allow them to deeply relax their body and their mind. They are being trained in the use of the Relaxation Response as well as a technique called creative imagination, by which they learn to enhance their mental images of healing. The hope is that these images of healing will strengthen their immune systems.

These cancer patients are participants in the Mind/Body program, a program staffed by biologists, psychologists and oncologists from the Division of Behavioral Medicine at Beth Israel Hospital at Harvard Medical School in Boston.

Three thousand miles west, another group of cancer patients is also meeting. This time, the setting is UCLA and the lesson being taught is how positive attitudes might affect the quality, and perhaps the quantity, of life.

These two programs are not rarities—a growing number of cancer centers have added some form of mind/body therapy to their conventional treatments. What sets these programs apart, though, is that they are part of controlled scientific studies, studies which could very well prove the mind's role in boosting the immune system, with the ultimate goal of healing cancer.

Why have we included this information about cancer patients in a book about preventing cancer—a book that's not so much for those who are ill as for healthy people who want to stay that way? Because experts say that the same attitudes, feelings and thought patterns that may help *cure* cancer may also help *prevent* it. There are emotions and personal values that may have the potential to create a stronger immune system and a healthier response to stress—two musts for fighting *or* avoiding cancer. One of the best ways to learn about these methods of personal change and growth is to look at the people who *have* learned them—the cancer patients who, in their response to this health crisis, have created happier, calmer and more purposeful lives. People who know that well-being is truly a state of mind.

PARTNERS IN HEALING

There is at least one doctor who doesn't need the results of tests to convince him of the important part the mind plays in healing cancer. Why? He has seen it work in his own practice with cancer patients. His name is Bernard S. Siegel, M.D. ("Bernie" to his patients), and he is attending surgeon at Yale-New Haven Hospital as well as assistant clinical professor of surgery at Yale Medical School.

As Dr. Siegel tells it, the basis of his belief came about after he had provided a group therapy situation for his cancer patients so that they could learn how to live with their illnesses. He was astonished by what he observed. "As I saw people learning how to live with their illnesses, I saw them having incredible control over their wellness." Sometimes their cancers disappeared, says Dr. Siegel, "They were getting better and I didn't lift a finger."

That's when Dr. Siegel decided that one of the best things he could do for cancer patients was to make the mind/body methods accessible. He established ECaP (Exceptional Cancer Patients), a program that uses a combination of stress reduction, conflict resolution and positive reinforcement (in the form of visualizations and positive emotions such as hope and love)—things he believes can stimulate the immune system and allow healing to take place.

"The body responds to the mind's messages, whether conscious or unconscious," says Dr. Siegel, explaining the mind/body approach in his book *Love, Medicine and Miracles* (Harper & Row). "In general, these may be either 'live' or 'die' messages. I am convinced we not only have survival mechanisms, such as the fight or flight response, but also a 'die' mechanism that actively stops our defenses, slowing the body's functions and bringing us toward death when we feel our life is not worth living."

Dr. Siegel recalls one patient named Irving, a financial advisor who invested people's life savings according to statistics and who came to see him with liver cancer. "His oncologist told him what statistics said about his chances, and from then on he refused to fight for his life," explains Dr. Siegel. "He said, 'I've spent my life making predictions based on statistics. Statistics tell me I'm supposed to die. If I don't die, my whole life doesn't make sense.' And he went home and died."

But then there was Jim, continues Dr. Siegel, a patient with colon cancer. "I told his family he had six months at most—this was back when I still predicted how long patients would live—but he proved me wrong," recalls Dr. Siegel. Every time Jim returned, Dr. Siegel was convinced that, at last, the cancer had recurred. "But," he says, "it was always some minor unrelated problem. Every time I offered follow-up therapy for his cancer, he refused. He was too busy living and had no time for my treatments. Jim has been healthy for well over a decade now."

Was Jim's story a miracle? A case of spontaneous remission? Dr. Siegel prefers to call what Jim experienced "self-induced healing." And it's often something that happens to people he calls exceptional patients. "They are people who, when confronted with illness, are willing to take responsibility for it and redirect their lives accordingly. They also are willing to participate in their own recovery . . . and to seek out all available resources (medical, psychological, spiritual, etc.) to give themselves the best chance for getting well. These are the people who are really willing to fight for their lives."

THE FAITH FACTOR—
THE NEW, OLD MEDICINE

And these are also the people, Dr. Siegel points out, who have *hope.* "If there's one thing I learned from my years of working with cancer patients, it's that there is no such thing as false hope. Hope is real and physiological. Hope acts as a placebo."

A placebo is a fake pill, "medicine" the patient only thinks is the real thing. But that doesn't mean the pill is worthless. Just the opposite. Placebos are so powerful that studies have shown that of patients who see their doctors, three-fourths will get better if they are given a placebo and only a placebo. "Even in the other 25 percent, medical treatments may be enhanced by the placebo effect." says Herbert Benson, M.D., of the Harvard Medical School.

Perhaps a more accurate way of explaining the placebo effect is "the healing power of expectant faith," suggests Jerome D. Frank, M.D., Ph.D., Professor Emeritus of psychiatry at Johns Hopkins University School of Medicine in Baltimore. After all, it's not the placebo that creates the cure, it's the patient.

To illustrate his point, Dr. Frank tells the story of how a physician asked a faith healer to try to cure three of his women patients from a distance, without their knowledge. The first patient had gallbladder inflammation with stones, the second was recovering poorly from abdominal surgery and the third was dying of cancer.

Nothing happened until the women were told of the faith healer who, they were led to believe, was capable of miraculous cures and would perform them at a particular time. At the correct time all three women "improved dramatically." The cancer patient recovered enough to return home, the gallbladder patient lost her symptoms, and the woman who had undergone surgery was permanently cured.

What healed them? Not the faith healer but their belief.

THE KEY IS CONTROL

The other "medicine" the pioneer mind/body programs are dispensing is assistance in how to avoid being a helpless victim. "An important goal of the program is to teach patients that they have some control in a disease that feels so without control," says Stephen Maurer, associate director of Beth Israel Hospital's Mind/Body Program.

Perhaps another phrase for being in control is active, optimal coping. And that's a term that is beginning to have special meaning to many cancer researchers. Why? Recent evidence is mounting that suggests that knowing how to cope effectively with life's crises (big and small) could blunt the effects of stress on the immune system and play an important role in controlling cancer.

The idea that cancer could be influenced by our coping style—our behavior—is replacing the theory set forth by many earlier researchers, who suggested that the disease may be brought on by something in our personality or by something traumatic that happened to us early in life.

One such early researcher was psychologist Lawrence LeShan, whose interviews with cancer patients led him to conclude that people who were depressed, despairing and cut off from loved ones were likely cancer candidates. Other researchers found that people prone to cancer were apt to have neglectful parents or to keep their emotions under wraps.

The problem with these early studies, say critics, is that they provided only a backwards look at cancer victims. Because they looked at people who already had cancer, they failed to answer the classic chicken/egg question. In other words, which came first—the personality or the disease (which may have altered the personality)?

To get closer to the answer, other researchers looked at long-term studies. Among them was the one conducted by Caroline B. Thomas, M.D., Professor Emeritus of Johns Hopkins University School of Medicine. Dr. Thomas evaluated a number of medical school students with psychological tests and followed them to see what kinds of illnesses they developed. What she found was that a major difference between those who later developed cancer and the rest of the group was a poor relationship with their parents. Thirty percent of those in the cancer group said they were "neither admiring of, nor comfortable with, their father or mother."

In another long-term study, which followed about 2,000 industrial employees for more than 20 years, epidemiologist Richard B. Shekelle, Ph.D., at the University of Texas Health Science Center, discovered that those who scored highest on depression were more than twice as likely to die of cancer than the rest of the group.

THE "TYPE C" PERSONALITY

Still, these past studies were not enough to convince all doctors that lack of control, helplessness, depression or any other long-term emotional states, for that matter, made certain people prone to cancer. Bernard Fox, Ph.D., professor of psychiatry at Boston University School of Medicine, says, "Recent studies have suggested that a hopeless, helpless attitude in cancer patients forecasts a shorter survival than a fighting spirit. Further, there is a suggestion that patients who suppress negative emotions tend to have shorter survival."

By that, Dr. Fox means that people who seem to be cheerful or happy, but who underneath are really angry, don't survive long.

Psychologist Lydia Temoshok, Ph.D., assistant professor of medical psychology in the Department of Psychiatry at the University of California in San Francisico, says, "The Type C coping style is theorized to be the polar opposite of the Type A behavior pattern," she explains. Type A behavior has been identified as striving, even driven, with a suppressed sense of hostility. "The Type Cs are actually undercontrolling, cooperative, self-sacrificing and polite. They have difficulty expressing negative emotions." In short, she says, people with the Type C coping style are perfect patients. The problem is, they may be worse off when it comes to surviving cancer.

When Dr. Temoshok evaluated videotaped interviews of patients with malignant melanoma, she found that those patients who were

Type Cs had thicker tumors, which indicates a poorer prognosis. In another study, Dr. Temoshok found that "Those who had trouble expressing negative emotions had tumors that were dividing at a higher rate and weakened immune response at the tumor site."

TYPE C MAY SUPPRESS IMMUNITY

What's even more convincing about this new area of study is that some researchers have been able to show that patients displaying the Type C personality traits have weakened immune systems.

In a National Cancer Institute study, University of Pittsburgh psychologist Sandra Levy, Ph.D., looked at 75 women with breast cancer. Half who were treated with mastectomy, while the other half had undergone lumpectomy, which removed only the tumor, plus radiation treatment. Five to seven days after surgery, a blood sample was taken to measure natural killer (NK) cell activity (white blood cells that are the first line of defense against tumor cells) to see how their immune systems were responding. At the same time, the women were evaluated for mood and personality, rating their overall adjustment to the illness.

Dr. Levy found that the patients who were rated as relatively undisturbed but who nevertheless complained about a lack of family support had lower natural killer cell activity than the patients who were rated as more disturbed but who had a good social support system. To Dr. Levy, the results suggested that those who outwardly displayed negative emotions and had good social support may be better off with regard to resisting tumor growth.

THE EMOTIONS/BRAIN/CANCER LINK

These studies could very well provide an important piece of the cancer personality puzzle, says Steven Locke, M.D., associate director of the Psychiatry Consultation Service at Beth Israel Hospital and coauthor of *The Healer Within* (Dutton). "Even though there have been studies linking emotions and personality to cancer, the data is inconclusive. What's been missing up until now is just how it affects the immune system—the physiologic link to cancer."

Dr. Locke explains that studies like Dr. Levy's are part of the new science of psychoneuroimmunology (PNI)—the study of the physiologic link between the brain, the nervous system and the immune stystem. "A premise of PNI is that the immune system does not operate in a biological vacuum but in fact is sensitive to outside influences," he writes. Moreover, he continues, "Certain states of mind and feelings can have powerful biochemical aftershocks."

Not only can things like genetics and diet influence the immune system, says Dr. Locke, "but there are more subtle influences, too, that can affect the immune system, including . . . a person's moods, feelings, states of mind, behavior, attitudes and his coping ability."

In his own studies, Dr. Locke found that healthy college students who reported many symptoms of depression had a diminished tumor-killing ability of their white blood cells in the laboratory.

And now studies are revealing that a person under stress releases biochemicals known as corticosteroids, which can inhibit the immune system, including the action of the macrophages—cells that fight tumors. Finally, research on coping and stress indicates that people who do not cope well in stressful situations show diminished activity of their natural killer cells in comparison to other individuals who appear to be coping better with comparable amounts of stress.

Until all studies are completed, it is too early to predict which personalities get cancer and which emotions affect it, concludes Dr. Locke.

A PSYCHOLOGICAL PREVENTION PLAN

And what, if anything, can we do emotionally and mentally to protect ourselves from cancer? "It's impossible to come up with a definite psychosocial prevention prescription until the mind/body code to cancer is broken," he says. His only suggestion, not surprisingly, has to do with learning how to be in control. "Learn how to resolve problems," he advises. "Don't permit them to go on forever. If you habitually respond to life stresses with feelings of helplessness and hopelessness or are prone to depression or anxiety when under stress, seek professional help."

Finally, he says, don't let the notion of the cancer-prone personality distract you from avoiding known carcinogens like cigarettes and excessive sunlight or from early detection techniques. "The important thing is to learn how to improve your quality of life, not how to avoid cancer."

On the subject of psychosocial prevention of cancer, Bernie Siegel's book reminds us, "Not everyone who suffers a tragic loss or stressful change in lifestyle develops an illness. The deciding factor seems to be how one copes with the problem.

"Many people don't make full use of their life force until a near-fatal illness goads them into a 'change of mind,' " he says. "But it doesn't have to be a last-minute awakening. The mind's power is available to us all the time, and it has more room to maneuver before disaster threatens."

The advice, then, is don't sit and stew over crises and calamities. Design a prevention plan and stick to it for life.

PATHS TO STRESS RESISTANCE

Avoiding the stresses of life—whether it's the good kind like getting married, getting promoted or having a baby, or the bad kind like contracting an illness, getting a divorce or losing a job—won't protect you from cancer. But learning how to diffuse the *effects* of stress and gain control just might.

One way to gain control is by developing a "hardy" personality, suggests Suzanne Ouellette-Kobasa, Ph.D., a professor of psychology at the City University of New York's graduate school. In her studies with executives, she observed that what got executives through stresses were three basic attitudes that she labeled *hardiness*: commitment to what they did, feeling in control of their lives and seeing change as challenge rather than a threat.

To trade hardiness for helplessness, says Dr. Ouellette-Kobasa, first focus on your body signals. Notice the pressure in your temples, the knotting in your stomach, the stiffness in your neck. Your body is giving you clues that you may be in a stressful situation. So stop and ask yourself, "What's keeping me from feeling good today?" This is a quick way to focus on your stress and increase your sense of control over it. Then you can start thinking about changing your unhealthy responses into "feel good" ones.

Another way to develop healthy coping skills is to "play back" a recent stress episode in your head. Then, write down three ways it could have gone better and three ways it could have gone worse. (You may want to recall someone who handles stress well and imagine yourself doing the same.) Soon you'll begin to realize that you can think of better ways to cope with life's hassles.

Finally, there's no need to collapse in the face of certain intense stress situations such as illness or divorce. Instead, try to take control. Failing that, you can at least learn the art of compensation. Regain your grip on life by taking up a new challenge such as swimming or teaching someone to read. Mastering a new task will reassure you that you can still cope.

MINDING YOUR BODY

You've got to learn to communicate with your body to tap the healer within, says psychologist Dennis T. Jaffe, Ph.D., of the Saybrook Institute in San Francisco. One way is through imagery. "Our bodies respond to pictures when they don't or can't respond to words," says Dr. Jaffe.

Most anticancer imagery is based on a technique made famous at the Simonton Cancer Institute, Pacific Palisades, California, where patients are taught to visualize the cancer cells in their bodies being overwhelmed by their treatment and flushed from their body. Then they imagine good cells taking over and picture themselves as healthy and free of disease.

To help you focus on your inner healer, all you need do is choose a soothing image—a mental film that makes you feel peaceful, calm and relaxed. Then your body will be ready to receive any positive, healthful messages you may want to send it.

Your imagery film, for example, might open with a scene of you lying on a soft, sandy beach beside gently rolling waves. Watch the palm trees slowly swaying as warm breezes lull you with their soothing massage.

While you are in this relaxed state, gently turn your attention to your body. Picture your skin as being clear and smooth; your internal organs—your heart, your lungs—as being strong and healthy. Get a close-up of your circulatory system and immune system. Picture your red blood cells coursing through your veins carrying their life-giving oxygen, while your white cells efficiently carry off toxins.

By "seeing" yourself in this way, say experts, you are communicating with your body and helping it to progress toward health.

One neuroendocrinologist found that cancer patients who used the imaging technique had a larger number of T-lymphocyte cells, which might help boost their ability to fight cancer.

TUNING OUT TENSION

There is some research that suggests that relaxation—in particular the technique called Progressive Relaxation, may result in more active natural killer cells in the blood. The beauty of the technique is that you don't have to be a Zen monk to learn it.

To try the technique yourself, take a comfortable position in a chair with your hands resting in your lap, or lie down on your bed with your feet against a wall or a heavy piece of furniture. Close your eyes and follow these steps.

1. Clench your right fist and tighten the muscles in your wrist and forearm. Hold for five seconds, feeling the tension. Then unclench your fist, letting the tension drain from your forearm, wrist and fingers. Note the difference between how your arm feels now and how it felt when it was tense. Repeat. Relax.
2. Clench your left fist and tense your left forearm. Note the difference between how your left arm feels and how your relaxed right arm feels. Relax, letting the tension slowly drain out through your fingertips.
3. Next, tense your upper arms and shoulders. Hold for a few seconds, then relax, again noting the difference between how your muscles feel when tense and how they feel when relaxed.
4. Now tense your neck. Hold for a few seconds, then relax. Your entire upper body should feel considerably more at ease than before you started.

5. Make a frown, scowling as hard as you can. Relax. Try to feel the tension drain out of your eyes, cheeks and lips.
6. Raise up on your toes, or push against the wall if you're lying down, to create some tension in your legs. Hold for a few seconds, then relax. Again, try to notice the tension draining away. Now your entire body should feel more at peace.
7. Your breathing should be normal and rhythmic. When you finish, take a deep breath, feeling the tension in your chest. Exhale. Breathe in again, hold, and let it out, saying to yourself, "I'm calm." Concentrate on your calmness.
8. Conclude by slowly counting to four, gradually becoming more alert. Open your eyes.

LEARNING THROUGH LOSS

Doctors have known that stressful events, such as losing a loved one, can increase susceptibility to a wide variety of diseases, including cancer. Now there's research that would seem to indicate that a "broken heart" could damage the immune system. Marvin Stein, M.D., and his associates at the Mount Sinai Medical Center in New York City studied the effects of bereavement on the immune function of men whose wives died of breast cancer. Months after the wives died, the men showed a striking decline in white-blood cell function.

Apparently, it's not the grief itself that's harmful but how you deal with your loss—whether or not you fully express yourself in the grieving process.

"To fully recover and move forward past the immediate loss, we must affirm and acknowledge our feelings," says Glen Davidson, Ph.D., professor of psychiatry at Southern Illinois University School of Medicine. That means openly and honestly voicing feelings of fear, sorrow, guilt, anger, depression, loneliness, anxiety and shame. "Only through telling our story over and over again do we clarify in our own minds what has happened and how we really feel about it. Through that, we come to accept the reality of the loss so we can go on living."

GETTING A LITTLE HELP FROM YOUR FRIENDS

When it comes to preventing cancer, your social life may be a factor. Epidemiologist Peggy Reynolds, Ph.D., of the California State Department of Health Services, looked at a study of nearly 7,000 people living in Alameda County, California who were followed for 17 years. None had a previous diagnosis of cancer and other cancer risks, such as smoking, were accounted for. What turned up was that the women who reported no or few social contacts were almost twice as likely to die of all cancers. Not too surprising.

But what did come as a surprise, says Dr. Reynolds, is that women who did have many social contacts but who nevertheless felt lonely were more than twice as likely to die from hormone-related cancers. Dr. Reynolds is unclear about what the connection is, but it may have something to do with the effect of emotions on hormone regulation. (Men, by the way, rarely get hormone-related cancers.) Apparently, just feeling socially isolated may put women at risk for cancer.

One antidote for alienation is to turn your attention to other people, suggests one doctor. "Get in contact, pay attention, listen, and be aware." says Allan Dye, Ph.D., associate professor of mental health counseling and personnel services and director of the counseling and guidance center at Purdue University, West Lafayette, Indiana. "You become more attractive to others when you pay attention to them and that leads to more affection directed at you."

DON'T REPRESS—EXPRESS!

Keeping anger inside could put you at risk for cancer. One study of the life history of cancer patients has found that many seemed unable to express anger or hostility in defense of themselves.

But that doesn't mean you should blow your top. Another study indicates that women who were highly volatile (as well as those who were very seldom angry) are more likely to have malignant tumors than women who have an appropriate expression of anger.

Yet a third study, this one done by Marjorie Brooks, Ph.D., formerly an assistant professor at Jefferson Medical College in Philadelphia, showed that women with breast cancer were more likely to apologize for their anger—even when they were right! "Women in normal health were more likely to get angry and forget about it," says Dr. Brooks. "They redirected their attention and energies to more pleasant things."

The best way to resolve anger and conflict is to ask, Why? Once we understand the motive behind an aggressive action, we can better come to terms with our feelings. But to get to that point we must first be willing to confront our true feelings and discuss them openly in a manner that's likely to bring about a satisfying resolution. "The purpose of anger is to make a grievance known," says social psychologist Carol Tavris, Ph.D. "If the grievance is not confronted, it will not matter whether the anger is kept in, let out or wrapped in red ribbons and dropped in the Erie Canal."

Radiation Therapy

R adiation.

Since science let that genie out of its bottle less than 100 years ago, we have seen a lot of horror, from Hiroshima to Chernobyl. Sometimes it seems as though humanity's command over radiation's deadly power is much too tenuous for our own safety. But if radiation is a killer, it can be a saviour as well.

More than half the people diagnosed with cancer receive radiation at some point in their therapy. Most often it is paired with either surgery or chemotherapy, or all three are combined in a ferocious campaign against cancer. But cancer is eradicated in more than 100,000 people a year by radiation treatment alone. Cancer cells' vulnerability to radiation was discovered long ago. Today, sophisticated, computer-guided equipment helps highly trained radiation therapy teams seek and destroy tumors with minimal damage to healthy tissue. Thousands of people are alive and well today because of radiation treatment.

HOW RADIATION WORKS—AND WHY

Radiation kills cancer cells by disrupting the DNA, the blueprint by which it reproduces itself. Luckily, the DNA in cancer cells is more susceptible to radiation than that of normal ones. Cancer cells are most vulnerable when they are getting ready to divide and multiply. Since that time varies in the cancer cells that make up a tumor, radiation treatments are spread out over days and weeks to increase the chance of destroying all the cancer cells.

There are two ways to receive radiation therapy—externally or internally. External radiation is still the more common of the two—this is the kind lay people often refer to as "cobalt" or "x-ray" treatment. In fact, there are three kinds of external radiation used in cancer therapy, explains William Hendee, Ph.D., a radiation physicist who is vice president for science and technology of the American Medical Association: electron beams, x-rays and gamma rays. The latter two are quite similar, differing only in the way they are produced. Gamma rays come from radioactive cobalt, while x-rays are produced by high energy x-ray machines. X-rays are produced by the same kind of machine used to detect broken bones, except that they have higher energy and therefore are more penetrating. Both gamma rays and x-rays can be targeted to cancers that are well below the surface of the skin, or in a rather dense part of the body like a bone or muscle. X-rays that can penetrate to very deep-seated tumors are produced with machines called high-energy linear accelerators. This high-tech equipment is usually found only in major cancer research centers, says Dr. Hendee.

The third kind of external radiation is electron beam therapy. These beams can't penetrate very deeply. Therefore, they are used on tumors located in easy-to-reach areas of the body, for instance near the skin's surface or near a body cavity. This kind of radiation is sometimes used during cancer surgery as well, when it can be aimed right at cancer cells through a surgical incision. Its advantage is that it can be given in very high doses—in one or a few treatments—since electron beams have a very selective range they're unlikely to damage healthy tissue under and around a tumor.

Many people are surprised, and a bit uneasy, to learn that radiation therapy can be carried on *inside* a patient as well. This treatment is done by means of implants—tiny rods, needles or "seeds" of radioactive material that give off high doses of gamma rays. Removable implants, used mostly in cancers of organs such as the cervix, uterus, tongue, prostate and bladder, let doctors deliver a lot of radiation right to a tumor. Because of the amount of radiation involved, some implants are left in for only a few days, and the patient must be somewhat isolated to avoid radiating healthy people. But once the therapy is over and the implants removed, the patient is no more radioactive than any other normal person. Other implants can be left in permanently because the radioactivity decays in a few days and what is left is harmless.

The decision about what kind of radiation therapy is best for you will be made by your doctor. That choice of therapy can affect where you will be treated. "Many local hospitals can handle all but the most difficult cases," says Dr. Hendee. "The advantage of using one near your home is that you can remain in familiar surroundings, supported by family and friends, and maintain your normal lifestyle as much as possible." But some high-energy radiation treatments can only be administered at big research centers. "American doctors have access to all sorts of information about treatment. If your doctor urges you to go to such a center," recommends Dr. Hendee, "don't hesitate to take that advice."

THE REWARDS—AND RISKS— OF RADIATION THERAPY

"In radiation treatment, success is measured by a different standard for each patient," says JoAnn Manning, M.D., of the Howard University Hospital Department of Radiation Therapy in Washington, D.C. "In one, it may be a total cure, in another, a few more years of productive life. Sometimes radiation is used to shrink a tumor before surgery, other times to ensure that all the cancerous cells left behind after a tumor is removed surgically are wiped out." Radiation is also used to relieve pain or stop bleeding, so a person whose outlook is poor can still be made more comfortable. "Every case of cancer is different," maintains Dr. Manning, "and every course of treatment is unique to that patient."

Some tumors respond to radiation better than others. When they are caught early enough and treated (often with surgery and drugs, as well as radiation) cancers such as Hodgkin's disease, one type of testicular cancer, larnyx and prostate cancers and tumors of the tongue and mouth are often cured. Lumpectomy followed by radiation for treating breast cancer is still being evaluated, but there are indications that in many cases this procedure can save both a woman's life and her breast, sparing her the trauma of mastectomy.

When both surgery and radiation promise to produce the same results in selected patients, radiation is often chosen because the patient's breast is saved, Dr. Manning explained. Radiation is also preferred to surgery in treating head, face, mouth and neck cancers. "The cosmetic outcome with radiation is much better, and the patient is spared reconstructive surgery later," she says.

But some organs are too sensitive to treat with radiation. Organs such as the stomach, kidneys and liver are very sensitive to radiation.

They must be protected both by lead shields and precise aiming of the beam when tumors in their vicinity are being irradiated. The bone marrow, also, is especially vulnerable to radiation. In fact, some cases of leukemia can be traced to earlier radiation therapy. "But the risk of developing a later tumor is so small that it is something you don't really worry about," says Dr. Manning.

RECEIVING RADIATION THERAPY

It's natural to feel apprehensive about radiation treatment. After all, you read almost every day about the hazards of radiation. The idea of lying still while radiation is shot right into you—even in a controlled dose, even if it's *good* for you—is not very appealing.

Knowing what to expect during your treatment—and after it—should help reduce your fears. Your best source of that information will be your radiation therapy team, the doctors, nurses, physicists and technologists who will all take part in your treatment.

The doctor is most likely to be a "radiation oncologist" with specialized training and several years experience in treating tumors with radiation. He or she will decide on the best way to give the radiation, where to aim the beam and how long and how frequently you should be treated. The radiation oncologist will have consulted your other physicians about your condition, but more tests or x-rays to locate the tumor as precisely as posible may be necessary. According to the AMA's Dr. Hendee, many cancer centers are using sophisticated equipment such as CAT scanners to locate a tumor, and feeding that information into a computer which calculates the dosage and the path of the radiation to the cancer.

The radiation therapy nurse is specially trained to help you throughout your treatment. In addition to working closely with the oncologist, the nurse will be able to offer information on possible side effects and advise you of ways to cope with them.

The radiation therapy technologist will administer the actual treatment, according to your doctor's instructions. Though not doctors, technologists have had at least three years of training in radiology and radiation therapy, and are licensed. The technologist and the nurse are the health professionals you will see at each treatment session. Be sure to inform both of them of any side effects you experience from the therapy, and how you are feeling in general. They can decide if you need to see your doctor at any time during your treatment. Other persons involved in your treatment may include *dosimetrists*, who assist a physician in calculating the doses of radiation needed, and how they are delivered. You may also meet the craftspeople who make the plaster molds or braces specially designed to help you hold still during each treatment, and the lead alloy shields that protect healthy organs from the radiation.

Most likely, your first meeting with the radiation therapy team won't include treatment. The nurse and technologist may show you the equipment and may even take you through a dry run so you know what to expect. This "simulation" also lets the team set up all the conditions needed for an actual treatment. They will mark your skin with an indelible pencil to designate the area the beam will be targeted. (Don't wash these marks off—the beam must reach the same spot each time to be effective.) You may have to partly or completely undress for treatment, so be sure to wear clothes you can get in and out of easily.

After the discussions with the radiation oncologist and the rest of the therapy team, you will be asked to sign a form stating that you have been informed about your treatment and give your consent to it.

WHAT TO EXPECT DURING TREATMENT

After all the preparation and build-up, radiation therapy patients are often surprised to find that each actual treatment is quite brief, usually no more than two to five minutes long. During that time it is necessary to hold absolutely still, so the radiation reaches its target without damaging healthy tissue.

Like getting any x-ray, there is no pain or sensation of any kind during the treatment. The days of severe skin burns from radiation therapy are long gone, although the treatment does usually cause some skin redness by about the third week. You will not have any awareness that the tumor is shrinking either, although some large tumors near the skin's surface, as in Hodgkin's disease, may get larger and cause pain in the early stages of radiation therapy.

It isn't unrealistic to try to live as normally as possible during your treatments. Keeping a regular daily routine is an effective way of coping with your illness. Usually the daily radiation session can be scheduled at your convenience, and having it set for the same time each day allows you to construct your life around it. Some people even find it possible to work during therapy, but don't push yourself too hard.

SIDE EFFECTS

Some uninformed people think radiation therapy is devastating, saying "the cure is worse than the disease." Dr. Manning, however, offers some reassurance. Many people who undergo radiation therapy suffer no severe side effects, she reports. Advances in radiation technology and in medical knowledge about how the body reacts to radiation have made it possible to kill cancer cells while minimizing damage to the healthy parts of the body. CAT scans and other sensing devices can now locate the precise site of most tumors, thus eliminating the need to radiate a bigger area in the hope of hitting all the cancer cells. Computers have made dosages more precise, too, so there is less chance of getting more radiation than is needed to do the job. Precise targeting and dosage mean less chance of damage to healthy tissue, and fewer side effects.

But radiation *is* powerful treatment, and it is unrealistic to expect it to affect only the cancer and not the rest of you, too. Nearly everyone who has radiation therapy experiences fatigue and some skin reactions. Beyond that, it is difficult to predict who will suffer side effects and how severe they may be. Much depends on the location of the tumor, the strength and duration of the treatment and the patient's general health. Eating well and taking care of yourself during radiation therapy are keys to regaining good health. And knowing that side effects may occur and what they may be, can make them easier to deal with.

FATIGUE AND EXHAUSTION

Fatigue, sometimes utter exhaustion, is one of the most commonly reported side effects of radiation therapy. This debilitation may be due to the illness itself, or to the stress and depression of coping with cancer. To compound that, waste products from the radiation's destruction of the cancer cells accumulate in your system, and your body's efforts to eliminate them are tiring, too. For any and all of these reasons, you should expect to feel tired, even exhausted, during your treatment. When it is finished, the fatigue will gradually go away.

In the meantime, you can cope with fatigue by getting more sleep at night, and scheduling naps either before or after treatments. Try to pace yourself in your everyday life, too. Don't give up doing things around the house or garden—keeping active is a good way to keep your spirits up—but don't try to do as much as you did before your illness began. Try to delegate some household tasks to family members or friends, or look for outside sources of help like homemakers or visiting social workers. Most likely you'll be able to resume your regular lifestyle after the therapy is over.

Other fatigue fighters include moderate exercise (consult your doctor first) and drinking eight to ten glasses of water a day to help flush those cellular waste products from your system. A well-balanced, nourishing diet will help counter exhaustion as well.

GASTROINTESTINAL PROBLEMS

Another misconception about radiation therapy is that it invariably causes severe vomiting and/or debilitating diarrhea. But Dr. Manning says she has never had a patient with problems so severe their treatment had to be interrupted. Changes in diet, and medications like anti-diarrheals almost always are enough, she says.

Radiation's effects on your gastrointestinal system depend on what part of your body is being treated. Therapy for a tumor in an extremity like a leg is unlikely to cause nausea or diarrhea. But treatment of a tumor in the head, neck or trunk will probably cause some digestive problems, because the lining of the whole digestive tract, from the mouth through the esophagus, stomach and intestines, is easily affected by radiation.

If you develop diarrhea or nausea (they don't usually start until a few weeks into the treatment) be sure to tell your doctor, radiation technologist and nurse. Drugs called anti-emetics can be prescribed to control nausea and vomiting, and your team will advise you of other ways to cope with it. These may include:

- Avoiding fatty foods.
- Sticking to clear liquids like cranberry juice, bouillon, gelatin, tea or carbonated beverages.
- Eating frequent, small meals.
- Munching on crackers or dry toast.
- Eating foods that are cold or at room temperature, like sandwiches or cereals.
- Avoiding sweets, spices and things with strong odors, like cheese.
- Experimenting with various eating patterns to determine if eating before or after your treatment makes a difference.
- Sleeping through it, if nausea periods are predictable, like after a treatment.
- Getting fresh air, either from an open window or a walk outside, if possible.

Many of the recomendations listed above apply to controlling diarrhea as well. But a few more things may help:

- Avoiding milk and other dairy products if they seem to make diarrhea worse.
- Drinking eight to ten glasses of liquid a day to counteract dehydration and mineral loss. Include fruit juices or electrolyte replacement drinks like Gatorade.
- Including high-potassium foods like bananas, potatoes or fruit nectars to replace this vital mineral.

A preliminary study in Canada shows that enteric-coated aspirin (the kind with a hard coating on the tablet to keep it from upsetting your stomach) reduces some of the gastrointestinal side effects of abdominal radiation therapy. Dr. Charles Ludgate, of the Cancer Control

Agency of British Columbia, gave eight patients three daily doses of 325 milligrams of enteric-coated aspirin for two to six months. After one month of aspirin, all eight had at least some improvement in their cramps, diarrhea or pain. Dr. Ludgate says that the aspirin may work by preventing muscle spasms in the intestines caused by radiation.

MOUTH AND DENTAL PROBLEMS

Since the tissues of your mouth are at the same time among the most delicate and the most abused in your body, it's no surprise that they can be adversely affected by radiation. Treatment, especially to the head or neck, can cause dry mouth, sores, loss of taste, throat pain and difficulty in swallowing. Any or all of these side effects could make eating unpleasant, just at a time when eating well is particularly important for you. It's for this reason your radiation therapy team will probably advise you to have any dental work you need done before you begin radiation therapy. Good dental hygiene is more essential than ever for you now, too. Here are some tips for preventing and/or dealing with mouth and throat problems:

- Brush teeth gently, with a soft, child's toothbush.
- Use a gentle toothpaste, perhaps one for sensitive teeth, or baking soda.
- Be sure to brush after each meal.
- Rinse the mouth with half-strength hydrogen peroxide. Avoid mouthwashes containing alcohol, which are irritating and drying.
- Use cocoa butter, lubricating jelly or a commercial lip balm to keep the lips soft.
- Drink water or other nonirritating liquids like fruit juices to keep the mouth moist.
- Avoid alcohol and tobacco.
- Avoid spicy, very hot or very cold foods, food that is hard to chew or crunchy (like popcorn or pretzels) and acidic foods like citrus.
- Add more liquid or semiliquid foods, such as soups, creamed food or gravies.

SKIN PROBLEMS

It's almost impossible to avoid some skin side effects from radiation. After all, the beams have to pass through it to reach the tumor. But your radiation therapy team will try to pinpoint the cancer's location so the smallest bit of your skin as possible is exposed to the radiation. Like the other potential side-effects, skin problems are highly variable and depend on several factors.

One is your skin's sensitivity to radiation, which is usually similar to its reaction to the sun. That is, if you are fair and tend to sunburn easily, your skin will probably react more to your therapy than someone whose skin is darker and tans well. In fact, damage to the skin shows up like sunburn, and may leave you with a permanently tanned spot where the beam was aimed.

About two weeks into your treatment, the irradiated spot will become reddish and perhaps itchy or sensitive to the touch. Here are some general guidelines for skin care during your treatment.

- DO NOT put anything like a lotion or ointment on the patch without consulting your doctor.
- Keep the area dry.
- Wash it *very* gently, if at all, with lukewarm water and *pat* it dry with a soft cloth.
- Avoid anything that may irritate your skin, from household cleaners to perfumes to constricting clothing.
- Don't shave in the area, except with an electric razor and only if your doctor says you may.
- Stay out of the sun during your treatment.

You may be temporarily more likely to sunburn at this time. Be especially careful of the radiated area of your skin; not only is it especially sensitive right now, you may have to shield it from the sun from now on.

If your skin is especially sensitive, or if the therapy is powerful or protracted, you may develop small, weeping blisters because your skin is shedding its upper layers. Tell your therapy team right away if this occurs, because your treatment may need to be halted temporarily. Your doctor may prescribe an antibiotic lotion or cream for you to apply to your skin to prevent infection, and suggest that you expose the area to the air several times a day.

After your therapy is over, the darkened patch of skin may fade over time. Or it may not, serving to remind you that from now on you must be careful about exposing that particular spot to the sun. Cover the area with a sunscreen with a sun protection factor (SPF) of 15 or more before going outside. In fact, with what we know now about the role sun plays in the development of skin cancer, you may want to apply sunscreen all over.

HAIR LOSS

Most people undergoing radiation therapy to the whole brain say this is the most upsetting side effect of all. Happily, it is also the most reversible.

Radiation causes hair to fall out because it interferes temporarily with follicle function. During radiation, the follicle produces either a weak, brittle hair which breaks easily, or no hair at all. Unlike chemotherapy, with whole-body effects that may cause total, though temporary baldness, radiation-induced hair loss is almost always confined to the area where you are being treated. So men may lose whiskers or chest hair if their treatment is aimed in that area. Radiation of the head may cause scalp hair to fall out.

The key to minimizing and managing hair loss is to be *gentle*. Handle your hair as little as possible during treatment and while it regrows. Here are some tips.

- Get a hairstyle that is easy to care for *before* treatment starts.
- Use a mild shampoo and conditioner, and only once or twice a week.
- Let your hair dry naturally; don't use electric blow dryers unless absolutely necessary.
- Don't comb or brush the hair too hard or too often.
- Avoid perms, hair dyes or hair spray. These can make hair dry and brittle and prone to breaking.
- Do not use rubber bands, hairpins, barrettes or electric rollers.

If you are faced with head radiation that may leave you completely bald for a while, choose a wig before your treatment starts.

THE FUTURE OF RADIATION THERAPY

Are there any breakthroughs on the horizon in radiation therapy? Both Dr. Hendee, the radiation physicist and Dr. Manning, the clinician, are optimistic.

At Howard and elswhere, Dr. Manning says, hyperthermia shows great promise. When cancer cells are at their most resistant to radiation, they are at their most vulnerable to heat. Once warmed to several degrees above body temperature and radiated, these resistant cells die. According to Dr. Manning, cancer researchers hope the one-two punch of heating a tumor by means of microwaves delivered through a needle and then treating it with radiation may prove devastating to cancers that are incurable now.

Dr. Hendee sees a future role for clones—synthetic cells—called monoclonal antibodies which can seek out only cancer cells and latch on to them. By attaching radioactive atoms to the antibodies, the radiation is delivered just to the tumor, bypassing healthy tissue in the process. This could eliminate the need for surgery in some cancer cases, and make it possible to treat heretofore unreachable tumors with radiation. He also says there are many investigations into other forms of radiation, such as neutrons, positive ions and pi-mesons, but such work is so preliminary and so expensive, he doesn't see it having a major impact on routine cancer treatment in the near future.

"The biggest breakthrough in cancer therapy may not to come from some new piece of machinery, though," Dr. Hendee suggests. "Learning how to harness and channel the power of each patient to help heal themselves—whether through guided imagery, relaxation therapy or some other sort of mental discipline—to me, that's one of the most exciting areas of investigation."

Surgical Treatment

No words had stunned Paul as much in his life. His doctor had just informed him that the lump on his prostate looked suspiciously like cancer—he would need surgery. His stomach tightened with fear; his mind filled with anxious questions. Would surgery really kill the cancer? Would his sex life end on the operating table?

During the weeks before further tests, Paul set out to learn all he could about prostate cancer and its treatment. He sent for brochures. He talked to men who had gone through prostate cancer surgery. He made a list of questions to ask his doctor.

This fact-finding flurry worried Paul's wife. She told him he was just working himself up unnecessarily and that he should leave everything to the "experts."

In fact, Paul's information quest was probably one of the best things he could do for himself. In fact, it's the "experts" who have found that knowledgeable patients have more successful operations and speedier recoveries. One study found that surgery patients shown a short slide and tape presentation about their operation needed less painkilling medication, and had less anxiety after the surgery than patients who didn't see the presentation.

516

"The body just works better if you know what is going to happen to it," explains W. Bradford Patterson, M.D., director of cancer control at the Dana-Farber Cancer Institute in Boston. "When you become informed about your surgery, you may be less tense, which means you are likely to breathe better. Better breathing helps fight infection in your lungs and generally helps you heal better."

Other experts believe that a feeling of control also may have an effect on the course of cancer, influencing the immune system and perhaps even helping the body resist a recurrence of the disease.

FIGHTING FEAR WITH FACTS

Perhaps the best reason for a fact-finding mission is this: It may ease the anxiety of undergoing surgery. "People fear cancer because they fear pain, disfigurement, disruption of normal activities and work, and ultimately, because they fear death," says Jeanne A. Petrek, M.D., breast cancer surgeon at Memorial Sloan-Kettering Cancer Center and author of *A Woman's Guide to the Prevention, Detection and Treatment of Cancer* (MacMillan). Yet, says Dr. Petrek, "even when these fears are realistic, information is helpful; the facts about diagnosis and treatment are more encouraging than might be supposed, due largely to recent dramatic advances."

You may be surprised, for example, to discover that 220,000 cases of cancer diagnosed each year are curable by surgery alone. Many operations are a lot less extensive than they used to be. Because cancer surgeons have employed new tools and added new therapies, often less tissue needs to be removed.

Take, for example, the use of the laser beam. The intense energy of this light is concentrated so that it can be used like a scalpel to remove tissue. It does not cut, however. It vaporizes. With lasers, surgeons can hone in on the troublesome tumor, even in hard-to-reach spots like the cervical canal. The laser will vaporize a tumor, leaving most of the surrounding tissue intact.

CELL SLEUTHING BEFORE SURGERY

If you are like most people, you may be more than a little worried that the discovery of a tumor will land you directly on the operating table. Not so. It takes a lot of sleuthing before the surgeon can even discuss treatment.

Why? Because, explains Robert McKenna, M.D., clinical professor of surgery at University of Southern California School of Medicine, in Los Angeles, no two cancers are alike. Some grow fast, some grow slow, some spread, and some stay put. That's why each cancer is treated differently. "One person may require one kind of surgery, while another may undergo surgery combined with radiation. Still a third may not be treated by surgery at all," he says.

What all this means is that before your surgeon knows which treatment is the best one for your cancer, you'll have to have your cells thoroughly scrutinized.

A biopsy provides the first examination of the suspicious cells. In this minor operation, a small amount of tissue is extracted from the tumor and placed on a slide for microscopic analysis. A pathologist then determines if the cells are benign, (which means they are from a noncancerous tumor) or malignant. Malignant cells signify cancer.

Other tests, such as bone and liver scans, can reveal whether cancer cells have spread to other locations. Additionally, your surgeon may remove and inspect some of the lymph nodes nearest the tumor. These are the structures which are believed to trap and destroy cancer cells and which may act as a barometer, foretelling microscopic invasion in the rest of the body. If the lymph nodes are found to be "negative," it means they contain no cancer, and that the disease probably has not spread from its original location. "Positive" nodes indicate the presence of cancer and probable spread.

BLUEPRINT FOR TREATMENT

Eventually, your condition is graded as being in one of four categories, according to how far it has advanced. Grades are A, B, C and D or Roman numerals I through IV. Cancer that is confined to the tumor site and has not spread is usually graded A or B (or I or II). The higher grades are usually assigned to cancer that has spread.

Once the status of the disease has been determined, the surgeon can then begin to select the treatment. If your cancer is in the early stages, (I, II or A, B) you will likely be treated locally by surgery, with or without radiation. Cancers in the later stages (III, IV or C, D) require chemotherapy, treatment with chemicals that go into the bloodstream to attack the cancer from within.

How does the surgeon know if the treatment will work? There are no guarantees, of course, but "cure rates" have been predicted for each treatment. That's the term for the percentage of people who have remained cancer-free after a number of years.

Aside from the stage of cancer, other factors help determine treatment. That's why there's no single "best" treatment for certain cancers, says Frederick Ames, M.D., associate professor of surgery at the University of Texas M.D. Anderson Hospital and Tumor Institute. "The deciding factor is often age, general health, lifestyle or even personal preference."

BREAST CANCER

Several years ago, the only treatment for breast cancer was radical mastectomy. This operation not only removed the breast and nipple, but the lymph nodes, chest muscle and most of the skin all the way down to the ribs. On occasion, women who went into the hospital for a biopsy awoke from anesthetic to discover their breast and muscles had been removed. Surgeons believed such quick and extensive surgery was best for stopping breast cancer in its tracks.

Today, partly because we have a better understanding of how breast cancer cells behave, the radical mastectomy is no longer the most common treatment. It's been replaced by less extensive operations, and some procedures simply remove little more than the lump itself.

Yet, the most important reason for the switch to more conservative surgery is this: Smaller tumors are being treated. "Thanks to earlier detection, women are coming in with lumps in earlier stages," reports Dr. Petrek. "Smaller lumps mean less radical treatment, and more chance that the breast can be spared."

Of course, treatment for breast cancer depends on your biopsy and tests results.

It's highly likely that the lump will be benign—the vast majority of all lumps biopsied are. If, however, it is found to be cancerous, those still in the early stages will have a choice of three surgical operations. Each of them has the same cure rate (about 80 to 90 percent). What differs about them is the amount of tissue taken out.

The surgery you and your doctor settle upon for the most part for early breast cancer, says Dr. Petrek, depends largely on your personal preference and lifestyle considerations.

To reach that decision, you'll need to gather information, weigh the pros and cons of the following operations and ask yourself questions. Fortunately, breast cancer is not likely to spread in the few weeks it takes for you to gather the information you need. So you will have time to, as one doctor put it, "accept the treatment that involves the least deformity, discomfort, disability, and risk of fatal complications—and gives the best chance of cure."

Modified radical mastectomy. This is now the most widely used surgical procedure. Like the radical version, it removes the breast tissue, nipple, and most or all of the lymph nodes under the arm. Unlike the radical mastectomy, it does not remove the chest muscle, so arm movement is spared. You may be relieved to know that breast reconstruction can be performed a few months after the mastectomy operation.

Simple mastectomy. In this procedure both muscle and lymph nodes are left in. This procedure is often chosen by doctors who be-

(continued on page 522)

FIVE SELF-CARE TIPS FOR BETTER SURGERY

"How well you weather the rigors of cancer surgery could very well depend upon how well you understand the procedure and how you have prepared yourself mentally and physically before the treatment," says Frederick Ames, M.D.

Here's a brief "to do" list that could help ensure successful surgery and recovery:

1. Seek a second opinion. "When there are several options to cancer surgery and your very life depends upon it, it only makes sense to seek a second opinon, a third and possibly a fourth," says Dr. Ames. But don't allow surgeon shopping to go on too long. "Accept the options offered, settle on a surgical team and trust that they are offering the best treatment available for your condition."

2. Don't sign until you're satisfied. Before you have any operation, you will probably be asked to sign an "informed consent" sheet, which lists the procedures, alternatives and risks. Being informed, though, is not the same as understanding. And the time to seek understanding is well before a paper is pushed under your nose.

   Make sure you understand what organs are being removed, what risks are involved and how it may affect your cancer, how it may affect your lifestyle, your looks, your sex life. Ask about your alternatives, and what happens if you don't have the surgery. What are the chances of the cancer recurring after surgery? What follow-up tests might you need? How long will your recovery take? What postoperative complications might you experience? How can you speed your recovery?

3. Stop smoking. Smoking puts a strain on your body's ability to recover from the trauma of anesthesia and surgery. Studies show that even quitting for 12 to 24 hours prior to surgery can make a difference in how fast you rally after an operation.

4. Stock up on nutrients. Your body needs all the nutrients it can get so that when the trauma of surgery occurs, you'll be able to withstand it, according to James L. Mullen, M.D., of the Hosptial of the University of Pennsylvania. "By getting the factory running at full speed—and

this takes from five to seven days—when the bomb hits, the body can handle it." A good diet, high in vitamins and minerals, should be one of your priorities before surgery.

The most important nutrients in terms of wound healing and infection fighting are vitamins A and C and the mineral zinc. The best food sources are yellow and orange vegetables and fruits, green leafy vegetables and liver for vitamin A; green peppers, citrus fruits, broccoli, Brussels sprouts and cantaloupe for vitamin C; and beef, lamb, chicken, cheese and pumpkin and sunflower seeds for zinc.

5. Seek psychological reassurance. "Cancer surgery may be more threatening, more anxiety provoking than other surgeries," notes Emily Mumford, Ph.D., professor of clinical sociomedical studies at Columbia College of Physicians and Surgeons, New York City. "You need to develop a coping style that will get you through it."

She suggests you do whatever it takes to help you manage the threat, so you may respond more appropriately to your treatment. "Do what you need to do to dispel awful fantasies which interfere with surgery and may prevent you from getting on with the business of treatment and healing."

For some, that may mean viewing an educational film about the operation. For the Scarlett O'Haras who would rather not think about it today, learning every squeamish detail may be a turn-off. They may prefer to be comforted by talking with someone who has had a similar operation.

Still others may find that they can ease their ordeal by practicing relaxation techniques, deep breathing, positive imagery or perhaps listening to a stress reduction tape.

According to Dr. Mumford, most patients recover better if they get a combination of education and emotional support. The point is, though, to choose a coping style that is reassuring.

lieve that allowing the lymph nodes to remain may help to fight cancer. That belief is backed by a recent study sponsored by the National Cancer Institute and the American Cancer Society. Researchers found that, after ten years, there were no differences in survival rates among women who were treated for breast cancer, whether the nodes were removed or not. Nevertheless, when the lymph nodes contained cancer and grew bigger, pain and swelling of the arms was the result.

Still, most doctors are not convinced that leaving in nodes won't provide a free ride for wandering cancer cells. In fact, almost half the women with breast cancer in the U.S. already have cancer in their lymph nodes. Others worry that failing to remove the nodes deprives surgeons of important information. "Knowing whether the lymph nodes are involved (in the cancer) is necessary for determining further treatment," says Dr. Petrek.

Lumpectomy, segmental or partial mastectomy. In this most sparing of all breast surgeries, only the tumor and a mimimum of surrounding tissue are removed, along with a few lymph nodes from the armpit. And to make sure that cancer is killed at its roots and that no stray cells are lurking elsewhere in the breast, surgery is usually followed by a series of radiation treatments for several weeks.

The radiation component can cut the chances of breast cancer recurring by nearly a third and may be one reason why studies have found that lumpectomy may even have a slight edge over mastectomy when it comes to killing cancer in its early stages.

In 1976, a study called the National Surgical Adjuvant Breast Project began to be conducted by Bernard Fisher, M.D. It involved nearly 2,000 women who had breast cancer tumors of about an inch and a half in size. Each woman was randomly assigned treatment either by total mastectomy, lumpectomy or lumpectomy with radiation.

What Dr. Fisher and his collegues discovered was that overall survival after lumpectomy with or without radiation was better than overall survival after total mastectomy. More than 92 percent of the women treated with radiation remained free of breast tumors after five years, while only 72 percent of the women without radiation were cancer-free at that time.

The advantage of the lumpectomy is obvious: Women get to keep their breasts. The disadvantage, though, is that not everyone is eligible, particularly those women who may have a large tumor or a small breast. Furthermore, some patients may wish to avoid radiation.

There is also the concern that radiation is expensive, time-consuming and may possibly induce a cancer down the road, especially for younger women. However, assures Dr. Petrek, "the benefits of killing local cancer today outweigh the possibility of promoting local cancer tomorrow."

These are important concerns which should be raised before the biopsy, not after. The reason? If you are eligible for breast conservation, it is possible for the doctor to perform it at the time of the biopsy. You need to go into the biopsy knowing as much as you can so there are no surprises when you wake up.

COLORECTAL CANCER

We can probably thank President Reagan for helping to bring colorectal cancer out of the closet and into the doctor's office. The news about his 1985 operation undoubtedly prompted countless people to seek treatment for their own symptoms, an action that might have saved more than a few lives.

According to LaSalle Leffall, M.D., professor and chairman of the department of surgery, Howard University College of Medicine, Washington, D.C., "if people get early treatment for colorectal cancer, they have an 80 to 90 percent chance of being cured." If treatment isn't received until the cancer has spread, only a third of the people will be cured.

Even so, many people have been scared off by colorectal surgery. One reason, perhaps, is that they may not be aware that, many times, removing colorectal cancer may be as uncomplicated as plucking off polyps that have grown like mushrooms along the colon. These tumors can be snared with the colonoscope, the telescopic instrument used to examine the colon.

If cancer is present, a colon resection [removal of a segment of the large intestine] is performed. This procedure is somewhat like removing the bad section from a pipeline. The part of the colon that contains the cancer is removed, along with the lymph nodes that drain this area. The healthy ends are rejoined. The colon may be shorter, but it is now cancer-free.

Only when the ends cannot be rejoined—usually because the cancer is located too low down in the rectum—is a colostomy performed. A colostomy creates an opening in the abdomen, through which waste is eliminated and collected in a bag worn outside the body.

Fortunately, this procedure is used much less frequently than in the past. A new device has made permanent colostomies unnecessary in about one in ten colorectal cancer patients. The device is a stapling instrument that allows the surgeon to reconnect the ends of the rectum where sutures couldn't reach. "If people learn that colorectal cancer can be cured without a colostomy, it may lead to earlier diagnosis and treatment," says Dr. Leffall.

Treatment doesn't end with the last stitch or staple, however. If you are at high risk for polyps—like President Reagan—you, too, may need to regularly have a colonoscopy, which allows a doctor to snip off any polyps before they grow into cancer.

GYNECOLOGICAL CANCERS

To understand the treatment options available for gynecological cancers, a brief anatomy lesson is in order. Picture the uterus as an upside down pear. The cervix is at the bottom, the top of the uterus lined with the endometrium is the bulging middle part, while the ovaries are perched at the end of the fallopian tubes, which sprout out near the top of the pear and branch out to both sides.

These sites can be host to the three kinds of cancer: cervical, endometrial and ovarian. Each cancer has its own treatment. In general, though, the farther up the pear the cancer is located, the harder it is to cure, and the fewer the treatment options.

Fortunately, the most common cancer—and the easiest to treat—is at the lowest level. In fact, cervical cancer is nearly 100 percent curable if the abnormal cells (called dysplasic) are in the precancerous, nonspreading or *in situ,* stage. Luckily, these cells are picked up by the Pap test most of the time.

Precancerous cells in the cervix are fairly easy to remove. They may be frozen off in the doctor's office or removed during a conization, an in-patient procedure which involves removing a cone-shaped wedge of the cervix containing the suspicious cells.

Precancerous cells in the endometrium may be scraped completely away during a procedure called a D and C, so nicknamed because it "dilates" the cervix and uses an instrument called a curette for scraping. This early treatment can result in a complete cure.

The treatment turns more serious the farther cells have spread. If cancer has reached up the cervical canal, for example, you may need to have a hysterectomy, the procedure which removes the cervix, the uterus, upper vagina, and possibly the lymph nodes.

While drastic, this procedure works. Hysterectomy cures cervical cancer that is confined to the cervical canal up to 85 percent of the time.

If you require a hysterectomy because of cancer in an ovary, it may be possible for the other, healthy ovary to remain intact. That way your estrogen supply is safeguarded.

Women should always ask about the possibility of sparing ovaries before being treated for cancer. In fact, it's a good idea to ask a lot of questions before any hysterectomy, since each procedure is different. Find out what's to be removed and if it can be removed through your vagina, rather than through an abdominal incision. "There is evidence that the procedure is just as effective, and it could spare you complications, as well as shorten your hospital stay," advise doctors.

LUNG CANCER

It's been called the cancer that may be the easiest to prevent but the hardest to conquer once you have it. Why? Because lung cancer is very aggressive and "silent"—it shows no symptoms until it has already spread. By that time, only about 13 percent of the people who have it live five or more years after diagnosis. And that's when all the big guns in the anticancer arsenal are used, including surgery, radiation therapy and chemotherapy.

The bright spot in this bleak picture is that if cancer is confined to the lung, it can be cured about 80 percent of the time. Other encouraging news is that surgeons no longer need to take large sections of the lung to kill the cancer. Studies have shown that it is possible in certain instances to remove just a wedge of the lung while conserving lung tissue. This procedure produces the same results as more extensive operations.

A new no-knife procedure may provide still another ray of hope for curing lung cancer. It's called photodynamic therapy and it uses a chemical and a laser beam. First, a photoactive chemical is injected into the bloodstream. When the laser beam strikes this substance, it turns into a poison that kills the cancer cells.

"Photodynamic therapy could turn out to be a very effective way to control very early cancers before they are visible and it may alleviate some of the symptoms in advanced cancer." says Stuart Pett, M.D., associate professor of surgery, University of New Mexico in Albuquerque. Another plus for the photo killers: They involve less pain and fewer side effects than standard surgery.

PROSTATE CANCER

Remember our friend Paul who worried that prostate surgery could end his sex life? He's not alone. Many men have shared this same fear, which is one reason why they may not dash to their doctors for a digital rectal exam.

But judging from the declining rates of deaths from prostate cancer, men have apparently gotten the good word: Prostate cancer can be cured 83 percent of the time if it's found before it spreads. The best part is that the surgical treatment need not mean a life of celibacy.

The credit for developing an operation which kills the cancer but spares the sexual plumbing goes to Patrick Walsh, M.D., chairman of the department of urology, Johns Hopkins University School of Medicine, Baltimore. Dr. Walsh discovered that he could treat prostate cancer by altering the radical prostatectomy technique. He removed the prostate gland, capsule, seminal vesicles and lymph nodes but found a way to do it without damaging the pelvic nerves that control erection. Then he studied his patients for a year.

What he found was that, after six months, 40 percent of the men were potent. After a year, all who were potent prior to surgery retained their ability to get an erection.

This nerve-sparing technique is good news, comments Robert P. Gibbons, M.D., professor of urology, and head of urology section at Virginia Mason Medical Center in Seattle. "Surgery provides the best chance of controlling cancer and now the odds are that it won't impair sexual functioning." If impotency does occur, it often can be successfully treated with a penile implant or injection, he adds.

Men found to have prostate cancer that is confined to the prostate usually have a 15-year survival rate following radical surgery. "Vigilance is the key to curing prostate cancer," says Dr. Gibbons. "All men over the age of 45 should have at least a digital rectal examination performed annually."

SKIN CANCER

If you've been staring at those strange spots that have cropped up on the backs of your hands or on your face, don't wait for them to go away. They probably won't. At least not without a little help. The grayish warts may be basal cell carcinoma; the red, crusty patches may be squamous cell carcinoma. Both are skin cancers.

And both can be cured if you have them removed when you first notice them. Best of all, most procedures are quick, painless and leave barely a scar.

Your doctor will numb your skin and remove the spot along with some surrounding tissue. If the tissue borders reveal cancer cells, more tissue will be taken until there is no trace of cancer.

Larger spots—over half an inch—require a little more surgery. The tumorous tissue is scraped out using a ring-shaped instrument, called a curette, while an electric needle burns a safety margin of normal skin around the tumor.

Tumors located in taut areas like the eyelids where skin can't be spared will need to be frozen off via a procedure called cryosurgery. Cancerous tissue is destroyed by the application of intense cold from liquid nitrogen and then slowly thawed. The tumor is destroyed and falls off within 24 hours.

Sometimes, it's impossible to figure out just where the borders are on skin cancer cells or just how far down into the skin the cancer has extended. Without removing the roots, the cancer can grow back.

Dermatologist Frederick Mohs found a way to solve that problem. He developed a procedure (now aptly dubbed, Mohs Surgery) which involves applying strong chemicals directly on the cancer and then cutting off a layer of skin about one-tenth of an inch thick. Each layer is checked immediately under the microscope for malignant growth and for the presence of a tumor. Shaving continues until the tissue is tumor-free.

The plus for this procedure is that it traces the cancer to the core but spares healthy tissue, which is especially important for those tight spots like the curve of the ear, reports B. Dale Wilson, M.D., assistant professor of dermatology, and clinician in Mohs Surgery at the Roswell Park Memorial Institute.

As effective as Mohs Surgery may be, the control of skin cancer once you're cured is up to you, reminds Dr. Wilson. "Don't even think of going into the sun without a sunscreen."

Glossary

Sarcoma, carcinoma. Colonoscopy, cystoscopy. Antibody, antigen. These words and others like them, scientific and medical terms that seem to be part of any discussion of a major health issue like cancer, may confuse and frustrate you if you are trying to learn about the factors that affect your health. In order to help you benefit from the information in this book, this section presents a list of many of the most frequently used terms (in alphabetical order, of course) and their meanings. In some definitions, a word or words are printed in italic type to signal that these words can also be found as a main entry.

Acute myelocytic leukemia (AML). Cancer of the white blood cells. It occurs mostly in adults and, if untreated, progresses rapidly. In people with Hodgkin's disease, it may result from a cancer treatment using *alkylating agents.*

Adenoma. A *tumor* that is *benign* and grows on the surface of an organ or a gland.

Alkylating agent. A synthetic compound used in cancer *chemotherapy* to destroy *malignant* cells, apparently by altering the *DNA* in the cell nuclei. These drugs can also destroy healthy cells and have been shown to increase the risk of other types of cancer.

528

Allergy. A sensitivity to a specific substance that produces any of a number of symptoms, commonly respiratory (sneezing, coughing) or skin reactions (hives, rashes). People with some allergies seem to have increased resistance to cancer because their immune systems are extrasensitive.

Amino acids. Chemical substances that form the basis of protein and occur naturally in plant and animal tissue. There are 20 amino acids necessary for the production of protein; the body can make 11 of them, but the remaining 9 must be obtained from food.

AML. See *Acute myelocytic leukemia.*

Amyldimethyl PABA. A form of *para-aminobenzoic acid* that, in combination with other screening agents, is an ingredient in sunscreens; also called padimate A.

Anthranilates. Ingredients in sunscreens that can screen both types of *ultraviolet light.*

Antibody. Antibodies are produced by white blood cells in response to specific foreign substances. They circulate in the bloodstream to fight off these foreign organisms. If the same alien substance attacks again, the white blood cells are able to recognize it sooner and reproduce the specific antibody to deal with it.

Antigen. Any substance capable of triggering the production of *antibodies.*

Antioxidant. A substance that has the ability to prevent or delay deterioration caused by the action of oxygen. In the body, antioxidants such as vitamin E may prevent the formation of *free radicals,* substances linked to cancer.

Artificial sweeteners. See *Aspartame; Cyclamates; Saccharin; Sorbitol.*

Aspartame. A synthetic compound of two *amino acids* that is used as a low-calorie *artificial sweetener.* It is 180 times as sweet as sugar.

Asthma. A respiratory condition that is characterized by recurrent attacks of breathing difficulty and wheezing, caused by spasms of the air passages in the lungs. It appears that some people who have asthma may have increased resistance to cancer.

Ataxia telangiectasia. A *hereditary* condition that causes nerve damage, lesions on the eyes and respiratory difficulties. People with this condition are at high risk for various forms of cancer.

Atrophy. The degeneration of a body part due to lack of activity.

Basal cell carcinoma. The most common type of skin cancer, usually caused by overexposure to the sun. It is usually localized but can spread if not treated.

Benign. The term used to describe a noncancerous *tumor* or condition.

Benign breast disease. The presence of noncancerous growths in the breast tissue. See also *Fibrocystic disease.*

Benzophenones. Ingredients that, in combination with forms of *para-aminobenzoic acid,* are used in sunscreens.

Benzopyrene. A cancer-causing *hydrocarbon* found in coal tar and cigarette smoke.

Beta-carotene. A yellow-red pigment found in some fruits and vegetables. It is a *precursor* of vitamin A, to which it converts in the body, and is thought to have a protective effect against cancer.

Bile. A greenish yellow fluid secreted by the liver and stored in the gallbladder until needed for digestion. It promotes digestion by creating an alkaline environment in the intestines and aiding in the absorption of fats. However, it is possible that excess fat and excess bile may contribute to intestinal cancer. See also *Bile acids.*

Bile acids. Acids derived from *cholesterol.* Some bile acids are carcinogenic and may play a part in the development of intestinal cancer.

Bioflavonoids. A group of components, found mainly in the white peel of citrus fruits, that have been shown to increase the absorption of vitamin C. They may also have a protective effect against cancer.

Biopsy. A procedure used to obtain a tissue sample for the diagnosis of cancer. It may involve taking the sample surgically or using a needle to draw tissue from the area.

Boil. A painful but noncancerous lump on the skin caused by staphylococcus bacteria. A boil usually has a "core" that contains pus and is surrounded by an area of inflammation.

Breast self-exam (BSE). The process by which a woman examines her breasts each month to detect suspicious lumps or changes in the skin.

BSE. See *Breast self-exam.*

Carbon monoxide. A colorless, odorless, tasteless gas formed by burning carbon or organic fuels in the presence of very little oxygen. It is a harmful component of cigarette and marijuana smoke.

Carcinoembryonic antigen (CEA). An *antigen* that is secreted into the bloodstream when certain types of cancer are present. By monitoring the quantity of CEA in the blood, doctors can detect the presence of these cancers and/or assess the progress of treatment.

Carcinogen. Any substance capable of causing cancer.

Carcinogenesis. The development or production of cancer.

Carcinoma. A *malignant* growth that tends to spread to surrounding areas and lead to *metastasis.* The majority of cancers of the breast, uterus, intestinal tract, skin and tongue involve carcinomas.

Carcinoma *in situ.* A *malignant* growth that is confined to the surface cells of the affected area.

CEA. See *Carcinoembryonic antigen.*

Cell. The basic structural unit of living organisms.

Cellulose. The most prevalent type of *fiber,* found in fruits, vegetables, nuts and bran. It helps relieve constipation and may help flush out *toxins* from the body and modulate blood *glucose* levels.

Cervical dysplasia. The presence of abnormal, possibly precancerous, cells in the cervix.

Cervical intraepithelial neoplasia. Abnormal growth and multiplication of cells on the surface of the cervix, which can lead to cancer if undetected.

Cervicography. A diagnostic test for cervical abnormalities in which a photographic instrument is used to obtain a photograph of the cervix. The slide, or cervigram, can then be read like an x-ray.

Chemotherapy. A method of cancer treatment that uses any of a number of drugs, or a combination of drugs, to destroy and/or retard the growth of *malignant* cells.

Cholesterol. A fatlike substance found in the body in the brain, nerves, blood and *bile*. It is manufactured by the liver and is necessary for various body functions. However, excess dietary cholesterol, obtained from animal fats and oils, has been implicated in heart and circulatory disease and may be a risk factor for bowel cancer.

Chromosome. A structure in the nucleus of animal and human cells. It contains the *DNA* of the cell.

Cilia. Tiny hairlike structures in the respiratory tract whose function is to sweep out impurities. If they are damaged, as they can be by various pollutants or cigarette smoke, the lungs are more vulnerable to disease.

Cinnamate. A substance that, in combination with *benzophenones* and forms of *para-aminobenzoic acid,* is used as an ingredient in sunscreens. Also called Octyl methoxycinnamate.

Cocarcinogen. A noncarcinogenic substance that increases the effect of a *carcinogen.*

Colonoscopy. Examination of the colon with a long, flexible, lighted instrument.

Colostomy. A surgical procedure in which an artificial opening is created in the intestine and extended to the abdomen for removal of body wastes. It is sometimes necessary after the removal of a diseased section of the large intestine.

Condyloma virus. See *Human papilloma virus.*

Contaminant. A substance that causes another substance to become impure. Environmental contaminants can be health hazards, contributing to many diseases, including cancer.

Cortisol. An adrenal *hormone* that turns body fat into *glucose* for energy.

Cyclamates. *Artificial sweeteners* that have been banned because of their possible cancer-causing effects.

Cyst. A closed sac or capsule that contains liquid or a semisolid substance. Cysts are usually harmless, but they should be removed to avoid possible infection or cell changes that could lead to cancer.

Cystoscopy. Examination of the bladder with a hollow metal tube that has a lighted end to allow a view of the inside of the organ.

Deoxyribonucleic acid (DNA). The basic component of all living matter. It occurs in the *chromosomes* and controls and transmits the *hereditary, genetic* code.

Dermatology. The medical specialty that deals with the diagnosis and treatment of skin diseases.

DES. See *Diethylstilbestrol.*

DHA. See *Docosahexaenoic acid.*

Diethylstilbestrol (DES). A synthetic form of *estrogen* that has been linked to incidence of cancer in children of mothers who were given the hormone to prevent miscarriage.

Diuretic. A medication or any other substance that increases the excretion of body fluids, especially urine.

DNA. See *Deoxyribonucleic acid.*

Docosahexaenoic acid (DHA). One of the *omega-3 long-chain fatty acids,* found in fish oils, that are believed to help protect against the artery-blocking and carcinogenic effects of other fats.

Dysfunction. The disturbance, impairment or abnormality of function of an organ.

Dysplasia. Abnormal development or changes in cells, sometimes an indication of the future development of cancer.

Eicosapentaenoic acid (EPA). One of the *omega-3 long-chain fatty acids,* found in fish oils, that are believed to help protect against the artery-blocking and carcinogenic effects of other fats.

Endocrine glands. Glands that secrete *hormones* to control digestion, reproduction, growth, metabolism and other body functions. The pituitary gland, thyroid gland, ovaries and testes, for example, are endocrine glands.

Endocrinology. The medical specialty that deals with the functions of the *endocrine glands* and the *hormones* they produce, as well as the diagnosis and treatment of endocrine disorders.

Endoscopy. Examination of interior body structures with an endoscope, an instrument designed to allow examination of hollow organs or body cavities. Types of endoscopes include the cystoscope (for the bladder) and proctoscope (for the colon).

Enzyme. A substance, usually a protein, that causes a chemical reaction in the body. Some enzymes may be involved with the action of *carcinogens*.

EPA. See *Eicosapentaenoic acid.*

Epidemiology. The medical specialty that deals with finding the causes of specific occurrences of diseases, toxic poisonings and other such occurrences that may be confined to a specific geographical area or segment of the population.

Essential fatty acids. Unsaturated *fatty acids* that cannot be formed in the body and must be provided from dietary sources. Excess intake of fatty acids, as from vegetable oils, may contribute to the development of cancer by promoting the formation of *prostaglandins*.

Estrogen. The female sex *hormone,* which controls the development of physical sexual characteristics, as well as menstruation and pregnancy. Synthetic forms of estrogen are used in *oral contraceptives* and in various therapies. They have been implicated in the development of some types of cancer.

Familial polyposis. A *hereditary* condition in which members of the same family develop intestinal *polyps*. Also called *Gardner's syndrome,* it is considered a risk factor for colorectal cancer.

Fanconi's anemia. A rare *hereditary* condition that leads to the development of cancer by making body cells more vulnerable to the action of *carcinogens*.

Fats. Animal or vegetable products that are eaten in many forms— butter, margarine, oils, dairy products, meats—and are essential to many body processes. Excess fat intake, however, has been implicated in various health conditions, including heart disease and cancer. See also *Lipids.*

Fat-soluble. Capable of being dissolved or released in the presence of fat. Fat-soluble substances, such as vitamins A, E, D and K, are stored in the body and not excreted, so an excess can be harmful.

Fatty acid. A compound of carbon, hydrogen and oxygen that combines with another chemical substance to form a fat. Some fatty acids are necessary for growth and metabolism, others may have a protective effect against cancer, and still others may contribute to the development of cancer.

Fiber. The indigestible portion of vegetables and fruits. Different types of fiber perform different functions in the body, including softening stools and adding to their bulk and absorbing wastes and *toxins* and carrying them from the body. See also *Cellulose; Pectin; Hemicellulose; Lignin; Gums/mucilages.*

Fiberoptics. The transmission of an image along flexible bundles of glass or plastic. Fiberoptics are used in some diagnostic instruments for examinations using *endoscopy.*

Fibrocystic disease. A condition in which fluids normally absorbed by breast tissue become trapped and form *cysts,* which may come and go in relation to the menstrual cycle. There may be a link between fibrocystic disease and the risk of breast cancer.

Five-year survival rate. A term used for those who have lived five years after being diagnosed with cancer. At this point, if the diagnosed cancer has not reappeared, and no new cancer has developed, doctors consider the patient recovered, or on the way to total recovery.

Free radicals. By-products of *oxidation* that damage body cells and thus leave the cells vulnerable to the effects of *carcinogens.*

Fumigant. A substance (smoke, gas or vapor) used to destroy pests. The use of some fumigants on food crops can lead to harmful effects when the food products are eaten.

Fungicide. A substance that destroys fungi or inhibits their growth. If residues remain on food crops, they can be toxic.

Gardner's syndrome. See *Familial polyposis.*

Gastroenterology. The medical specialty that deals with the diagnosis and treatment of diseases of the stomach and intestines.

Gene. A biologic unit of heredity that makes up segments of *DNA* and determines all inherited characteristics.

Genetic engineering. The process of changing certain *hereditary* traits, including predisposition to some types of cancer, by altering genetic makeup.

Genetic predisposition. A *hereditary* tendency to disease.

Genetics. The study of heredity and the factors that affect it.

Glucose. A simple sugar that is the main source of energy for living organisms. The body produces glucose as the end product of carbohydrate digestion.

Gums/mucilages. Forms of *fiber* used as thickening agents in foods. Gums can help lower *cholesterol* and modulate blood *glucose* levels.

Gynecology. The medical specialty that deals with the diagnosis and treatment of diseases of the female reproductive system.

HDL. See *High-density lipoproteins.*

Hemicellulose. A form of *fiber* found in fruits, vegetables and bran. Hemicellulose relieves constipation and may help flush *toxins* out of the body.

Herbicide. A chemical substance used to destroy or inhibit plant growth, as in weed killers. Exposure to some of these substances has been shown to increase cancer risk.

Hereditary. Genetically transmitted from parents to offspring. Hereditary material is contained in the ovum and sperm, so a person's inherited characteristics are determined at conception. See also *DNA; Gene.*

High-density lipoproteins (HDL). The type of fatty proteins in the blood that are believed to be beneficial because they carry *cholesterol* from artery walls and deposit it in the liver, where it is stored or excreted. A diet high in *polyunsaturated fats* increases HDL.

Hormone. A chemical messenger secreted by the *endocrine glands* and carried in the bloodstream to produce a specific effect on the body. Hormones control growth, metabolism, reproduction and other functions.

HPV. See *Human papilloma virus.*

Human papilloma virus (HPV). A sexually transmitted virus that causes genital warts. It is thought to be a cause of cervical cancer.

Hydrocarbons. A large group of compounds, composed of carbon and hydrogen, that are produced when meats are broiled or smoked and also are found in marijuana smoke.

Hysterectomy. Surgical removal of the uterus.

Immune system. The body mechanisms that resist and fight disease. The main defenders are white blood cells (*lymphocytes,* phagocytes, etc.) and *antibodies,* which, along with other specialized defenders, react to the presence of foreign substances in the body and try to destroy them.

Immunosuppressive drug. A drug that modifies the natural immune response so that it will not react to a foreign substance in the body. This type of drug is most commonly given after organ transplants so that the new organ will not be rejected. However, because they alter the immune response, these drugs can put patients at greater risk for cancer.

Insecticide. A chemical agent used to destroy insects. Exposure to some of these substances can increase cancer risk.

Insulin. A protein hormone, produced by the pancreas, that participates in carbohydrate and fat metabolism and controls *glucose* levels in the blood.

Internal medicine. The medical specialty that deals with conditions that do not require surgery.

Intradermal test. A diagnostic test for infectious disease and allergy in which a small amount of the suspected substance is injected between layers of the skin to see if a reaction occurs.

Invasive cancer. Cancer that spreads to the healthy tissue surrounding the original *tumor* site.

Ionizing radiation. A type of electromagnetic radiation, such as x-rays, that is capable of ionizing (altering the number of electrons) the atoms of body tissues. The process of ionizing may lead to *genetic* changes in the cells that may in turn lead to cancer.

Kaposi's sarcoma. A type of skin cancer that is associated with reduced immune response, as in people with acquired immune deficiency syndrome (AIDS) and those who are taking *immunosuppressive drugs.*

Lactobacillus acidophilus. A type of bacteria, found in the intestinal tract and in some kinds of yogurt, that may retard the activity of an *enzyme* believed to convert harmless substances into *carcinogens* in the digestive tract.

Lactose intolerance. The inability to digest milk and milk products due to a deficiency of or lack of the *enzyme* lactase.

LDL. See *Low-density lipoproteins.*

Lignin. A type of *fiber* found in fruits, vegetables and bran. It has the ability to help lower *cholesterol* levels in the blood.

Lipids. Forms of fats, such as *cholesterol* and *triglycerides,* that circulate in the bloodstream.

Lipoproteins. Compounds of proteins with fats that carry *cholesterol* in the bloodstream. See also *High-density lipoproteins; Low-density lipoproteins; Very low-density lipoproteins.*

Low-density lipoproteins (LDL). Fatty proteins that carry *cholesterol* to the body cells, including the blood vessels, where it can build up and cause circulatory and heart problems.

Lumpectomy. Surgical removal of a small, localized, *malignant* breast *tumor* and the surrounding tissue. It is a less radical procedure than *mastectomy,* and is usually followed by *radiation treatment.*

Lymph nodes. Small, oval-shaped organs, located throughout the body, that produce infection-fighting *lymphocytes* and filter germs and foreign substances from the lymph fluid.

Lymphocytes. Disease-fighting white blood cells that are produced by the *lymph nodes.*

Macrophages. White blood cells that destroy invading organisms by ingesting them.

Malignant. The term used to describe a cancerous *tumor* or condition.

Malignant melanoma. A cancerous skin *tumor* made up of *melanin*-producing cells anywhere on the body.

Malnutrition. Poor nutrition resulting from a deficiency in diet or an inability of the body to utilize food.

Mammography. A diagnostic x-ray of the breasts, used when suspicious lumps are found. It is also used as a screening procedure for women who are at high risk for breast cancer.

Mastectomy. Surgical removal of cancerous breast and nearby *lymph nodes.*

Melanin. Black or dark brown pigment in the skin.

Melanoma. A tumor that is usually *malignant* and has a dark pigment.

Metastasis. The spread of cancer from the primary site or organ to another site or organ. Specific cancers sometimes have somewhat predictable patterns of metastasis.

Methylxanthines. Ingredients in coffee and tea—caffeine, theobromine and theophylline—that have been studied for their possible relationship to *fibrocystic disease.* No increased risk was found.

Minipill. An *oral contraceptive* that contains only *progestin.* It is prescribed for nursing mothers, women over 35 and those who cannot tolerate *estrogen.*

Monoclonal antibodies. Highly specific antibodies that react to a specific *antigen.* They are used in diagnostic tests to detect the presence of cancer.

Multiphasic pill. An *oral contraceptive* that contains only enough estrogen to prevent ovulation and varying amounts of *progestin* to help control breakthrough bleeding and other side effects.

Multiple myeloma. A type of cancer in which bone is destroyed, resulting in fractures and bone pain. People with this type of cancer who are being treated with *alkylating agents* are at greater risk for leukemia within four to five years after treatment.

Mutagen. A substance that accelerates the normal rate of *mutation* in genetic material.

Mutation. The process by which a *gene* undergoes a permanent change that will affect its heredity.

Neoplasia. The formation of a *tumor.*

Nitrate. A substance that is present in water and some foods and is converted to *nitrite* in storage, during cooking or during digestion.

Nitrite. A substance that occurs in foods, either as a product of *nitrate* breakdown or when added artificially as a preservative, that reacts with other substances in the body to produce *nitrosamines.*

Nitrosamines. Powerful *carcinogens* formed in the stomach when a food containing *nitrate* or *nitrite* is eaten.

Node. A small mass of tissue that contains *lymphocytes.*

Nodule. A small, solid mass of tissue.

Occult. Hidden, as occult blood in the stool.

Octyldimethyl PABA. A form of *para-aminobenzoic acid* that, along with other screening agents, is an ingredient in sunscreens; also called padimate O.

Octyl methoxycinnamate. See *Cinnamate.*

Omega-6 fatty acids. A type of *fatty acids,* found in vegetable oils, that have been linked to the production of harmful *prostaglandins* and the development of cancer.

Omega-3 long-chain fatty acids. A type of *fatty acids,* found in fish oils, that are thought to neutralize the effects of the *omega-6 fatty acids* by inhibiting their ability to trigger the production of *prostaglandins.*

Oncology. The medical specialty that deals with the diagnosis, treatment, and study of cancer.

Oral contraceptives. Contraceptives containing *estrogen* and *progestin* that prevent conception by inhibiting ovulation and thickening cervical mucus so that sperm cannot penetrate.

Oxalic acid. A substance found in some vegetables that binds with calcium and prevents its absorption.

Oxidation. The action of oxygen on a substance, usually producing deterioration. The effect of oxidation on body cells produces *free radicals.*

Oxybenzone. See *Benzophenones.*

PABA. See *Para-aminobenzoic acid.*

Palpation. Examination by feeling an area of the body with the fingers to detect abnormalities.

Pap test. A diagnostic and screening test in which a scraping of cells is taken from the cervix. The Pap test can detect cervical abnormalities and precancerous conditions before any symptoms are evident.

Para-aminobenzoic acid (PABA). A B vitamin that, in several forms, is used as an ingredient in sunscreens.

Patch test. A diagnostic test for allergy in which a small patch impregnated with the suspected allergen is applied to the skin to see if a reaction occurs.

Pathology. The medical specialty that deals with the causes, nature and effects of diseases and abnormalities.

Pectin. A type of *fiber,* commonly known as fruit fiber, that is found in fruits and some vegetables. It does not affect constipation but does have the ability to lower *cholesterol* levels.

Pharmacology. The medical specialty that deals with the nature and properties of drugs.

Phytate. A substance in *fiber* that can bind with calcium and prevent its absorption.

Polyp. A growth that protrudes from mucous membrane. Polyps may be found in the nose, ears, mouth, lungs, heart, uterus, cervix, rectum, bladder and intestine. Polyps that occur in the cervix, intestine, stomach, or colon can eventually become malignant and should be removed.

Polyunsaturated fat. The type of fat, found in vegetable oils such as corn oil and safflower oil, that has been associated with lower cholesterol levels and with a higher ratio of *high-density lipoprotein* to *low-density lipoprotein* cholesterol.

Precancer. A condition that tends to become *malignant,* such as intestinal polyps.

Precursor. A substance from which another substance is formed, such as *beta-carotene,* which is a precursor of vitamin A.

Preinvasive. A term used to describe abnormal tissue that has not yet invaded the area outside the original site of growth.

Procarcinogen. A chemical substance that becomes carcinogenic only after it has been altered during body processes such as digestion.

Proctology. The medical specialty that deals with disorders of the rectum and anus.

Proctosigmoidoscopy. Examination of the rectum and sigmoid colon with a sigmoidoscope. See also *Sigmoidoscopy.*

Progesterone. The female sex *hormone* that causes the buildup of the uterine lining in preparation for conception and performs other functions prior to and during pregnancy.

Progestin. A synthetic form of *progesterone,* used in combination with *estrogen* in *oral contraceptives.*

Prognosis. A prediction of the probable course and outcome of an occurrence of disease, including the prospects for recovery.

Prostaglandins. Hormonelike substances formed from *essential fatty acids.* Prostaglandins affect the operation of the nervous system, reproductive system, circulatory system and metabolism. Depending on several factors, their effects on the body can be either beneficial or harmful.

Psychoactive. Affecting the mind and/or behavior.

Rad. An acronym for "radiation absorbed dose," a measurement of the absorbed dose of tissue by *ionizing radiation.* The term is used in assessing levels of radiation.

Radiation treatment. A type of therapy in which controlled doses of radiation are delivered to destroy or stop the growth of *malignant* cells.

Radioactive markers. Radioactive isotopes that are introduced into the body to help pinpoint areas where cancer exists.

Radiology. The medical specialty that deals with the use of radiation in the diagnosis of disease.

Radon. A colorless, odorless gaseous element, produced by the breakdown of radium, that has been found in the environment and is believed to be a cause of lung cancer.

Retinoblastoma. A rare, usually *hereditary,* form of eye cancer in children that is present at birth but may not produce symptoms until the age of 2 or 3.

Ribonucleic acid (RNA). A nucleic acid that is present in all cells and is similar to *DNA.* It controls the formation of protein by the cells.

RNA. See *Ribonucleic acid.*

Rodenticide. An agent that is used to destroy or repel rodents. Exposure to such substances may increase cancer risk in people.

Saccharin. An *artificial sweetener,* several hundred times sweeter than sugar, whose role as a possible *carcinogen* has been controversial and is as yet undecided.

Sarcoma. A *tumor,* often *malignant,* that is composed of cells of connective tissue such as bone, cartilage or muscle tissue.

Saturated fat. Solid fat, such as butter and the fat in meats, that is associated with high *cholesterol* levels.

Scratch test. A test for allergy in which very small amounts of the suspected substance are inserted into small scratches in the skin to see if a reaction occurs.

Sebaceous cyst. A noncancerous *cyst* of a sebaceous (skin) gland that contains the fatty secretion of the gland. Due to the possibility of infection, sebaceous cysts should be treated.

Sigmoidoscopy. Examination of the lower part of the colon with a sigmoidoscope, an instrument that allows an internal view of the organ.

Skin cyst. See *Sebaceous cyst.*

Sorbitol. An *artificial sweetener* used in some foods intended for people who cannot eat sugar. It is not lower in calories than sugar.

SPF. See *Sun protection factor.*

Squamous cell carcinoma. A type of skin cancer often caused by overexposure to the sun. It can also be caused by exposure to chemicals. It can be easily treated and is not usually life-threatening.

Sun protection factor. A measurement of the amount of sun exposure allowed by a sunscreen before burning occurs. An SPF of 15 means that a person who would normally burn in 15 minutes can apply the sunscreen and stay in the sun for four hours before burning (15 times the normal exposure).

Systemic. A term used to describe something that affects the whole body.

Testosterone. The male sex *hormone* that controls the development of physical sexual characteristics.

Titanium dioxide. An ingredient used in opaque sunscreen ointments.

Toxin. A poisonous substance.

Triglyceride. A type of fat that circulates in the bloodstream and is stored in body tissues. As with *cholesterol,* high blood levels of triglycerides are linked to heart disease.

Tumor. A swelling, enlargement or growth, *benign* or *malignant,* anywhere in the body. There are many types of tumors, classified according to their origin and makeup.

Ulcerative colitis. A condition in which there is chronic, recurring ulceration of the colon, with pain, bleeding and diarrhea. It is considered a risk factor for colorectal cancer.

Ultraviolet light. Light that has wavelengths shorter than those of visible light and longer than those of x-rays. Overexposure to the ultraviolet rays of sunlight is a major risk factor for skin cancer.

Urology. The medical specialty that deals with the diagnosis and treatment of diseases of the urinary tract in women and the genitourinary tract in men.

Very low-density lipoproteins (VLDL). Fatty proteins that are believed to carry the most *cholesterol* in the blood and contribute to the buildup of cholesterol on artery walls.

VLDL. See *Very low-density lipoproteins.*

Water-soluble. Capable of being dissolved or released in the presence of water. Water-soluble substances, such as vitamin C and the B vitamins, are used up quickly.

Wilms' tumor. A *malignant tumor* of the kidney that occurs in children and is possibly *hereditary*.

Xeroderma pigmentosum. A rare type of *hereditary* cancer that makes the skin and eyes extremely sensitive to light. It begins in childhood and is frequently fatal.

Xeromammography. A form of *mammography* that produces a positive image (instead of the negative x-ray image). It requires a slightly higher dose of radiation than traditional mammography.

Zinc oxide. An ingredient in opaque sunscreen ointments.

Index

Note: Page numbers for tables appear in *italic.*

A

Abdomen
    lump or fullness in, 26
    pain in, 56
        from chemotherapy, 461
        in colorectal cancer, 19, 101, 115
        in ovarian cancer, 40
        in pancreatic cancer, 43
    swelling of, in liver cancer, 31
Acidophilus, 413, 414
Acute lymphoblastic leukemia, 459, 460
Acute myelocytic leukemia, 285
Adrenal corticosteroid hormones, 286
Adrenal glands, 481, 483, 484
Adriamycin, 400, 401, 463
Adult T-cell leukemia, 196, 305, 312–313
Aflatoxins, 31, 164
Aging, vitamin D in, 392
AIDS, 195, 303–4, 305–7
Air cleaners, 213
Air fresheners, 213
Air pollution, 259–60
Alar, 275, 279, 281
Alcohol, 65–68
    in breast cancer, 9–11
    carcinogenic mechanism of, 67–68
    in esophageal cancer, 20–21
    in laryngeal cancer, 29, 117
    in liver cancer, 31, 32
    in oral cancer, 36, 38, 39, 118
    in pancreatic cancer, 43, 44
    tobacco and, 66, 67, 68
Aldicarb, 276
Aldrin, 280
Alkylating agents, 285
Allergies, 69–70
Alpha-tocopherol. *See* Vitamin E
Aminogluthethimide, 483, 484
Ammonia, 227
Anemia
    aplastic, 374
    from chemotherapy, 461
    in colorectal cancer, 101
    Fanconi's, 188, 191
    pernicious, 53, 54
Anthanilates, 328
Antibodies
    in immunity, 194–98
    monoclonal, 108–9, 489–91, 514
Antioxidants, 356, 376, 377, 385, 396
Appetite loss
    from chemotherapy, 462
    in colorectal cancer, 101
    in kidney cancer, 26

Cornbread with Cheese, Chilies and Beans, 428
Cranberry Pears, 447
Creamy Blueberry Breakfast Pudding, 423
Fruit Compote, 424
Lentils in the Round, 429
Prune Butter, 453
Raisin and Sweet Potato Scones, 425
Raspberry Bread Pudding with Sunshine Sauce, 451
Spinach, Mushroom and Cheese Panino, 432
Tangerine Raisin Butter, 452
Triple Wheat and Millet Bread, 433
Fibrocystic disease, 95–97
Fibroids, uterine, 124
Finding the Fiber You Need, *154*
Fish oil, 138, 158–60
Flatulence, in ovarian cancer, 40
Fluids, chemotherapy and, 463, 468
Flutamide, 485
Folate, 372–75
    cell changes and, 273
    in cervical cancer, 14, 252
    cervical dysplasia and, 311
    smoking and, 349
Food(s). *See also* Diet *and specific foods*
    barbecued, 71–73
    in cancer prevention, 419–53
    cholesterol in, *146–47*
    fat in, 139, *140–44,* 145
    fiber in, 153–56, *154, 155*
    frozen, 168
    nitrosamines in, 235–36
    pesticides in, 275–83
    pickled, 21, 53
    salt-cured, 293–94
    smoked, 238
    vitamins in, 169, 172–73
Food additives, 161–66
Food colorings, 161–66
Food preparation, 169–75
Food preservation, 53, 54
Food refrigeration, 380–81
Formaldehyde, 204–6, 342
Free radicals, 178, 299, 396
Friendships, and cancer, 474, 503–4
Fruit, 176–84

in cancer research, 176–77
fat in, *140*
fiber in, *155,* 180, *181*
juices, 180, 383
organically grown, 281–82
peeling, 183–84
pesticides on, 183–84, 280–81
in season, 183
vitamins in, 181, 383
Fucoidan, 359

G

Gamma rays, 506
Gardner's syndrome, 19, 105
Gas, in stomach cancer, 120
Gasoline, in pancreatic cancer, 44
Gastrointestinal problems, 510–11
Genes, 2, 188, 189
Genetic engineering, 189
Genetic registers, 192
Genital warts, 13, 308, 310
Glottis, cancer of, 28
Gold, radioactive, 219, 221
Goodness from Greens, *364*
Grains, fat content of, *141*
Groin ache, in testicular cancer, 56
Ground pollution, 262–63
Growths, bleeding or enlarged, 51
Gums (fibers), 153, *154,* 180
Gums (of mouth), 36, 38
Gynecological cancers, 287, 524

H

Hair dyes, 185–86
Hair loss, 467–68, 513–14
Hairy cell leukemia, 489
Hands, tingling in, 466
Hazardous wastes, 262–63
Headaches, 204, 205, 463
Head and neck cancer, alcohol and tobacco in, 66
Healing, 494–504
Heart problems, 124, 463
Hemicellulose, 152, *154,* 180
Hemochromatosis, 217
Hemoglobin, 216
Hemophilia, in liver cancer, 32
Hemorrhoids, 19, 102, 108
Hepatitis B, 31, 196, 313
Herbicides, in marijuana, 228

Rodale Press, Inc., publishes PREVENTION®, the better health magazine.
For information on how to order your subscription,
write to PREVENTION®, Emmaus, PA 18098.